Adverse Cutaneous Drug Reactions to Cardiovascular Drugs

Esen Özkaya • Kurtuluş Didem Yazganoğlu

Adverse Cutaneous Drug Reactions to Cardiovascular Drugs

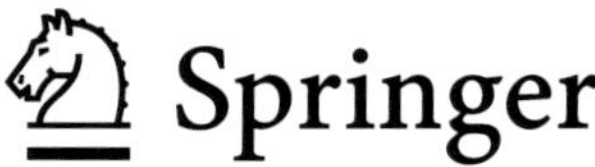

Springer

Esen Özkaya
Department of Dermatology
Istanbul University
Istanbul Medical Faculty
Istanbul
Turkey

Kurtuluş Didem Yazganoğlu
Department of Dermatology
Istanbul University
Istanbul Medical Faculty
Istanbul
Turkey

ISBN 978-1-4471-6535-4 ISBN 978-1-4471-6536-1 (eBook)
DOI 10.1007/978-1-4471-6536-1
Springer London Heidelberg New York Dordrecht

Library of Congress Control Number: 2014951704

Printed on acid-free paper

Springer is part of Springer Science+Business Media (www.springer.com)

To the memory of my beloved father
Prof. Dr. Muzaffer Özkaya and to my mother
Nesrin Özkaya,
To Meral,
To Mehmet Ali,
To Bora.

Esen Özkaya

To Kamuran and Kaan.

Kurtuluş Didem Yazganoğlu

Preface

Adverse cutaneous drug reactions are among the most frequent events in patients receiving drug therapy. Cardiovascular drugs are an important group of drugs with potential risk of developing adverse cutaneous drug reaction especially in the elderly as marketing of more new drugs and their prescription continue to increase. However, like with most other drugs, the exact incidence of cutaneous side effects from cardiovascular drugs is difficult to estimate due to sporadic reporting. Moreover, a reliable designation of a certain drug as the cause of a certain type of reaction can rarely be made. Apart from the well-known angioedema/urticaria from angiotensin-converting enzyme inhibitors, lichen planus/lichenoid reaction from beta adrenergic blockers, and photosensitivity from thiazid diuretics, adverse cutaneous drug reactions from cardiovascular drugs might be seen in a wide spectrum extending to rare but life-threatening conditions such as erythroderma, Stevens-Johnson syndrome, toxic epidermal necrolysis, or drug hypersensitivity syndrome.

This book is a practical guide on adverse cutaneous drug reactions to cardiovascular drugs. The reported types of adverse cutaneous drug reactions to cardiovascular drugs will be discussed comprehensively according to drug class and the type of dermatologic reaction with special emphasize on cross-reactions and the diagnostic procedure. It also features 116 images including clinical figures of common adverse cutaneous drug reactions and those showing diagnostic procedures mainly consisting of patch and photopatch testing with the suspected drugs.

The book is arranged in three main parts. The first part features general information on adverse cutaneous drug reactions; the second part includes adverse cutaneous drug reactions to specific classes of cardiovascular drugs arranged according to the type of dermatologic reaction; and the third part describes the role of patch testing in the diagnosis of drug eruptions. Complementary tables are included at the end of almost every chapter to make it easier for the reader to take a quick look at the major cutaneous drug reactions in each cardiovascular drug class. There are also tables summarizing the most commonly reported reactions according to the specific class of cardiovascular drugs and vice versa and showing the possible cross-reactions between the drugs, thus facilitating finding an alternative drug for therapy.

Management and therapy of the adverse cutaneous reactions is not the main subject of this book. It is also not intended to reflect a complete list of cardiovascular drugs and related adverse cutaneous drug reactions but rather to focus on major reactions and the main causative agents.

Adverse Cutaneous Drug Reactions to Cardiovascular Drugs will be of considerable importance to all dermatologists and medical professionals who manage the skin, while being an important reference resource for cardiologists in terms of identifying potential adverse reactions to the drugs they prescribe.

Istanbul, Turkey Esen Özkaya
Istanbul, Turkey Kurtuluş Didem Yazganoğlu

Acknowledgements

We thank our colleagues in the Dermatovenereology Department of İstanbul Medical Faculty, İstanbul University, for their contributions to the diagnosis of some cases included in this book.

Esen Özkaya and Kurtuluş Didem Yazganoğlu

Contents

Abbreviations

ACDR	Adverse cutaneous drug reaction
ACE	Angiotensin converting enzyme
ACEI	Angiotensin converting enzyme inhibitor
AGEP	Acute generalized exanthematous pustulosis
ANA	Antinuclear antibodies
ANCA	Antineutrophil cytoplasmic autoantibody
ARB	Angiotensin II receptor blockers
AT	Angiotensin
BS	Baboon syndrome
cAMP	Cyclic adenosine monophosphate
CCB	Calcium channel blocker
CD	Cluster of differentiation
COX	Cyclooxygenase
CTCL	Cutaneous T cell lymphoma
DHS	Drug hypersensitivity syndrome
DIF	Direct immunofluorescence
DMSO	Dimethyl sulphoxide
DNA	Deoxyribonucleic acid
DRESS	Drug rash with eosinophilia and systemic symptoms
dsDNA	Double-stranded deoxyribonucleic acid
EM	Erythema multiforme
EMPACT	Erythema multiforme associated with phenytoin and cranial radiation therapy
EN	Erythema nodosum
FasL	Fas ligand
FDA	Food and Drug Administration
FDE	Fixed drug eruption
GM-CSF	Granulocyte-macrophage colony-stimulating factor
HHV	Human herpes virus
HITT	Heparin-induced thrombocytopenia and thrombosis

HIV	Human immunodeficiency virus
HLA	Human leukocyte antigen
HMG-CoA	3-hydroxy-3-methylglutaryl coenzyme A
HSP	Henoch Schönlein purpura
IFN	Interferon
Ig	Immunoglobulin
IGDR	Interstitial granulomatous drug reaction
IIF	Indirect immunofluorescence
IL	Interleukin
kDa	Kilodalton
LAT	Lymphocyte activation test
LMWH	Low molecular weight heparin
LT	Leukotriene
LTT	Lymphocyte transformation test
MCD	Mast cell degranulation
MDA	Multiple drug allergy
MHC	Major histocompatibility complex
MIF	Macrophage migration inhibition
NPH	Neutral protamine Hagedorn
NSAID	Nonsteroidal antiinflammatory drug
p-i	Pharmacological interaction of drugs with immune receptors
PLS	Pseudolymphoma syndrome
PUVA	Psoralen + Ultraviolet A
SCLE	Subacute cutaneous lupus erythematosus
SCORTEN	Score for toxic epidermal necrolysis
SDRIFE	Symmetrical drug related intertriginous and flexural exanthema
SH	Sulphydryl
SJS	Stevens-Johnson syndrome
SLE	Systemic lupus erythematosus
SSA	Sjögren's syndrome A
SSB	Sjögren's syndrome B
SSLR	Serum sickness-like reaction
SSSS	Staphylococcal scalded skin syndrome
TEN	Toxic epidermal necrolysis
TNF	Tumor necrosis factor
Type A reactions	A for "augmented"
Type B reactions	B for "bizarre"
UV	Ultraviolet

Introduction

Adverse cutaneous drug reactions (ACDR) are among the most frequent events in patients receiving drug therapy. Cardiovascular drugs are an important group of drugs with potential risk of developing ACDR especially in the elderly as marketing of more new drugs and their prescription continue to increase. However, like with most other drugs, the exact incidence of cutaneous side effects from cardiovascular drugs is difficult to estimate due to sporadic reporting.

Moreover, a reliable designation of a certain drug as the cause of a certain type of reaction can rarely be made. Apart from the well-known angioedema/urticaria from angiotensin-converting enzyme inhibitors, lichen planus/lichenoid reaction from beta adrenergic blockers, and photosensitivity from thiazid diuretics, ACDR from cardiovascular drugs might be seen in a wide spectrum extending to rare but life-threatening conditions such as erythroderma, Stevens-Johnson syndrome, toxic epidermal necrolysis, or drug hypersensitivity syndrome.

In this book, the reported types of ACDR to cardiovascular drugs are discussed according to drug class and the type of dermatologic reaction highlighting the cross-reactions and the role of patch testing as an important diagnostic procedure.

A wide list of cardiovascular drugs is reviewed including angiotensin-converting enzyme inhibitors, angiotensin II receptor blockers, alpha-2 adrenergic receptor agonists, alpha-adrenergic receptor blockers, adrenergic neuron blockers, class I antiarrhythmics (sodium channel blockers), beta blockers (class II antiarrhythmics), class III antiarrhythmics, calcium channel blockers (class IV antiarrhythmics), diuretics, sympathomimetics, vasodilators, lipid-lowering drugs, platelet inhibitors, thrombolytics, anticoagulants, and miscellaneous drugs. However, it is not intended to reflect a complete list of drugs and ACDR but rather to focus on major reactions and the main causative agents.

A total of 116 images are included featuring the clinical appearance of common ACDRs and diagnostic procedures such as patch and photopatch testing with suspected drugs. Complementary tables may allow scanning the most common ACDR and the related cardiovascular drugs along with the possible cross-reactions at first glance, thus facilitating finding an alternative drug for therapy.

Part I
General Aspects of Adverse Cutaneous Drug Reactions

Chapter 1
General Aspects of Adverse Cutaneous Drug Reactions

Keywords Drug eruption • Cardiovascular drugs • Maculopapular • Erythema multiforme • Acute generalized exanthematous pustulosis • Photosensitivity • Hyperpigmentation • Vasculitis • Angioedema • Erythroderma • Stevens–Johnson syndrome • Toxic epidermal necrolysis • Drug rash with eosinophilia and systemic symptoms

Adverse cutaneous drug reactions (ACDR) or drug eruptions represent one of the most common types of adverse reactions to drug therapy. The overall incidence rate is estimated around 2–3 % in hospitalized patients [1–3]. Antibiotics, nonsteroidal antiinflammatory drugs (NSAIDs), and anticonvulsants are usually regarded as the most common inducers, but almost every drug may cause skin reactions. Advanced age, polypharmacy, and female gender are among the main factors predisposing to ACDR [4, 5].

ACDR cover a wide spectrum of reactions including mild to moderate eruptions such as maculopapular eruption, urticaria, eczematous eruption including drug-induced Baboon syndrome/SDRIFE (symmetrical drug-related intertriginous and flexural exanthema), lichenoid eruption, fixed drug eruption (FDE), erythema multiforme (EM)-like eruption, bullous eruptions like drug-induced pemphigus or pemphigoid, pustular eruption, acneiform eruption, photosensitivity, hyperpigmentation, purpura, vasculitis, and erythema nodosum; or severe eruptions such as angioedema, erythroderma/exfoliative dermatitis, Stevens–Johnson syndrome (SJS), toxic epidermal necrolysis (TEN), drug hypersensitivity syndrome (DHS)/drug rash with eosinophilia and systemic symptoms (DRESS), lymphomatoid drug eruption/pseudolymphoma syndrome (PLS), and skin necrosis. Drugs may also induce an activation of a preexisting dermatosis such as psoriasis, lichen planus, pityriasis rosea, or even a systemic disease, such as systemic lupus erythematosus (SLE), subacute cutaneous lupus erythematosus (SCLE), serum sickness-like reaction, or porphyria. Mucosal reactions like oral lichenoid lesions and gingival hyperplasia or adnexal reactions like alopecia, hypertrichosis, or nail disorders may also occur.

E. Özkaya, K.D. Yazganoğlu, *Adverse Cutaneous Drug Reactions to Cardiovascular Drugs*, DOI 10.1007/978-1-4471-6536-1_1

Characteristic Features of Adverse Cutaneous Drug Reactions

Maculopapular Drug Eruption

Maculopapular eruption, also known as morbilliform eruption or exanthema, is the most common type of cutaneous drug reactions. It is characterized by small, distinct, bright-red maculopapular lesions with a symmetrical distribution. The eruption often shows a morbilliform pattern resembling measles, but unlike measles and other viral eruptions, which characteristically starts on the face, it usually starts on the trunk, subsequently involving the face and the extremities (Figs. 1.1, 1.2, 1.3, 1.4, and 1.5). Lesions may coalesce to involve large areas. They might be accentuated on intertriginous or pressure areas. Palmoplantar involvement might also occur (Fig. 1.6). The eruption might have a purpuric character on the lower extremities. In rare cases, it may evolve into erythroderma/exfoliative dermatitis.

Maculopapular drug eruption might be accompanied by a mild pruritus. Fever and systemic symptoms are usually absent.

Histopathology shows perivascular lymphocytic infiltration with or without eosinophils with minimal epidermal changes [4].

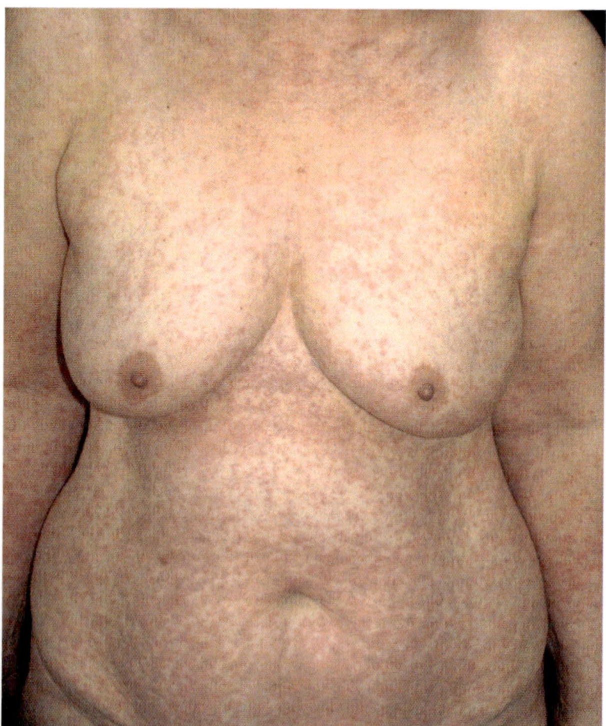

Fig. 1.1 Maculopapular/morbilliform drug eruption on the trunk and upper extremities showing confluent lesions on the abdominal skin

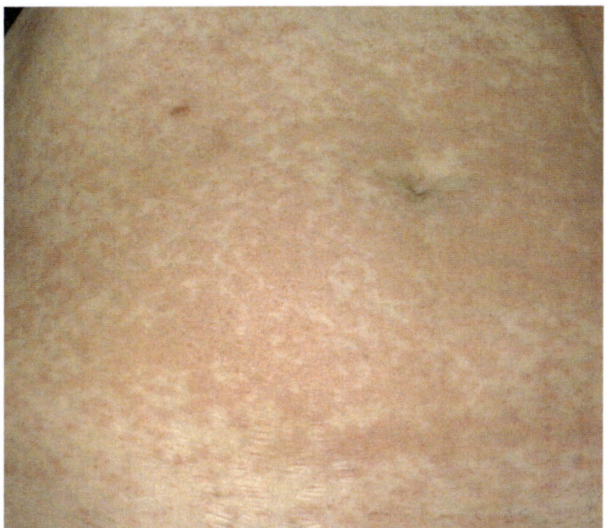

Fig. 1.2 A close-up of confluent maculopapular lesions on the abdominal skin shown in Fig. 1.1

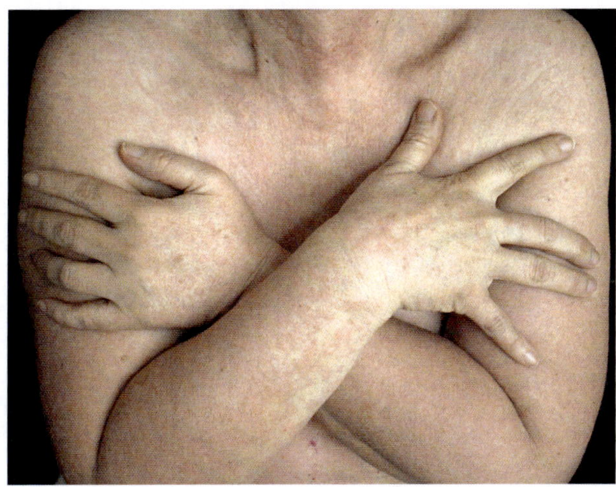

Fig. 1.3 Maculopapular drug eruption on the trunk and upper extremities including the dorsum of the hands

Beta-lactam antibiotics such as amoxicillin and ampicillin are the main inducers of this type of drug eruption. Cephalosporins, antiepileptics, sulfonamide antibiotics, and allopurinol may also be frequently associated with maculopapular drug eruption [6]. The eruption usually starts within a few days to a few weeks of drug therapy. Ampicillin-induced exanthema in patients with infectious mononucleosis might be regarded as a prototype of this eruption. Regarding cardiovascular drugs, maculopapular eruption is seen with angiotensin-converting enzyme inhibitors (ACEIs) (mainly captopril), angiotensin II receptor blockers (ARBs), calcium channel blockers (CCBs), class I antiarrhythmics, diuretics, platelet inhibitors, and aminocaproic acid.

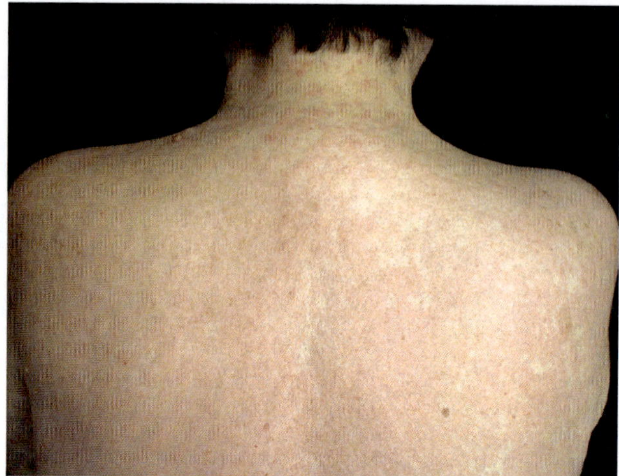

Fig. 1.4 Maculopapular drug eruption on the back skin showing confluence of the lesions

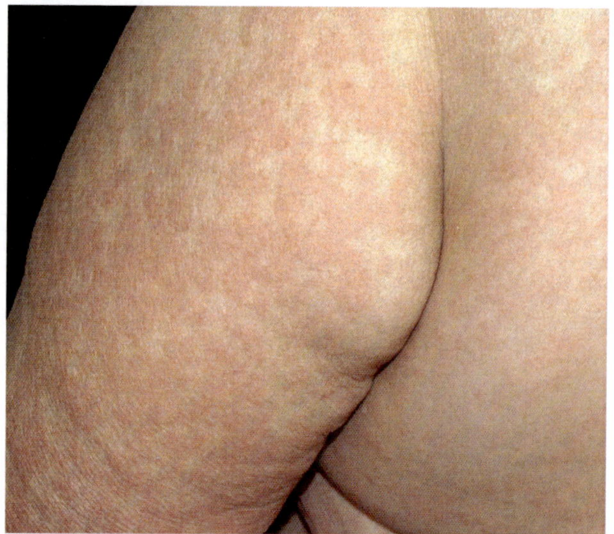

Fig. 1.5 Maculopapular drug eruption on the outer part of the upper arm and the back skin

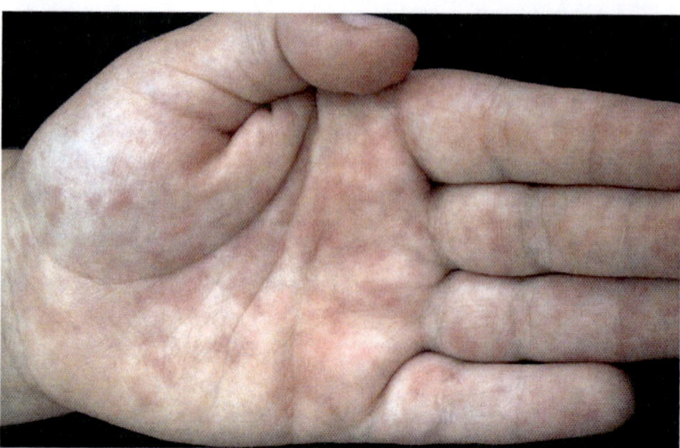

Fig. 1.6 Maculopapular drug eruption involving the palms

Differential diagnosis should include viral exanthemas and syphilitic roseola. Viral exanthema characteristically starts from the face, and it is usually associated with fever and enlarged lymph nodes. Syphilitic roseola are rich on spirochetes.

Cessation of the causative drug and treatment with topical corticosteroids, systemic antihistamines, and if necessary systemic corticosteroids usually result in recovery of the condition.

Drug-Induced Angioedema/Urticaria

Urticaria is the second most common type of cutaneous drug reactions that is characterized by sudden occurrence of red to pale itchy wheals (Fig. 1.7). The eruption usually starts within minutes or a few days of drug therapy. An individual lesion usually disappears within 24 hours. Urticaria can be seen in association with angioedema or anaphylaxis. Angioedema resulting from edema of the deep dermis (Fig. 1.8), hypodermis, and submucosa usually presents with sudden swelling of the lips (Fig. 1.9), eyelids, tongue, or genitalia as deep urticarial papules and plaques. Acute anaphylaxis, and anaphylactoid reactions typically present with angioedema, urticaria, dyspnea, and hypotension.

Histopathology of drug-induced urticaria is usually consistent with classic urticaria, showing vasodilatation and dermal edema and perivascular lymphocytic infiltration occasionally with a few eosinophils [4].

Drug-induced urticaria may be immunologic or non-immunologic. The main inducers of an immunologic urticaria that is frequently associated with type I hypersensitivity reaction are beta-lactam antibiotics. Immunologic urticaria might also be associated with type III hypersensitivity. The main inducers of non-immunologic drug-related urticaria include acetylsalicylic acid, other NSAIDs, radiocontrast media, opiates, and ACEIs. According to a meta-analysis, there is also risk of angioedema with ARBs in patients with prior angioedema associated with ACEIs [7].

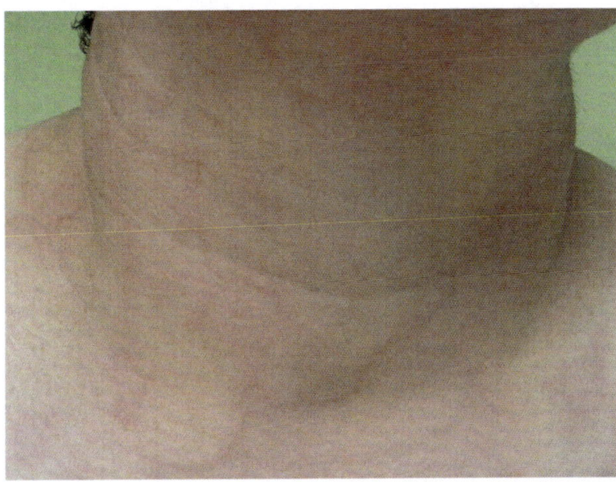

Fig. 1.7 Pale, itchy wheals with erythematous borders on the neck in urticarial drug eruption

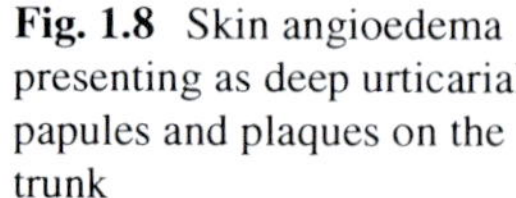

Fig. 1.8 Skin angioedema presenting as deep urticarial papules and plaques on the trunk

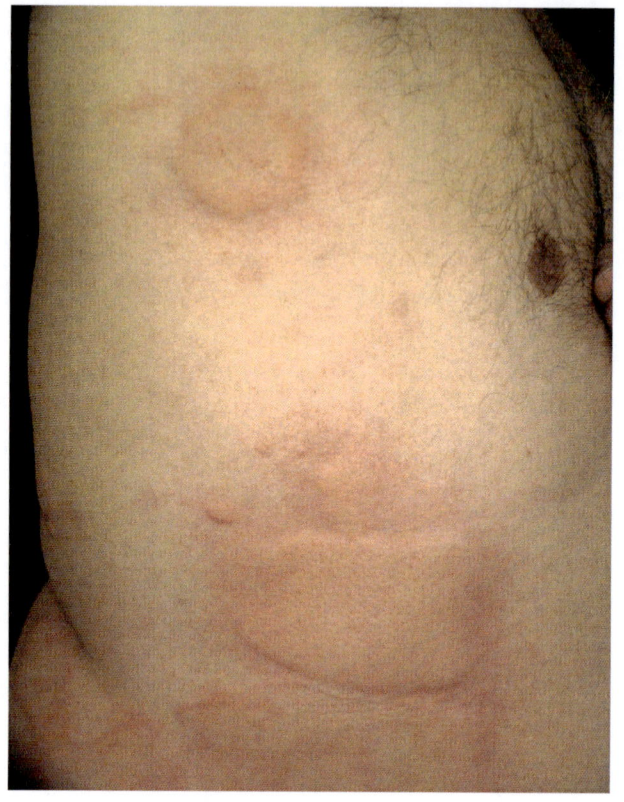

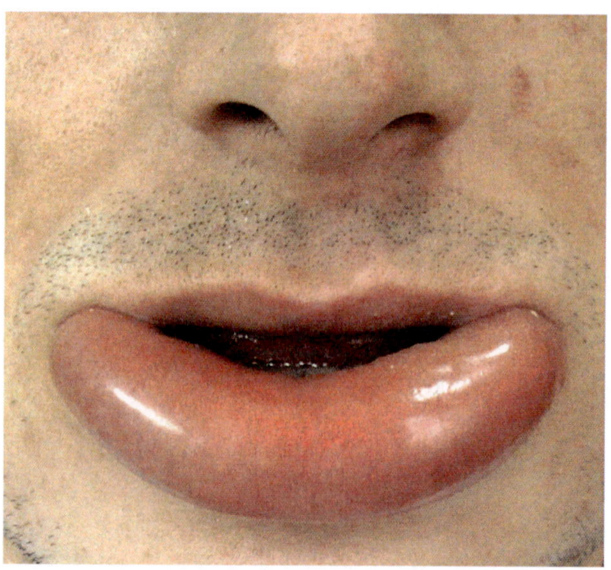

Fig. 1.9 Angioedema of the lower lip

Withdrawal of the causative drug and treatment with systemic antihistamines, and if necessary with systemic corticosteroids, usually result in recovery of the condition.

Eczematous Drug Eruption

Eczematous eruption induced by drugs resembles acute eczema on the trunk and extremities clinically presenting with widespread erythema, edema, vesicles (Figs. 1.10, 1.11, 1.12, and 1.13), and weeping, and in the healing phase with desquamation. The eruption usually starts symmetrically on flexural and intertriginous areas, subsequently evolving into a generalized pattern. In rare cases, it may evolve into erythroderma/exfoliative dermatitis.

Histopathologically, spongiosis in the epidermis is the hallmark for acute eczema. Eczematous drug eruption usually occurs with systemic use of contact allergenic drugs or their cross-reactants in patients previously sensitized by topical use of these drugs. However, according to a recent knowledge on the immunopathogenesis, namely, the newly introduced "p-i concept" (pharmacologic interaction of drugs with immune receptors), it might also be induced by direct systemic use of noncontact allergenic drugs, hence by direct systemic sensitization [8]. Apart from the well-known hapten concept, the p-i concept is a novel pathomechanism that may be involved in direct recognition of some chemically inert molecules, particularly certain small-sized drugs, by T cells [8].

A distinct clinical variant characterized by acute onset of diffuse bright-red erythema on the gluteal and anogenital area (Figs. 1.14 and 1.15), usually demarcated by sharp, well-defined borders, resembling the hairless red rump of the baboons (African Old World monkeys belonging to the genus *Papio*), is known as Baboon syndrome (BS) [9]. There is often additional symmetrical erythema on the groins and the upper inner surface of the thighs in a V-shaped pattern (Fig. 1.16), and on other intertriginous (axillae) or major flexural (antecubital/popliteal) areas. Lesions are sometimes accompanied by papules, pustules, vesicles, bullae, petechiae, or pustules, the latter raising the question as to whether acute generalized exanthematous pustulosis (AGEP) and BS should not be regarded as variants of a continuous spectrum of possible clinical manifestations [10, 11]. Itching and burning are usually the accompanying symptoms [10].

Systemically administered contact allergens, e.g., mercury and nickel, are the main inducers of BS. However, contact allergenic drugs or noncontact allergenic drugs might also induce BS. SDRIFE (symmetrical drug-related intertriginous and flexural exanthema) was recently proposed as another kind of drug eruption to replace the term BS in cases induced by systemically administered noncontact allergenic drugs [12]. Specific site involvement presenting as symmetrical lesions on the gluteal and/or major flexural and intertriginous skin (Fig. 1.17) is clinically characteristic for SDRIFE. The five diagnostic criteria of SDRIFE include (1) exposure to a systemically administered drug that is not a contact allergen, first or repeated doses, (2) sharply demarcated erythema of the gluteal/perianal area and/or V-shaped erythema of the inguinal/perigenital area, (3) involvement of at least one

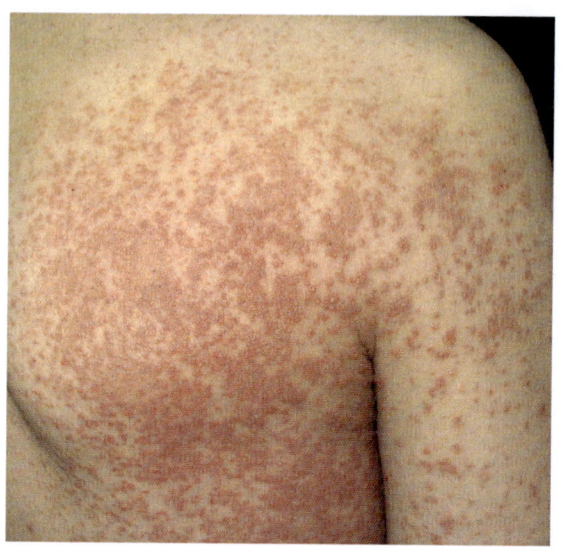

Fig. 1.10 Eczematous drug eruption on the back skin and the outer part of the upper extremity showing widespread erythematous, edematous, and vesicular lesions

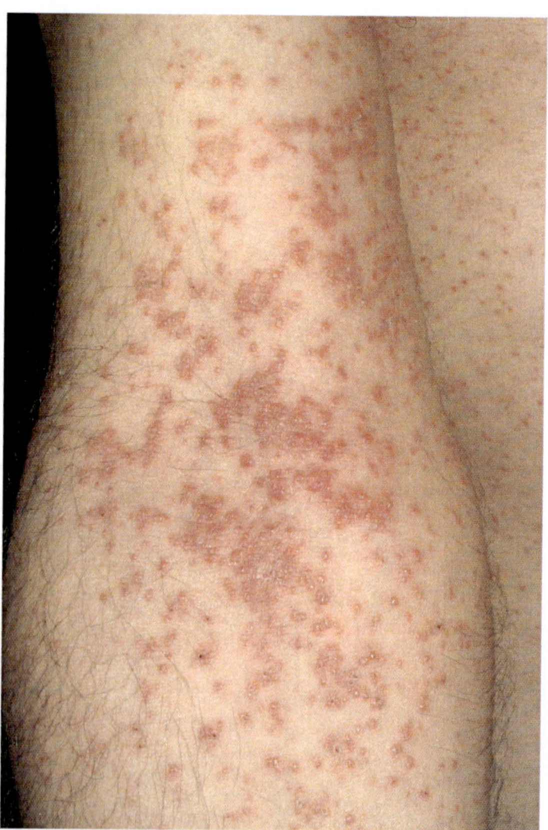

Fig. 1.11 Eczematous drug eruption on the flexural part of the upper extremity and on the trunk showing erythematous, edematous, and vesicular lesions

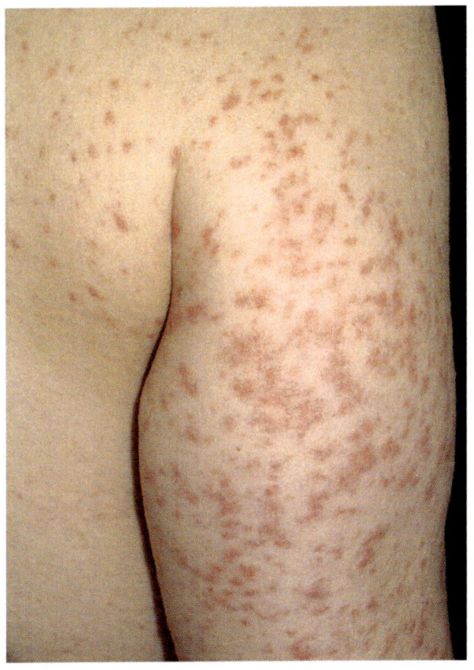

Fig. 1.12 Eczematous drug eruption on the upper arm with erythematous, edematous, and vesicular lesions

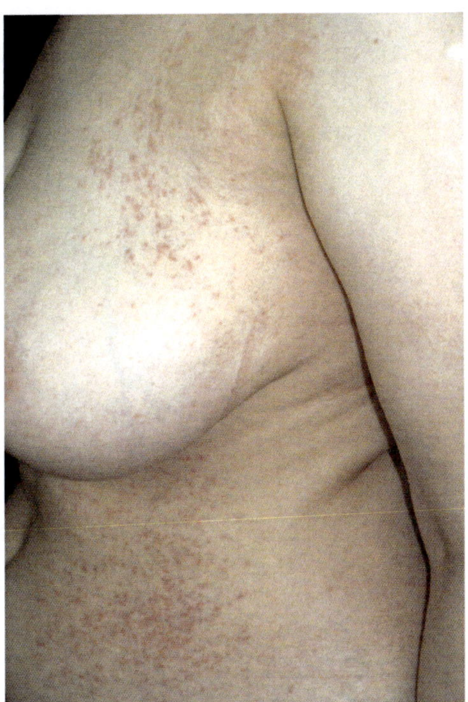

Fig. 1.13 A mild eczematous drug eruption on the trunk

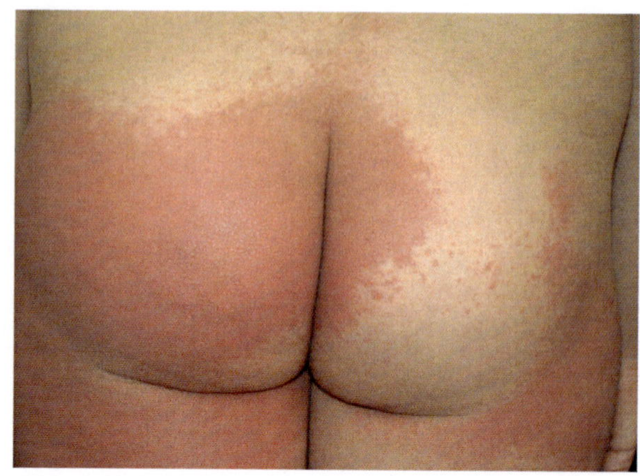

Fig. 1.14 Baboon syndrome with the characteristic, bright-red erythema on the gluteal area

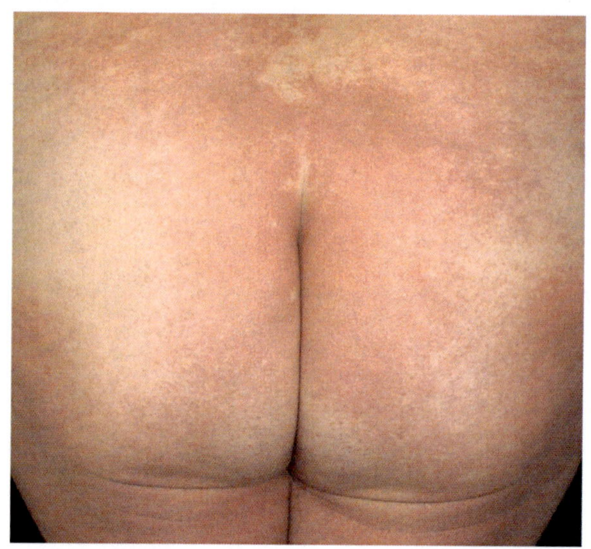

Fig. 1.15 Baboon syndrome with the characteristic, bright-red erythema on the gluteal area

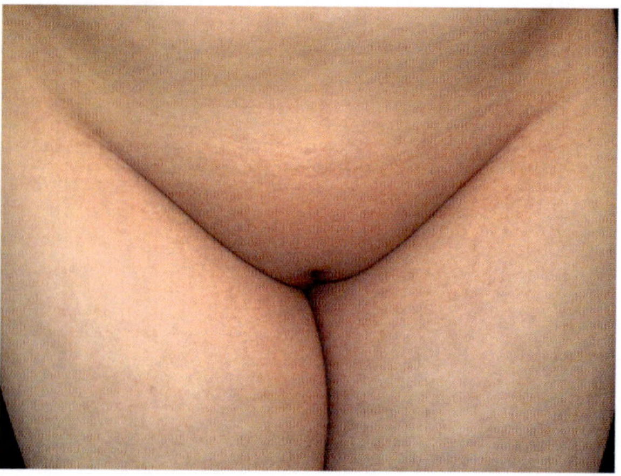

Fig. 1.16 Symmetrical erythema on the groins and the upper inner surface of the thighs in a V-shaped pattern in Baboon syndrome

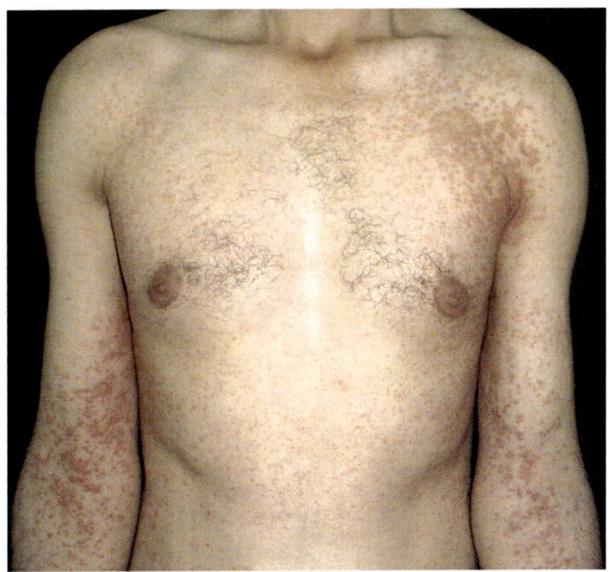

Fig. 1.17 Symmetrical lesions on major flexural and intertriginous areas such as the axillae and antecubital fossae in SDRIFE (symmetrical drug-related intertriginous and flexural exanthema)

other intertriginous/flexural fold, (4) symmetry of affected areas, and (5) absence of systemic symptoms and signs [12].

Beta-lactam antibiotics such as amoxicillin and ampicillin are the main inducers of eczematous drug eruption. Cardiovascular drugs such as anticoagulants, methyldopa, statins, CCBs, and thiazides were also found to be associated with eczematous drug eruptions [13]. Heparin and telmisartan–hydrochlorothiazide have been reported to induce BS/SDRIFE [14, 15].

Lichenoid Drug Eruption

Lichenoid drug eruption resembles idiopathic lichen planus that is characterized by pruritic, small, shiny, reddish to violaceous polygonal papules with white scaly appearance on the surface caused by Wickham's striae (Figs. 1.18, 1.19, and 1.20). Linear lesions due to isomorphic Koebner phenomenon may be seen. Idiopathic lichen planus is often affecting the flexor surfaces of the wrists, forearms, and legs. Although the clinical patterns of lichen planus and lichenoid eruptions are similar, the lesions in lichenoid eruptions are usually more confluent on the trunk and extremities usually lacking Wickham's striae on their surface (Figs. 1.21 and 1.22) [4].

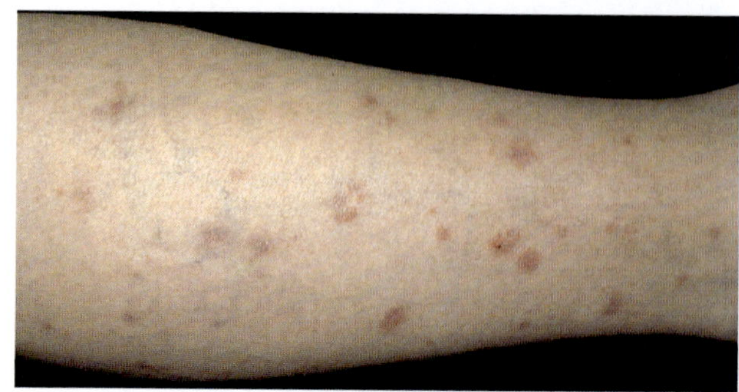

Fig. 1.18 Lichenoid eruption on the lower extremity showing small, shiny, reddish to violaceous polygonal papules with fine scales on the surface (Wickham's striae)

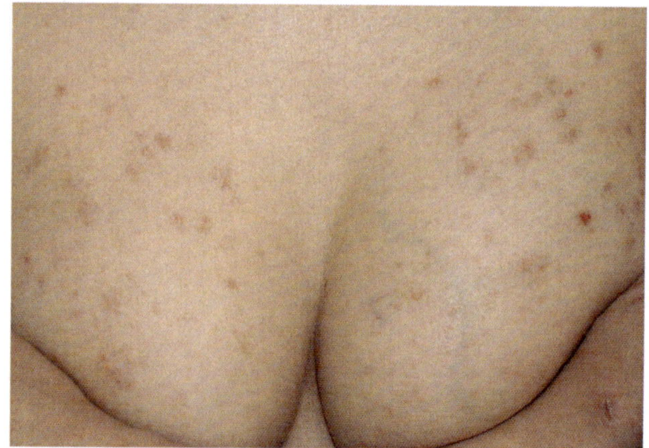

Fig. 1.19 Lichenoid eruption on the upper trunk showing small, shiny, reddish brown, polygonal papules with fine scales on the surface

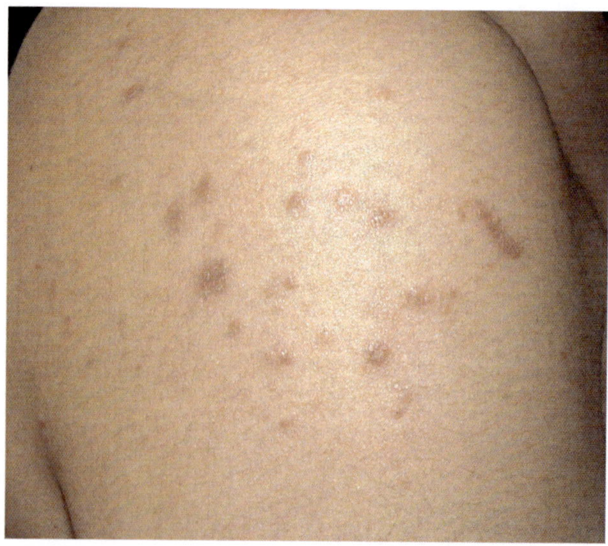

Fig. 1.20 Lichenoid eruption on the outer part of the upper arm showing small, shiny, reddish brown, polygonal papules with fine scales on the surface (Wickham's striae)

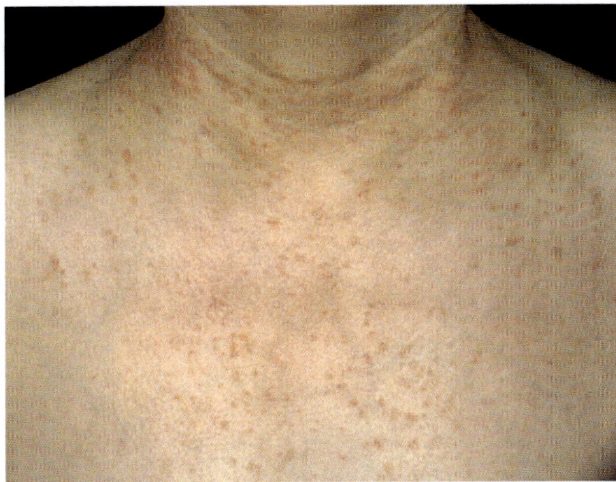

Fig. 1.21 Lichenoid eruption on the neck and the upper trunk showing small, reddish brown papules

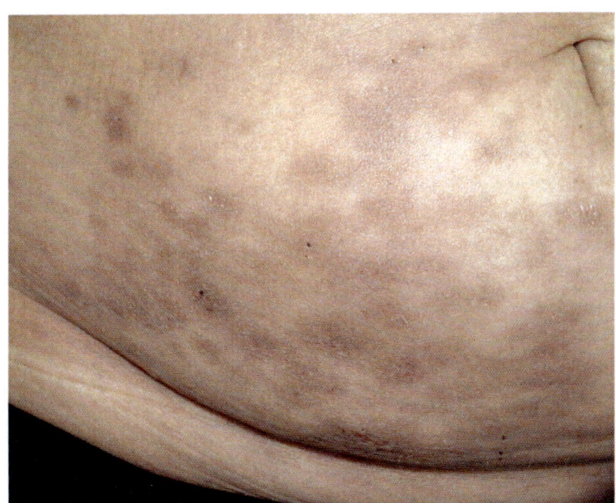

Fig. 1.22 Reddish brown to violaceous lichenoid lesions on the abdominal skin

Lichenoid drug eruption may also resemble the acute eruptive form of lichen planus, characterized by acute onset of numerous lichenoid lesions, symmetrically distributed on the trunk and extremities. It may take weeks or months for the eruption to develop following exposure to the causative drug [4]. Sometimes there might be an atypical distribution such as on sun-exposed areas suggesting a lichenoid photosensitivity reaction (Fig. 1.23). The mucosa or the nails are usually not affected [16], but there might be exceptional cases of oral lichenoid drug eruption [17]. In rare cases, lichenoid eruption may evolve into erythroderma/exfoliative dermatitis.

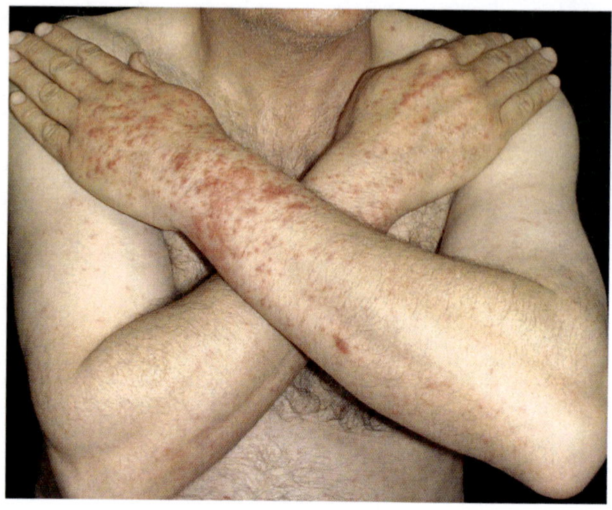

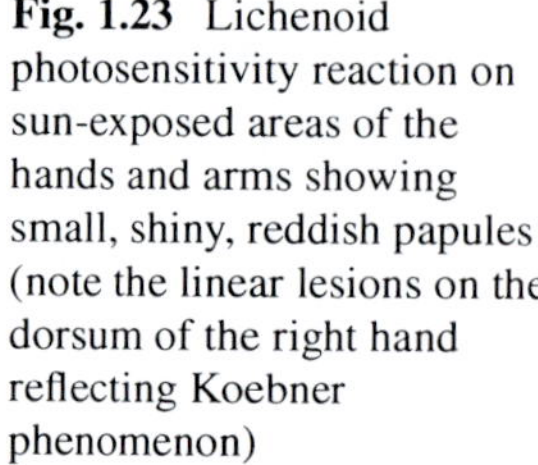

Fig. 1.23 Lichenoid photosensitivity reaction on sun-exposed areas of the hands and arms showing small, shiny, reddish papules (note the linear lesions on the dorsum of the right hand reflecting Koebner phenomenon)

Cardiovascular drugs such as beta-blockers [18], ACEIs, furosemide, methyldopa, diuretics, statins, platelet inhibitors, and other drugs such as gold salts and antimalarials are among the main inducers of lichenoid drug eruption [4].

Fixed Drug Eruption

FDE is characterized by solitary (Fig. 1.24) or multiple (Figs. 1.25 and 1.26), round- to oval-shaped, reddish to dusky purple-colored plaques on the skin or mucosae, sometimes surmounted by vesicles or bullae (Figs. 1.27 and 1.28). As a unique feature, lesions in FDE recur on exactly the same site upon readministration of the causative drug. Lesions start usually within minutes up to several hours (about 30 minutes to 8 hours) after the intake of the offending drug [19]. Symptoms like burning and itching may accompany. Lesions usually heal with residual hyperpigmentation (Fig. 1.29). The lips (Figs. 1.30 and 1.31), hands, and genitalia (especially male genitalia) are frequently involved sites. FDE on the lips might be difficult to differentiate from herpes simplex infection. Mucosal lesions are usually bullous/erosive (Fig. 1.32) but they may also present with aphthous or erythematous morphology [20]. Bullous/erosive mucosal lesions might be difficult to differentiate from pemphigus vulgaris, EM major, or SJS [20]. Aphthous mucosal lesions should be differentiated from aphthous stomatitis, herpes simplex infection, and Behçet's disease. There is an uncommon maximal variant of generalized bullous FDE, which might sometimes be difficult to differentiate from TEN. The main differential diagnostic finding of FDE is the site-specific recurrence of the lesions by therapeutic or diagnostic rechallenge [20].

Lichenoid or EM-like changes are seen in the histopathological examination of FDE in the acute phase that is characterized by dyskeratosis, hydropic degeneration of the basal cells, dermal edema, and a perivascular lymphocytic infiltrate of the upper dermis [19]. Residual pigmentation in the healing phase is accompanied by hyperpigmentation of the basal layer and pigment-laden macrophages in the upper dermis [19].

NSAIDs, antibiotics, and hypnotics are among the most frequent inducers, but cardiovascular drugs such as platelet inhibitors, class I antiarrhythmics, and beta-blockers might also cause FDE.

Withdrawal of the causative drug and treatment with topical corticosteroids will usually result in the recovery of the lesions.

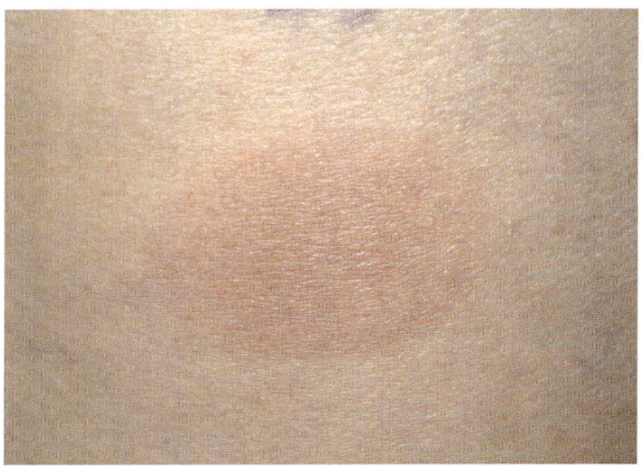

Fig. 1.24 Fixed drug eruption: solitary, oval-shaped, reddish-colored plaque on the trunk

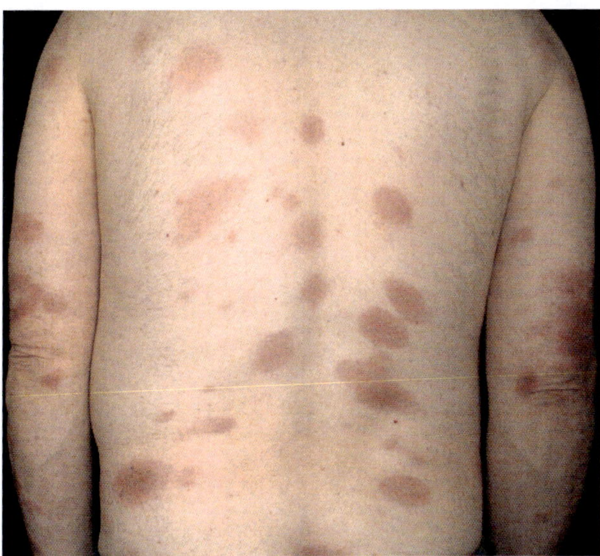

Fig. 1.25 Fixed drug eruption: multiple, round- to oval-shaped, dusky red-colored plaques on the trunk

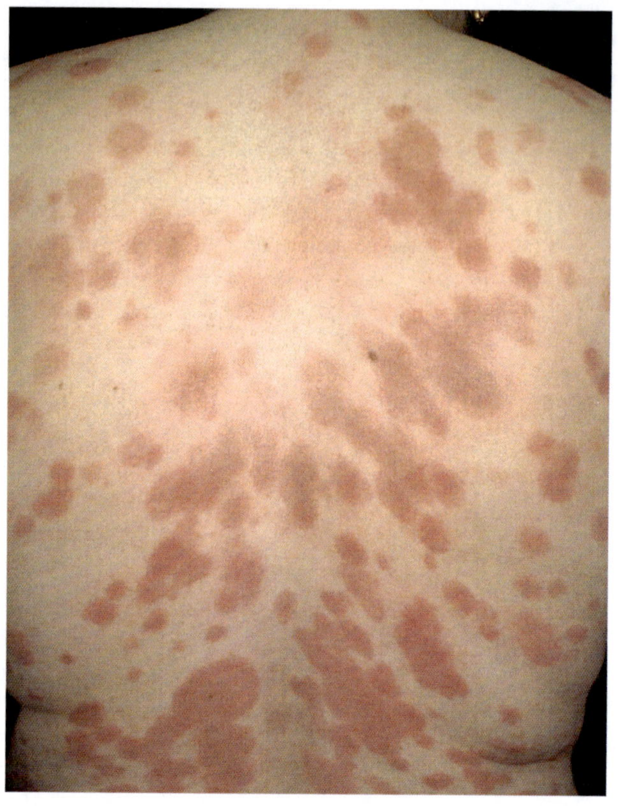

Fig. 1.26 Fixed drug eruption: multiple, round- to oval-shaped, bright-red-colored plaques on the trunk

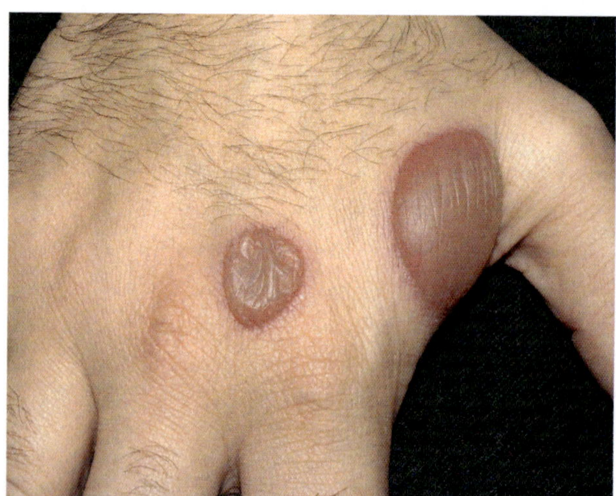

Fig. 1.27 Fixed drug eruption: round- to oval-shaped, dusky purple-colored plaques on the dorsum of the hand surmounted by bullae

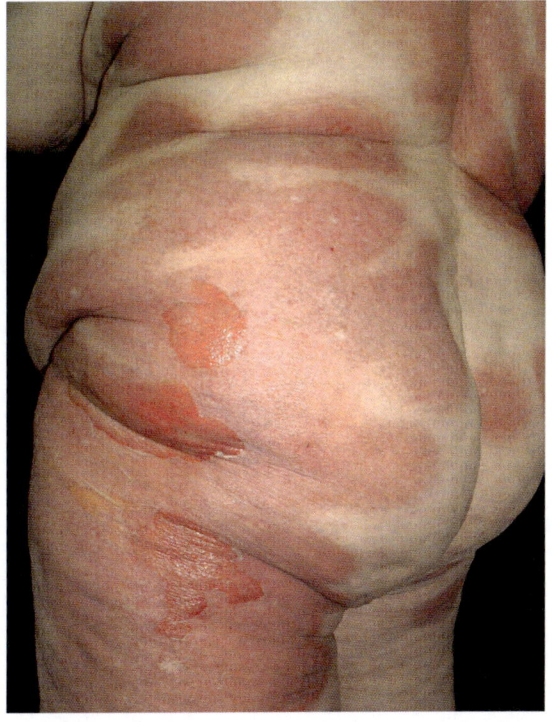

Fig. 1.28 Fixed drug eruption: dusky red-colored, large, confluent plaques on the trunk and lower extremities, partially surmounted by bullae and erosions

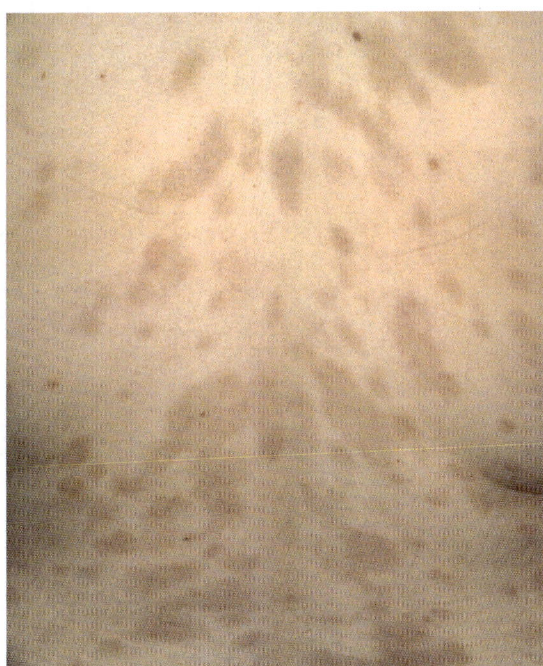

Fig. 1.29 Fixed drug eruption: healing phase of the lesions showing residual hyperpigmentation

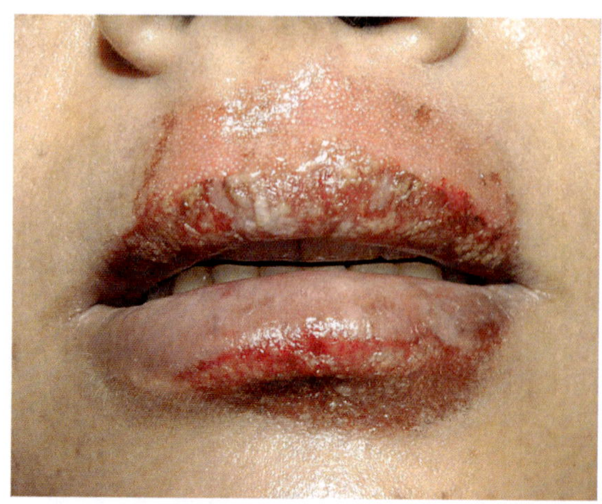

Fig. 1.30 Fixed drug eruption (FDE): involvement of lips. Well-defined plaques with vesicles and erosions. FDE on the lips might be difficult to differentiate from herpes simplex infection

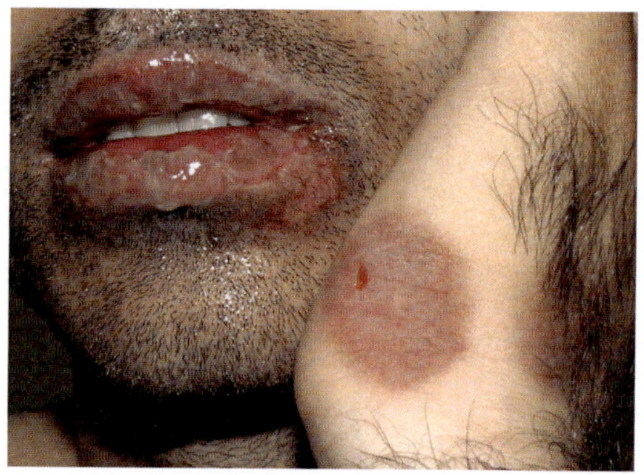

Fig. 1.31 Fixed drug eruption: involvement of the lips showing bullae and erosions. Bullous/erosive mucosal lesions might be difficult to differentiate from pemphigus vulgaris, erythema multiforme major, or Stevens-Johnson syndrome. Accompanying recurrent, site-specific lesions on the hand is a helpful differential diagnostic clue in this patient

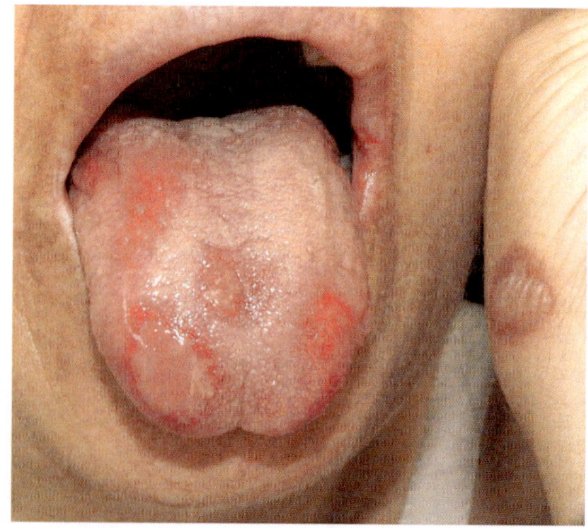

Fig. 1.32 Fixed drug eruption: multiple, reddish-colored plaques surmounted by bullae on the dorsum of the tongue. Bullous/erosive mucosal lesions might be difficult to differentiate from pemphigus vulgaris, erythema multiforme major, or Stevens-Johnson syndrome. Accompanying recurrent, site-specific bullous lesion on the hand is a helpful differential diagnostic clue in this patient

Erythema Multiforme-Like Drug Eruption

Classical EM that is usually associated with herpes simplex and other infections is characterized with dusky red, targetoid papular lesions and no mucosal involvement. Acral parts of the body such as the hands (Fig. 1.33) and feet including palmoplantar areas, distal parts of the extremities, face, and neck are most frequently involved in classical EM. EM-like drug eruption, however, is mainly located symmetrically on the trunk and extremities (Figs. 1.34 and 1.35). Targetoid appearance of the lesions might be less prominent or even absent in EM-like drug eruption. Histopathological examination showing dyskeratosis and hydropic degeneration of the basal cells is necessary to confirm the diagnosis.

NSAIDs, antiepileptics, phenothiazines, penicillins, and sulfonamides are among the inducers of EM-like eruption. Cardiovascular drugs such as diuretics have also been reported to be associated with this type of drug eruption.

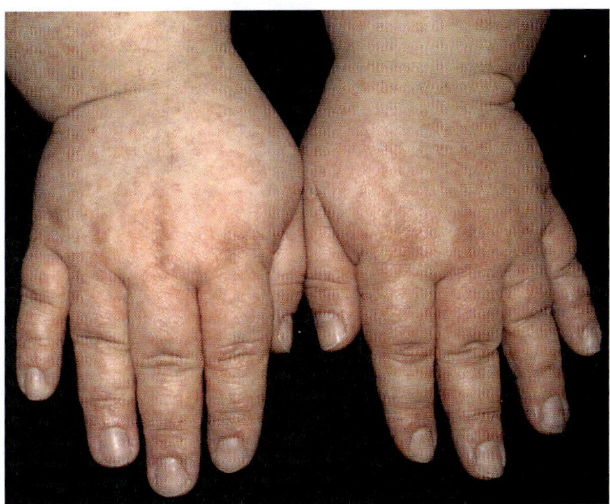

Fig. 1.33 Dusky red-colored, targetoid papules on the dorsum of the hands in erythema multiforme

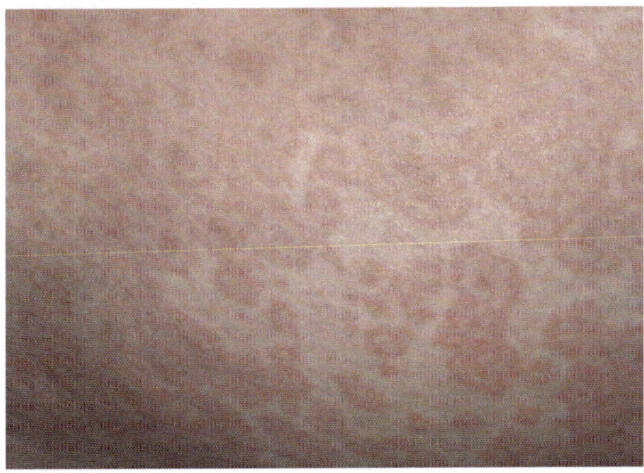

Fig. 1.34 Dusky red-colored, confluent targetoid lesions on the trunk in erythema multiforme-like drug eruption

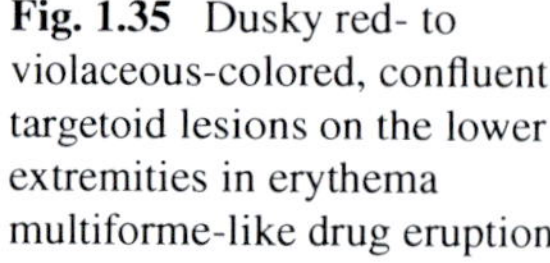
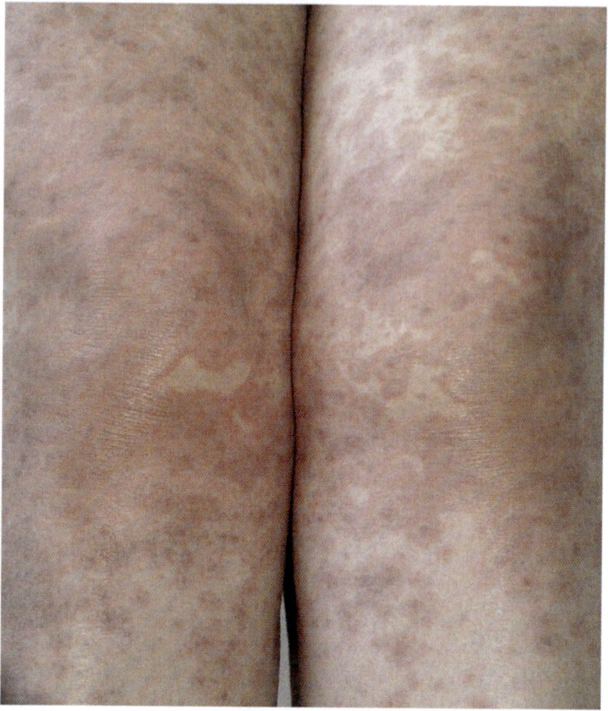

Fig. 1.35 Dusky red- to violaceous-colored, confluent targetoid lesions on the lower extremities in erythema multiforme-like drug eruption

The development of EM confined to the radiation field during or following cranial radiation in patients receiving prophylactic anticonvulsant therapy with phenytoin was recently defined as EMPACT (Erythema Multiforme associated with Phenytoin And Cranial radiation Therapy) [21, 22]. Phenobarbital has also been reported to cause EMPACT [23].

Bullous Drug Eruptions

Bullous drug eruptions include drug-induced pemphigus, bullous pemphigoid, linear IgA dermatosis, or pseudoporphyria closely resembling the characteristic clinical features of the related dermatoses [4, 24].

Pemphigus vulgaris is characterized by flaccid intraepidermal bullae, rapidly covered with crusts, erosions of the skin (Fig. 1.36), and accompanying or preceding erosions of the mucous membranes. Nikolsky's sign is present. There might be a chronic urticarial/eczematous preblistering prodrome in drug-induced pemphigus which may help in differentiating it from idiopathic pemphigus [4, 25]. Also, there is lack of strong positivity rates in direct immunofluorescence (DIF) in drug-induced pemphigus [4, 25]. Similar to idiopathic pemphigus, mucosal involvement is also common in drug-induced pemphigus.

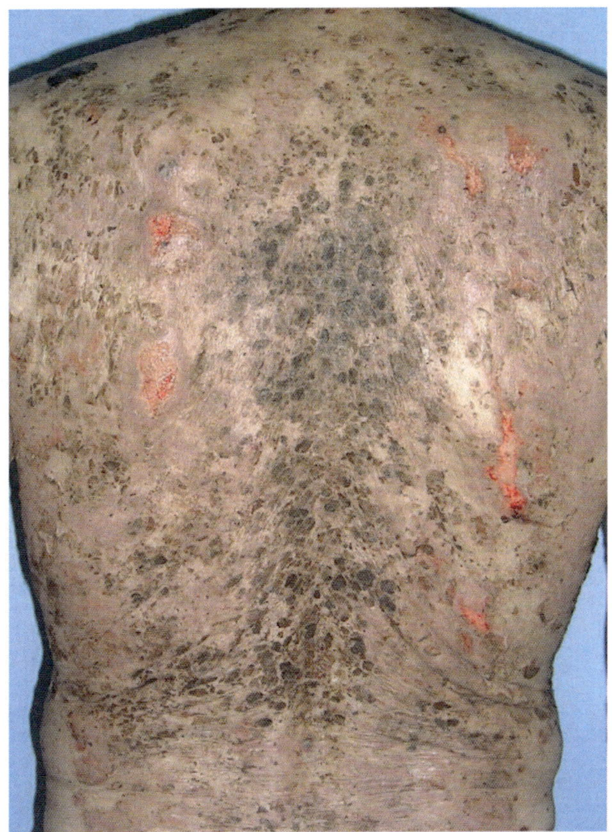

Fig. 1.36 Erosions and crusts resulting from rupture of flaccid bullae on the trunk of a patient with pemphigus vulgaris

Clinical findings of drug-induced pemphigoid are usually indistinguishable from the idiopathic form showing tense, subepidermal bullae, either on an erythematous or normal skin (Fig. 1.37). However, the young age of patients should raise suspicion of drug-induced pemphigoid [4]. Lichen planus pemphigoides may also occur with certain drugs that might be difficult to differentiate from bullous pemphigoid.

Drug-induced linear IgA dermatosis is usually characterized with a vesiculobullous eruption in annular arrangement on the trunk and pelvic area that may resemble the idiopathic form (Fig. 1.38) [4].

Drug-induced pseudoporphyria is characterized with skin fragility and blistering mainly on sun-exposed areas, resembling porphyria cutanea tarda [4]. Lesions heal with hyperpigmentation, scarring, and formation of milia. In contrast to porphyria cutanea tarda, porphyrin levels are normal in drug-induced cases [26].

The latency period between exposure and onset of a bullous drug eruption may be prolonged, and the diagnosis might be therefore challenging. The in vitro interferon-gamma (IFN-gamma) release from lymphocyte test [25] and immunostaining with antibodies to desmoglein were found useful for diagnosing drug-induced pemphigus, the latter suggested as an indicator of a good prognosis [27]. Drug-induced linear IgA dermatosis was found to be more severe than the spontaneous form in a study, with lesions mimicking TEN [28].

Drugs that can cause pemphigus are divided into three groups, namely, thiol drugs (containing sulfhydryl radical) such as captopril, penicillamine, and gold sodium thiomalate; then phenol drugs such as aspirin, rifampin, levodopa, and heroin; and nonthiol nonphenol drugs such as NSAIDs, ACEIs, CCBs, glibenclamide, and dipyrone [25]. Thiol drugs may cause acantholysis via various proposed mechanisms [25]. Phenol drugs lead to the release of cytokines like tumor necrosis factor-alpha (TNF-alpha) and interleukin-1 alpha from keratinocytes which are involved in acantholysis [29, 30]. Among nonthiol nonphenol drugs, CCBs may cause pemphigus due to the fact that desmogleins are calcium dependant [31].

Regarding cardiovascular drugs, ACEIs (captopril, enalapril) and CCBs (nifedipine) are well known to induce drug-induced pemphigus, whereas furosemide, spironolactone, and clonidine may induce pemphigoid [4]. Linear IgA dermatosis is mainly associated with vancomycin and also with other drugs such as ciprofloxacin, beta-lactams, diclofenac, and granulocyte colony-stimulating factor [4]. Furosemide and thiazide diuretics as well as NSAIDs are among the inducers of pseudoporphyria [4].

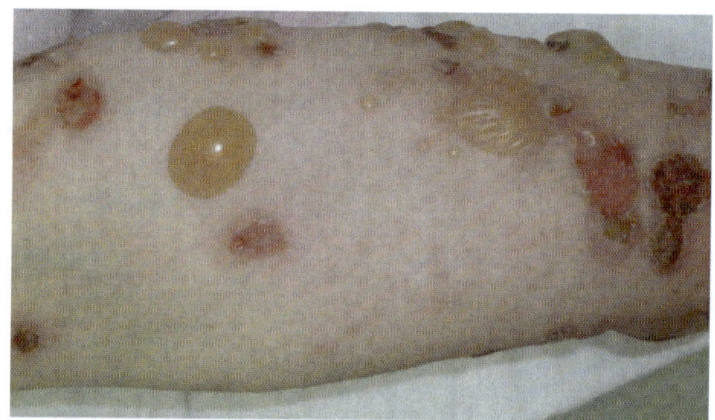

Fig. 1.37 Tense bullae, erosions, and crusts on the arm of a patient with bullous pemphigoid

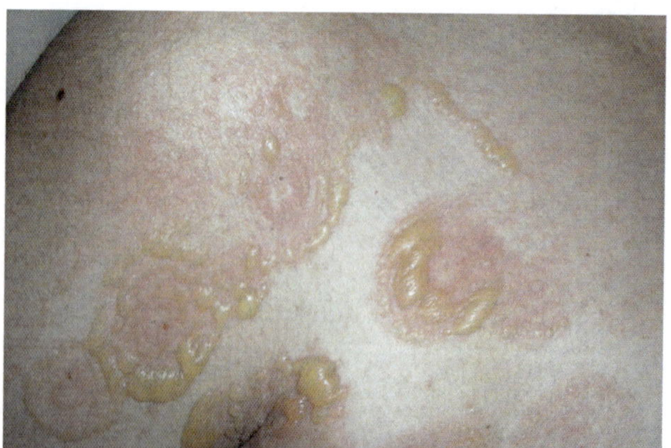

Fig. 1.38 Vesiculobullous eruption in annular arrangement on the upper trunk and arm in a patient with linear IgA dermatosis

Pustular Drug Eruption/Acute Generalized Exanthematous Pustulosis

Pustular eruption induced by drugs may be localized or generalized. It is characterized by rapid development of tiny, superficial, sterile pustules on an erythematous base. Its localized form presents with lesions in intertriginous areas. The generalized form of pustular eruption characterized by acute extensive formation of sterile small superficial pustules on an erythematous base, often accompanied by a high fever and peripheral blood leukocytosis, is called AGEP (Figs. 1.39, 1.40, and 1.41). It usually starts within 3–5 days of therapy with the causative drug [32]. There is typically no mucosal involvement. Diagnostic criteria and a scoring system based on the morphological and histopathological features and the course of disease have been defined for the diagnosis of AGEP [33, 34].

Histopathology shows subcorneal epidermal pustules, mild spongiosis, few necrotic keratinocytes, and superficial dermal edema with a lymphocytic infiltration occasionally including eosinophils [4].

Beta-lactam antibiotics such as amoxicillin and ampicillin, hydroxychloroquine, sulfonamides, terbinafine, and the cardiovascular drug diltiazem are the main inducers of pustular drug eruption/AGEP [32].

The reaction usually resolves within 2 weeks after stopping the causative drug, and in severe cases with treatment of systemic corticosteroids.

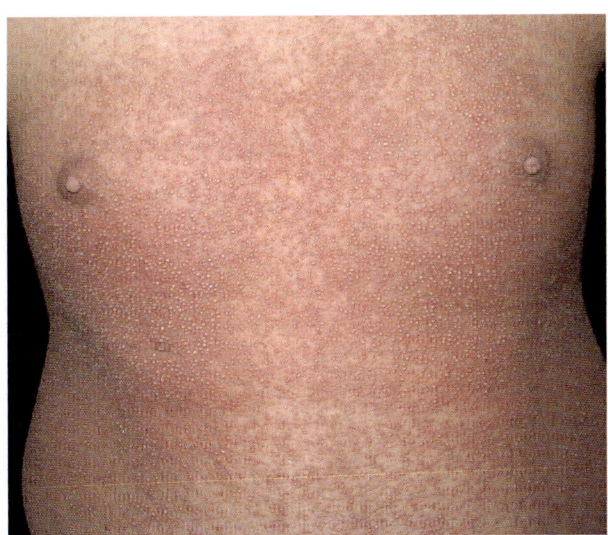

Fig. 1.39 Widespread, tiny, superficial, sterile pustules on an erythematous base on the trunk of a patient with acute generalized exanthematous pustulosis

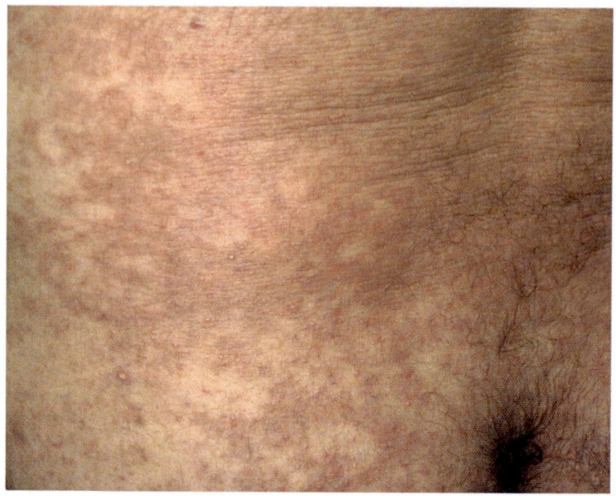

Fig. 1.40 Acute generalized exanthematous pustulosis (early stage) showing tiny, superficial, sterile pustules on an erythematous base on the trunk

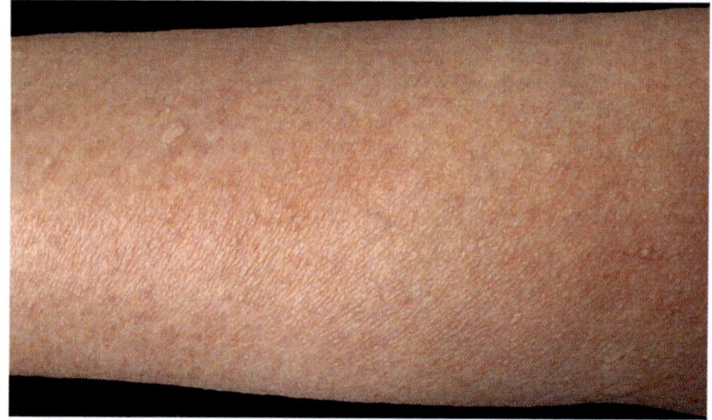

Fig. 1.41 Acute generalized exanthematous pustulosis (early stage) showing tiny, superficial, sterile pustules on an erythematous base on the forearm

Acneiform Drug Eruption

In contrast to acne vulgaris, acneiform eruption is characterized with sudden onset of monomorphic papulopustular eruption on normal-appearing skin without comedones, nodules, or cysts (Figs. 1.42, 1.43, and 1.44). Some drugs have been reported to exacerbate acne vulgaris. Corticosteroids, epidermal growth factor receptor inhibitors, anticonvulsants, antipsychotics, antidepressants, lithium, TNF-alpha inhibitors, anabolic steroids, danazol, antituberculosis drugs including isoniazid, oral contraceptives, and halogenated drugs are among the main inducers of acneiform drug eruption [35]. Regarding cardiovascular drugs, quinidine may also be associated with acneiform lesions [35]. The condition usually resolves after withdrawal of the causative drug and treatment with appropriate topical and/or systemic drugs such as tetracyclines.

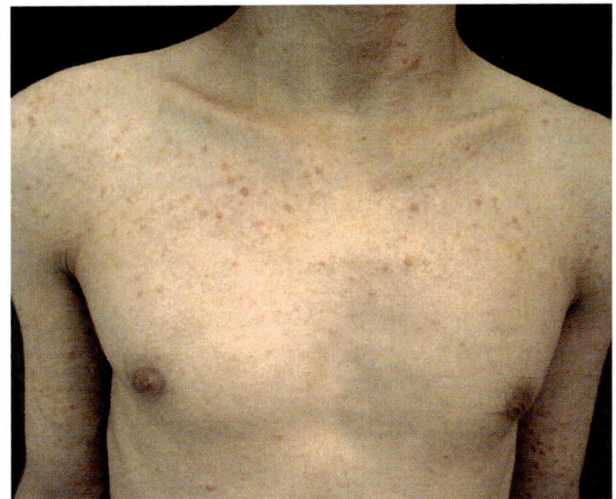

Fig. 1.42 Mild acneiform drug eruption showing monomorphic papules and pustules on normal-appearing skin in a patient receiving systemic corticosteroids

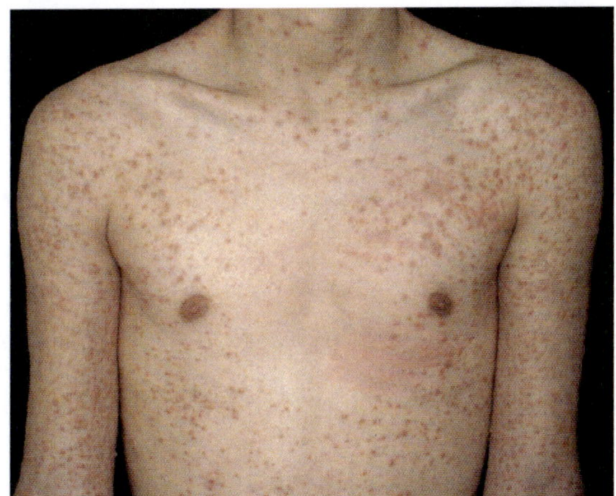

Fig. 1.43 Severe acneiform drug eruption showing monomorphic papules and pustules on normal-appearing skin in a patient receiving systemic corticosteroids

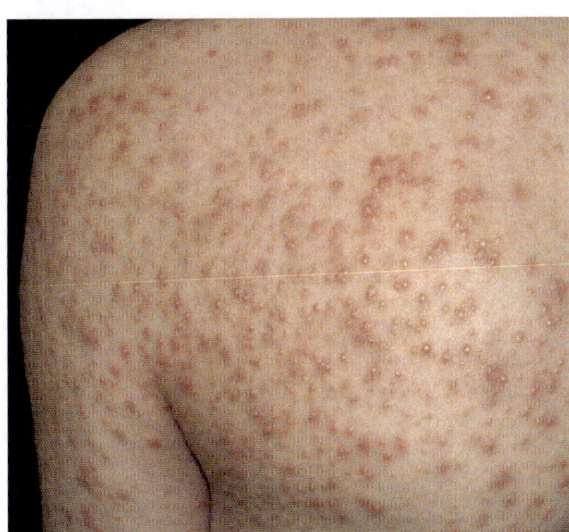

Fig. 1.44 A close-up of monomorphic papules and pustules on normal-appearing skin in a patient with severe acneiform drug eruption shown in Fig. 1.43

Drug-Induced Photosensitivity

Photosensitivity induced by the combination of drugs and ultraviolet (UV) radiation may be most frequently phototoxic or rarely photoallergic, or both, occurring in sun-exposed areas of the skin such as the face, neck (usually in a V-shaped pattern), and extensor sites of the forearms and hands (Figs. 1.45, 1.46, 1.47, 1.48, and 1.49) [36]. UVA (320–400 nm) is most often implicated [4]. Sun-protected areas such as the upper eyelids and submental and retroauricular regions are spared.

Phototoxic drug eruption resembles an exaggerated sunburn reaction characterized with sharply defined erythema, edema, blistering, weeping, and desquamation, usually resolving with postinflammatory hyperpigmentation [1]. The reaction is dose dependent and can occur in any one receiving high doses of the inducer drug and the corresponding UV radiation [4]. It usually starts within hours following the ingestion of the phototoxic drug and exposure to a relevant UV radiation. Photo-onycholysis that is characterized by the separation of the nail from the nail bed induced by ultraviolet radiation may accompany [37]. Tetracyclines, isotretinoin, and psoralens are among the inducers of phototoxic drug eruption.

Photoallergic drug eruption, which is only seen in individuals with prior sensitization to the inducer drug, is characterized by an eczematous eruption showing erythema and vesiculation in the acute phase, often spreading beyond the irradiated areas. Lichenification, a diffuse thickening of the epidermis leading to exaggeration of the skin lines, frequently occurs from repeated rubbing of the photosensitive skin in the chronic phase (Figs. 1.45 and 1.48). A lichenoid eruption on sun-exposed areas would suggest a lichenoid photosensitivity reaction (Fig. 1.23). The reaction usually starts within 24–48 hours following reexposure to the previously sensitized photoallergic drug and the relevant UV radiation [4]. Thiazide diuretics, ACEIs (captopril), ARBs, CCBs, amiodarone, quinidine, cholesterol-lowering agents such as fibrates, NSAIDs (piroxicam), sulfonamides, sulfonylureas, fluoroquinolones, and phenothiazines are among the main inducers of photoallergic drug eruption [38].

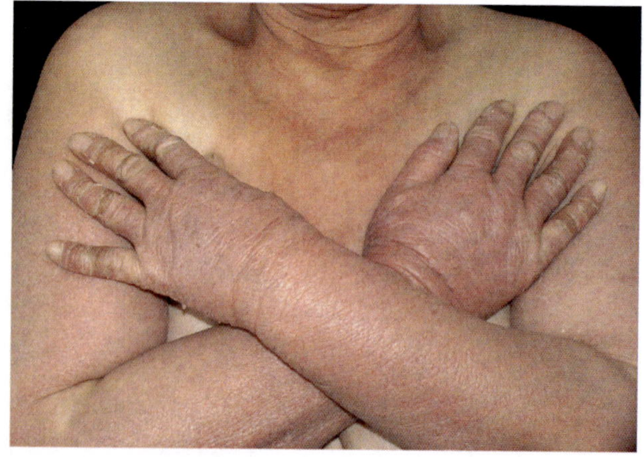

Fig. 1.45 Photosensitivity presenting with erythema, edema, scaling, and lichenification on sun-exposed skin of a patient receiving hydrochlorothiazide

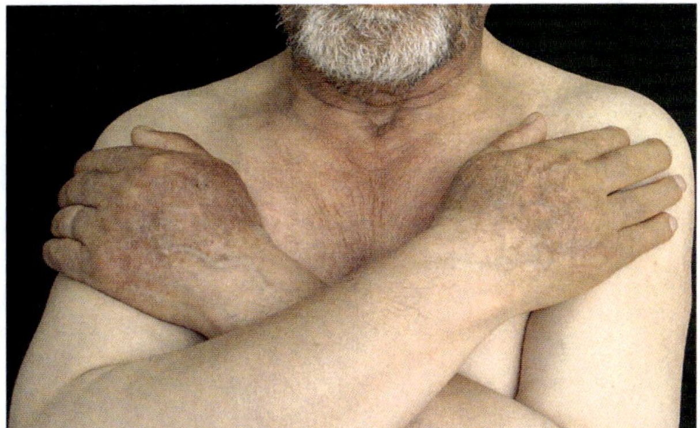

Fig. 1.46 Photosensitivity presenting with erythema, edema, and hyperpigmentation on sun-exposed skin of a patient receiving hydrochlorothiazide

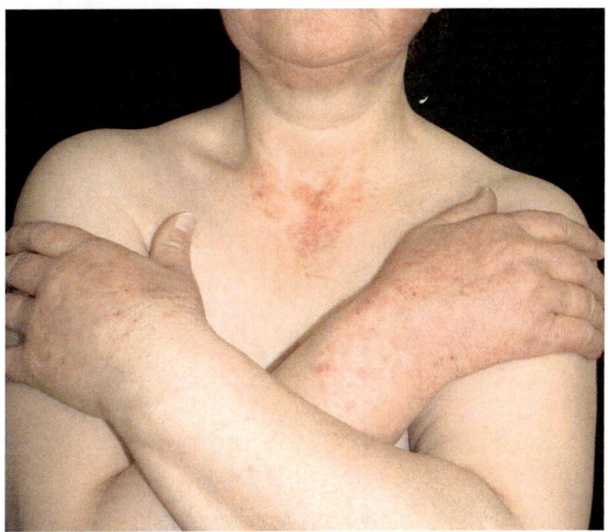

Fig. 1.47 Photosensitivity presenting with eczematous lesions on sun-exposed skin

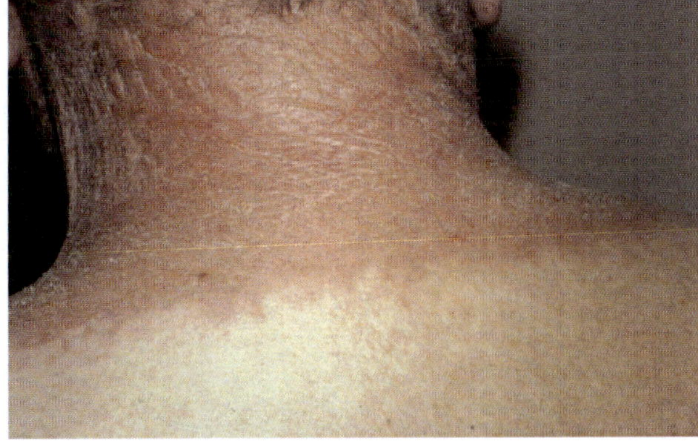

Fig. 1.48 Photosensitivity presenting with erythema, edema, scaling, and lichenification on the neck of a patient receiving hydrochlorothiazide. Note the cutoff between the lesional skin and the photo-protected areas covered by clothes

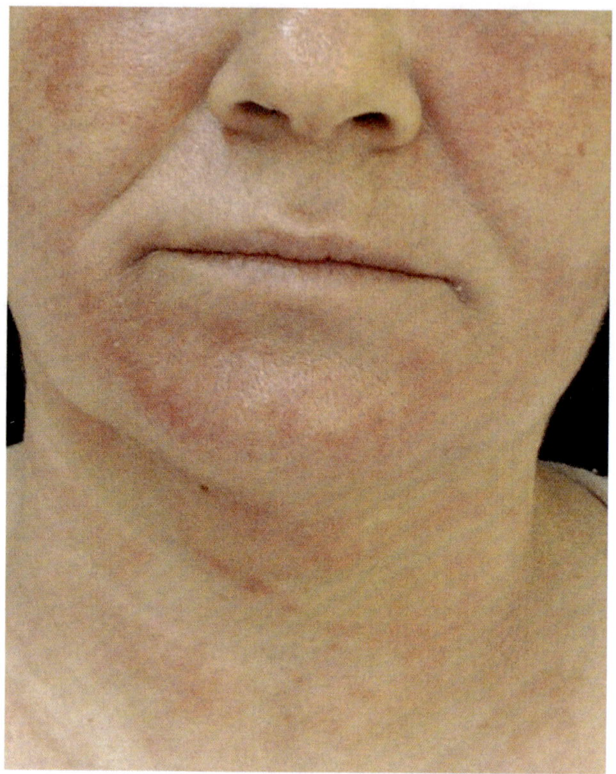

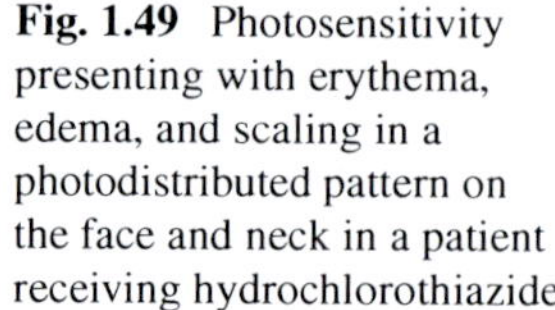

Fig. 1.49 Photosensitivity presenting with erythema, edema, and scaling in a photodistributed pattern on the face and neck in a patient receiving hydrochlorothiazide

Drug-Induced Hyperpigmentation

Hyperpigmentation induced by drugs may be widespread or localized, mainly confined to sun-exposed areas, sometimes resembling chloasma on the face. It may result from increased synthesis of melanin, or accumulation of the triggering drug or its metabolite, or deposits of iron following damage to the dermal vessels [39]. It is frequently associated with photosensitivity (Fig. 1.50). The main drugs inducing hyperpigmentation are amiodarone, minocycline, phenytoin, quinidine, antimalarials, oral contraceptives, cytotoxic drugs, heavy metals, and psychotropic drugs [39, 40]. The color of pigmentation may be variable such as blue gray with amiodarone and quinidine, and brown with phenytoin [1, 41].

Apart from amiodarone, diltiazem, phenytoin, and quinidine are other cardiovascular drugs frequently associated with hyperpigmentation.

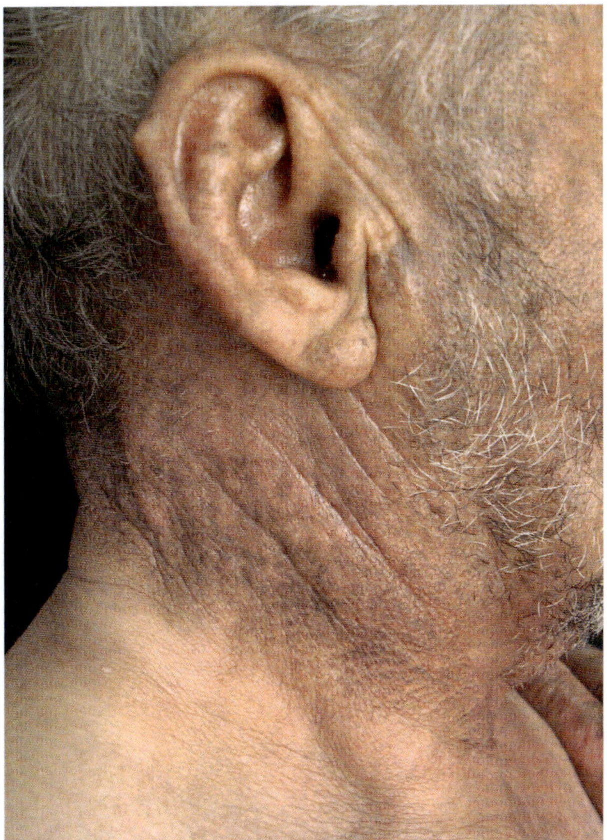

Fig. 1.50 Drug-induced hyperpigmentation on the face and neck, associated with photosensitivity in a patient receiving hydrochlorothiazide

Purpuric Drug Eruption

Purpura is characterized by dusky red to purple macules or patches, nonblanchable with diascopy, resulting from cutaneous extravasation of blood (Fig. 1.51). The term purpura covers three differently named lesions, i.e., petechiae (<5 mm), purpura (5–10 mm), and ecchymosis (>1 cm) according to their diameter. The main causes of drug-induced purpura are thrombocytopenia (<30,000/mm^3) and platelet dysfunction. Lesions usually start from the lower extremities. However, a similar picture can be caused by damage to small blood vessels, either by immunologic mechanisms or by changes in vascular permeability [1].

Acetyl salicylic acid (aspirin)-induced inhibition of platelet aggregation, anticoagulant-induced reduced blood clotting, and corticosteroid-induced vasculopathy are examples leading to purpuric drug eruption.

Among cardiovascular drugs, quinidine, diuretics, anticoagulants, platelet inhibitors, thrombolytics, and CCBs [42] are commonly associated with drug-induced purpura.

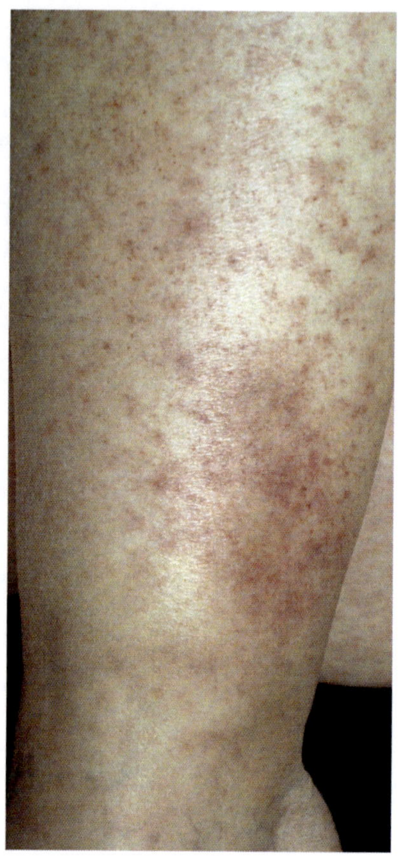

Fig. 1.51 Dusky red- to purple-colored, petechial purpuric lesions on the arm which are nonblanchable on diascopy

Drug-Induced Vasculitis

Vasculitis, associated with inflammation of blood vessels, may present as isolated cutaneous vasculitis or as a cutaneous manifestation of systemic vasculitis, e.g., renal involvement. The most common type of cutaneous vasculitis is leukocytoclastic. Leukocytoclastic vasculitis commonly presents with purpuric macules and raised, purple-colored papules or plaques with irregular margins (palpable purpura) (Figs. 1.52 and 1.53), hemorrhagic blisters, and ulceration, also known as necrotizing vasculitis, such as in Henoch–Schönlein purpura (HSP). Histopathology and DIF microscopy, the latter showing deposition of IgA in the walls of involved blood vessels as a diagnostic hallmark, will confirm the diagnosis of HSP. Leukocytoclastic vasculitis may also present as urticarial vasculitis (Fig. 1.54) showing wheals resembling classical urticaria but with duration of an individual lesion more than 72 hours, often accompanied by burning or pain and residual purpura or hyperpigmentation. The presence of leukocytoclasia and fibrinoid necrosis in the histopathology of an urticarial lesion would lead to the diagnosis of urticarial vasculitis.

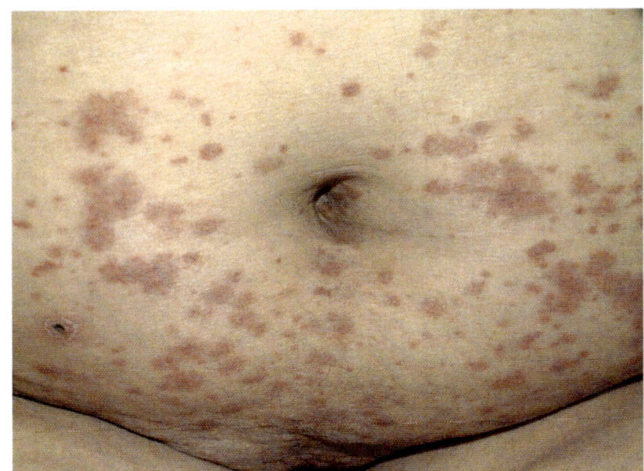

Fig. 1.52 Leukocytoclastic vasculitis showing purpuric macules and papules (palpable purpura) on the abdominal skin

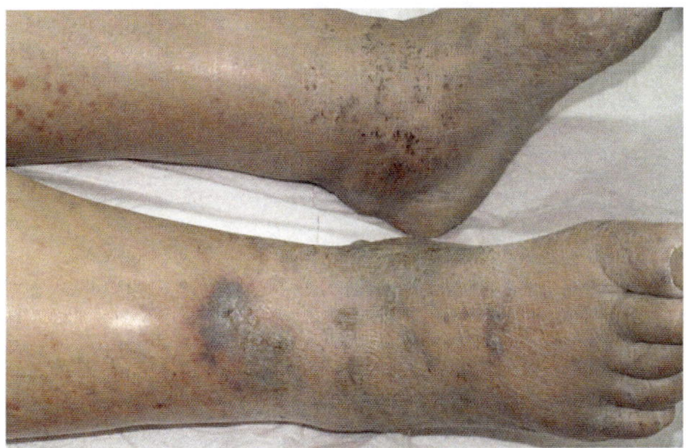

Fig. 1.53 Leukocytoclastic vasculitis showing reddish- to violaceous-colored macules, papules, and plaques (palpable purpura) with irregular margins, hemorrhagic blisters, and crusts on the lower legs and feet

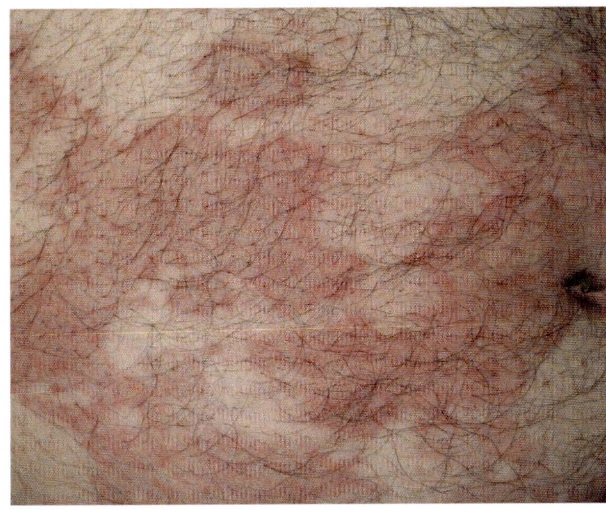

Fig. 1.54 Urticarial vasculitis presenting with purpuric wheals with duration of an individual lesion more than 72 hours, accompanied by burning or pain

Urticarial vasculitis accompanying systemic symptoms like fever and arthralgia/arthritis should raise the suspicion of serum sickness or serum sickness-like reaction.

Drug-induced vasculitis usually starts within 1–3 weeks following the administration of the causative drug. Lesions resolve after withdrawal of the drug and treatment with systemic corticosteroids. Among the cardiovascular drugs, ACEIs, hydralazine, amiodarone, diuretics, quinidine, beta-blockers, thrombolytics, anticoagulants may be associated with drug-induced vasculitis [4, 43]. Intravenous use of amiodarone might commonly induce thrombophlebitis as well [44].

Calcium channel blockers have been reported to cause nonvasculitic eruptive telangiectasia [45].

Hydralazine, minocycline, propylthiouracil, and levamisole-adulterated cocaine have been found to be associated with antineutrophil cytoplasmic autoantibody (ANCA) vasculitis [46].

Drug-Induced Erythema Nodosum

Erythema nodosum (EN) is a septal panniculitis clinically presenting with an acute, nodular, erythematous eruption that is usually localized on the extensor aspects of the lower legs. It may be idiopathic or related with several systemic diseases or drug therapies [47]. Oral contraceptives and sulfonamides are common inducers.

Drug-Induced Erythroderma/Exfoliative Dermatitis

Erythroderma/exfoliative dermatitis is characterized by widespread confluent erythema that is often associated with desquamation, involving more than 80 % of the body surface (Figs. 1.55, 1.56, and 1.57). It is a condition with a significant risk of morbidity and mortality. Drugs may cause erythroderma directly, or several drug eruptions, e.g., maculopapular, lichenoid, eczematous, may evolve into erythroderma during their course. It usually begins within a few weeks following treatment with the causative drug. Apart from the drugs, erythroderma may also be related with various dermatoses such as psoriasis or lichen planus, systemic diseases, or malignancies, e.g., mycosis fungoides.

Pruritus, high fever, and enlargement of the lymph nodes may accompany. The skin thermoregulation and the fluid/electrolyte balance are usually impaired. Hypoalbuminemia may occur. There is a tendency towards secondary infection.

Sulfonamides, allopurinol, barbiturates, hydantoin derivatives, phenylbutazone, carbamazepine, NSAIDs, gold salts, and lithium are among the common inducers

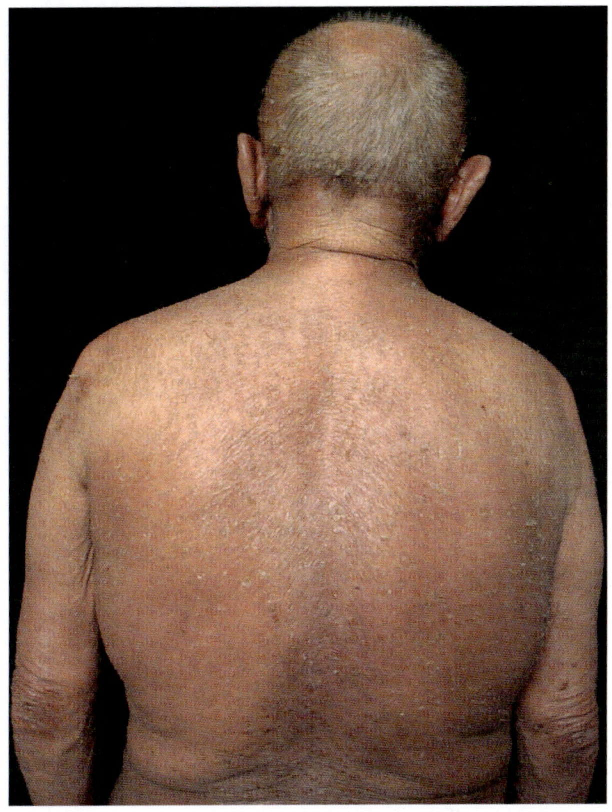

Fig. 1.55 Erythroderma/exfoliative dermatitis showing diffuse erythema and desquamation of the skin

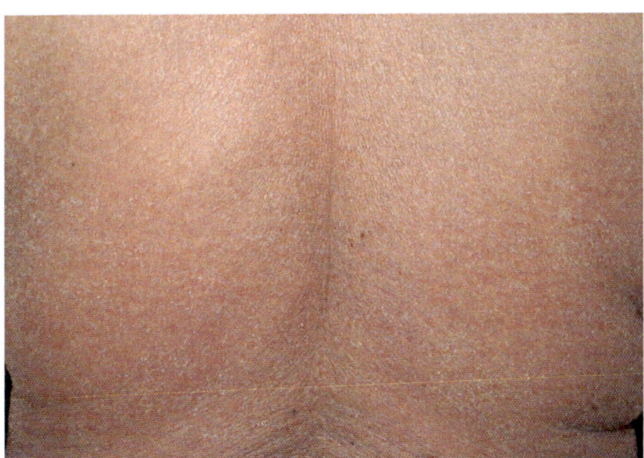

Fig. 1.56 Erythroderma/exfoliative dermatitis showing widespread confluent erythema and desquamation of the skin

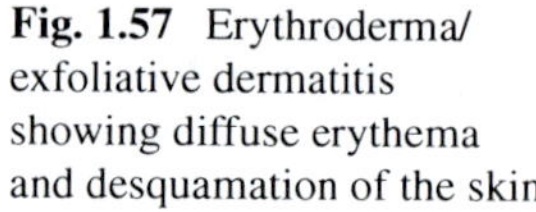

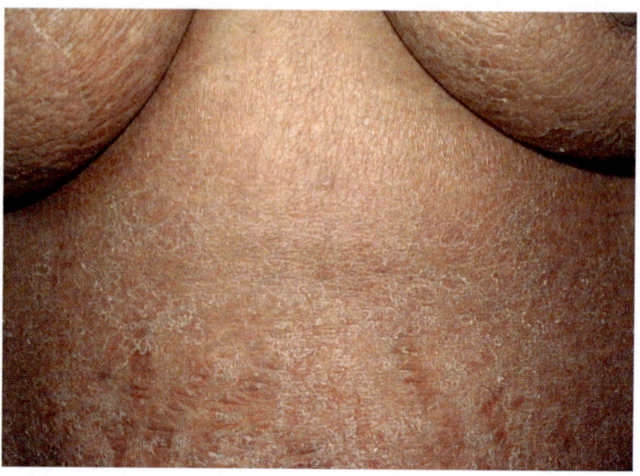

Fig. 1.57 Erythroderma/exfoliative dermatitis showing diffuse erythema and desquamation of the skin

of drug-induced erythroderma [4, 48]. Cardiovascular drugs such as captopril, CCBs, class I antiarrhythmics, and vasodilatory drugs may also be associated with erythroderma.

Stevens–Johnson Syndrome

EM, SJS, and TEN are considered to represent variants within a continuous spectrum of disease [1]. In SJS, there are mucosal erosions and skin blistering covering up to 10 % of the body surface area in addition to EM-like targetoid lesions (Fig. 1.58). It usually starts within 1–3 weeks of therapy with the offending drug, with prodromal symptoms like fever, headache, malaise, and myalgia. The face, neck, trunk, and extremities including the palms and soles are usually involved. Histopathology of bullous lesions shows full-thickness epidermal necrosis with subepidermal blistering. At least one mucosal area is involved such as oral, genital, conjunctival, pharyngeal, laryngeal, or perianal, showing painful hemorrhagic bullae and erosions. The lips are typically covered with hemorrhagic crusts (Fig. 1.59). Oral candidiasis may develop as a consequence of disturbed oral hygiene.

Bronchitis, pneumonia, pericarditis, glomerulonephritis, and hepatitis may develop. The mortality rate is approximately 5–10 % in SJS [49, 50]. Early therapy with systemic corticosteroids is usually effective.

NSAIDs, allopurinol, barbiturates, carbamazepine, sulfonamides, penicillins, and cephalosporins are among the most common inducers of SJS. Cardiovascular drugs such as phenytoin and diuretics have also been reported to be associated with SJS.

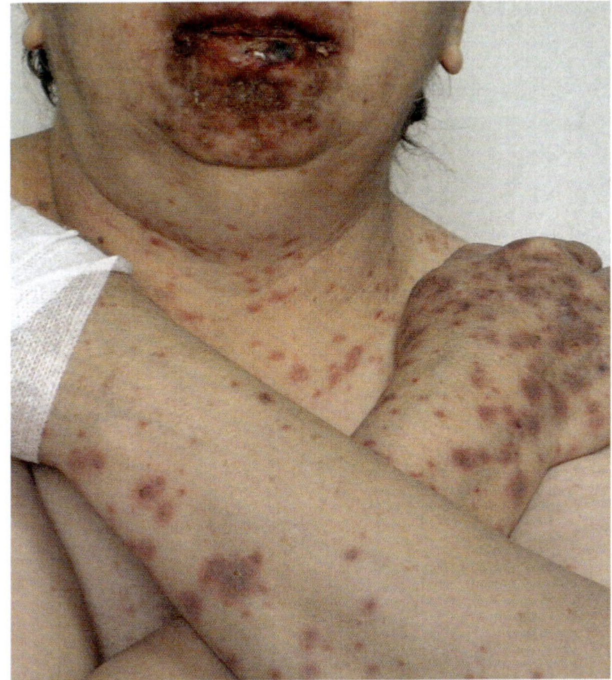

Fig. 1.58 Stevens–Johnson syndrome showing dusky red to violaceous targetoid lesions on the neck, arms and dorsum of the hands along with hemorrhagic blisters, erosions, and crusts on the lips and chin

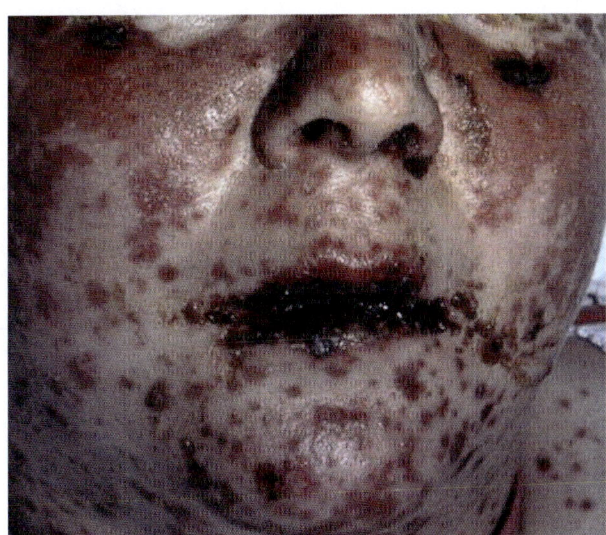

Fig. 1.59 Stevens–Johnson syndrome showing typical hemorrhagic crusts on the lips in addition to dusky red-colored papules and plaques with blister formation and crusts on the face and neck

Toxic Epidermal Necrolysis

TEN is the most severe cutaneous drug reaction with a high mortality rate over 30 % [50, 51]. Similar to SJS, it usually starts within 1–3 weeks of therapy with the offending drug, with prodromal symptoms like fever, headache, malaise, and myalgia. Initially, there is diffuse erythema (Figs. 1.60 and 1.61) and burning sensation, rapidly evolving into a generalized maculopapular eruption, and widespread bullae covering more than 30 % of the body surface area in addition to severe involvement of mucosae. Large areas of erosions have the appearance of a second-degree burn with a positive Nikolsky's sign. Nails may be lost. Conjunctival, gastrointestinal, and urogenital mucosae might be involved leading to keratoconjunctivitis, gastrointestinal bleeding, and urogenital problems like urethritis. Histopathology of bullous lesions shows full-thickness epidermal necrosis with subepidermal separation.

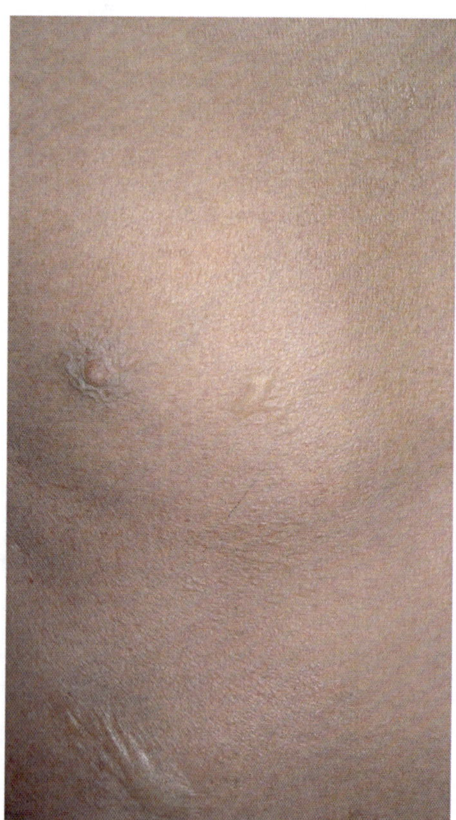

Fig. 1.60 Early-stage toxic epidermal necrolysis showing diffuse erythema and formation of bullae

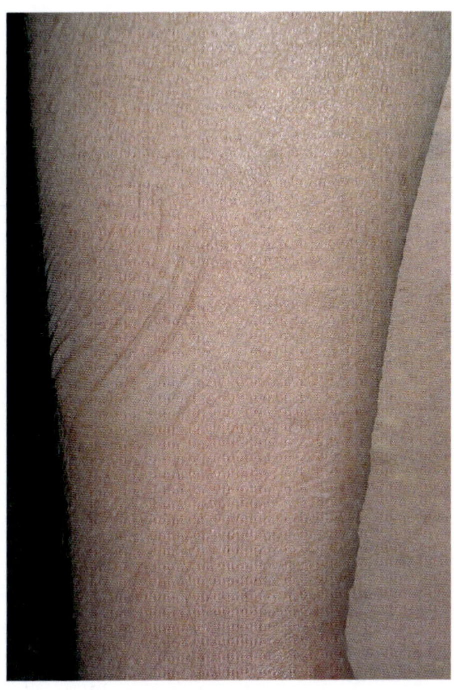

Fig. 1.61 Early-stage toxic epidermal necrolysis showing diffuse erythema and formation of bullae with Nikolsky's sign

The skin thermoregulation and the fluid/electrolyte balance are usually impaired. Mortality is mainly related to sepsis, fluid/electrolyte imbalance, or gastrointestinal hemorrhage. Bronchitis, pneumonia, and renal insufficiency may develop. The mortality rate can be predicted by using the severity-of-illness score named SCORTEN [52]. As patients are on high risk for sepsis, it is essential to transfer them to an intensive care burn unit [53]. Prevention of infection is essential as well as maintenance of fluid and electrolyte balance and nutritional support. Systemic corticosteroids, cyclosporine, and intravenous immunoglobulins are the mainstays of therapy depending on the case [54], but the effectiveness of these therapies and other alternatives such as plasmapheresis and biologics is uncertain [53]. Prompt withdrawal of the suspected drugs may decrease mortality [55].

NSAIDs, antiepileptics, sulfonamides, and allopurinol are among the inducers of TEN. Cardiovascular drugs such as phenytoin and diuretics have also been reported to be associated with drug-induced TEN.

Staphylococcal scalded skin syndrome (SSSS) should be regarded in the differential diagnosis. SSSS is mainly seen in pediatric patients and is characterized by widespread erythema and superficial (subcorneal) blisters induced by the exfoliative toxins of *Staphylococcus aureus*. It is usually successfully treated with antistaphylococcal antibiotics.

Drug Hypersensitivity Syndrome/Drug Rash with Eosinophilia and Systemic Symptoms

DHS/DRESS is an uncommon but severe, idiosyncratic drug reaction with a significant risk of morbidity and mortality [56]. It is defined by generalized, long-lasting maculopapular (Fig. 1.1) or any other skin eruption occasionally progressing to erythroderma, accompanied by fever up to 39 °C or higher, lymphadenopathy, and visceral involvement. Hepatic involvement is characterized by an acute elevation in serum transaminases up to five- to tenfold. Renal or hematological abnormalities may also occur. Atypical lymphocytes are commonly seen. Facial edema is often associating. Typically, fever precedes skin eruption, so an infectious etiology is usually suspected at first. A scoring system has been suggested for the diagnosis of DRESS [57].

Antiepileptics such as carbamazepine and lamotrigine, sulfonamides, allopurinol, terbinafine, vancomycin [58], and more recently new retroviral drugs [56] are among the main inducers of DHS/DRESS. The reaction has a long latency period up to 8 weeks after starting the responsible drug [4]. The long latency period and fever as the initial symptom may complicate the early diagnosis of the condition. Phenytoin when used as antiepileptic drug is frequently associated with DHS/DRESS.

Withdrawal of the offending drug and treatment with systemic corticosteroids are usually effective.

Lymphomatoid Drug Eruption/Pseudolymphoma Syndrome

Lymphomatoid drug eruption or PLS and DHS show some similar clinical and histological findings. Like DHS, PLS is another life-threatening reaction that presents with fever, generalized skin eruption, lymphadenopathy, and internal organ involvement. It may take a prolonged course even after the cessation of causative agents [59]. PLS may also give rise to harmful effects if misdiagnosed as malignant lymphoma, and patients with PLS are treated unnecessarily with chemotherapy, because it may mimic histologically other lymphomas, including mycosis fungoides [59]. Lymphomatoid drug eruption has been reported with ACEIs and ARBs [60]. Phenytoin and mexiletine were also reported to be associated with this type of drug eruption. Recently, amlodipine, a CCB, and metoprolol, a beta-blocker, were reported to cause CD30+ lymphomatoid drug eruption showing diffuse erythema in addition to macules, papules, and annular plaques [61].

Drug-Induced Necrosis

Necrosis may occur with anticoagulants such as warfarin and heparin, and with sympathomimetics. Warfarin necrosis occurs mainly in patients with protein C/S deficiency or a factor V Leiden mutation [62]. Cutaneous findings include petechiae that progress to ecchymoses, hemorrhagic bullae, and necrosis [62]. It is a condition with a high rate of morbidity and mortality. Other cardiovascular drugs such as beta-blockers and thrombolytics, the latter via cholesterol embolism, may also cause skin necrosis.

Drug-Induced Lupus Erythematosus

Some drugs are able to induce SLE or SCLE. Classical drug-induced lupus is characterized by the presence of antinuclear antibodies (ANA) and antihistone antibodies [63] although the latter is not pathognomonic for drug-induced lupus. Antihistone antibodies are also found in 75 % of the cases of idiopathic SLE [63]. Antibodies against double-stranded DNA are typically absent in drug-induced lupus [4]. Seroconversion to ANA does not require withdrawal of the drug unless systemic symptoms occur [4]. There are no pathognomonic cutaneous manifestations in drug-induced lupus. In comparison to idiopathic SLE, the incidence of malar rash, discoid rash, photosensitivity, alopecia, and oral ulcers are reported to be rare [63]. Symptoms may develop within a long period up to a year after the commencement of treatment [4]. Withdrawal of the causative drug usually results in resolution of the symptoms. Procainamide, hydralazine, isoniazid, minocycline, and recently the anti-TNF drugs are strongly associated with the development of drug-induced lupus [63–65].

Drug-induced SCLE may present with annular–polycyclic, papulosquamous, or psoriasiform lesions mainly on the upper trunk with involvement of the lower legs that are usually spared in idiopathic SCLE [65]. ANA, anti-Ro/SSA, anti-La/SSB antibodies may be found positive [66], whereas antihistone antibodies might be absent [65]. Among the cardiovascular drugs, thiazide diuretics, CCBs, and statins have been more commonly implicated to trigger SCLE [67, 68]. Recently, we saw a patient with SCLE-like eruption possibly induced by filgrastim, a granulocyte colony-stimulating factor [69] (Figs. 1.62, 1.63, and 1.64).

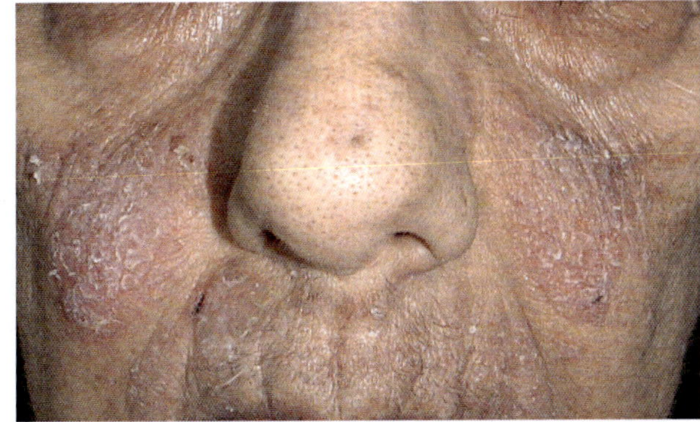

Fig. 1.62 Symmetrical erythemato-squamous plaques on the malar areas and above the upper lip in a patient with subacute cutaneous lupus erythematosus-like eruption possibly induced by filgrastim, a granulocyte colony-stimulating factor

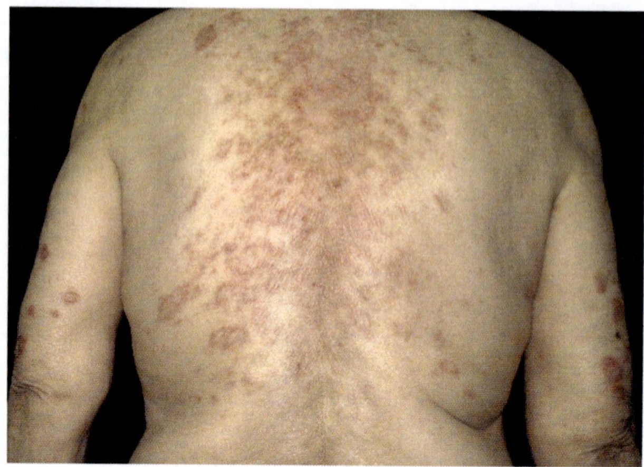

Fig. 1.63 Erythemato-squamous plaques on the back and symmetrically on the upper extremities, mainly in annular–polycyclic configuration, in a patient with subacute cutaneous lupus erythematosus-like eruption possibly induced by filgrastim, a granulocyte colony-stimulating factor

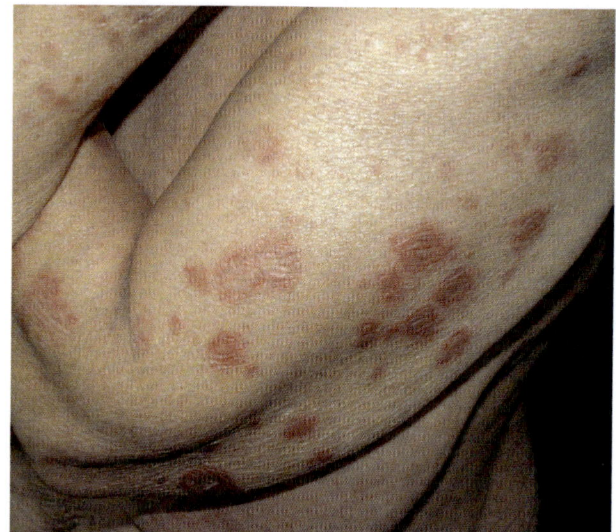

Fig. 1.64 Erythemato-squamous plaques on the arms, mainly in annular–polycyclic configuration, in a patient with subacute cutaneous lupus erythematosus-like eruption possibly induced by filgrastim, a granulocyte colony-stimulating factor

Drug-Induced Psoriasis/Psoriasiform Eruption

Psoriasis is a chronic inflammatory skin disease, usually characterized by red, scaly patches, papules, and plaques. Certain drugs such as lithium, gold salts, beta-blockers, antimalarials, NSAIDs, tetracyclines, adrenergic antagonists, interferon, gemfibrozil, iodine, digoxin and clonidine are capable to induce or exacerbate psoriasis [70, 71] or induce a psoriasiform eruption (Fig. 1.65). In contrast to many other drugs which may also induce psoriasis de novo, antimalarials were claimed only to trigger an existing psoriasis [72]. Among the cardiovascular drugs, ACEIs, ARBs, and CCBs may also trigger psoriasis or induce a psoriasiform drug eruption.

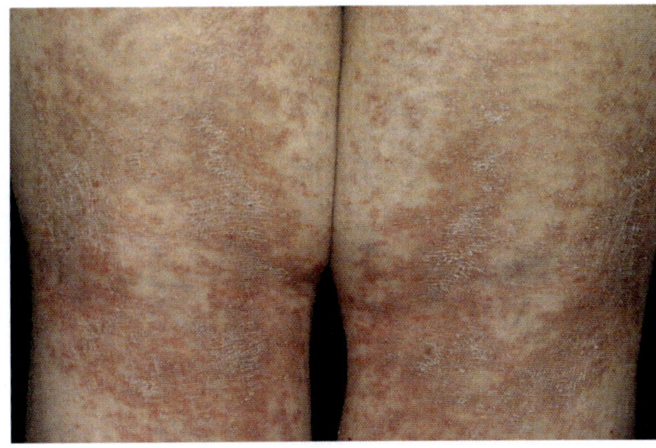

Fig. 1.65 Red, scaly psoriasiform plaques on the lower extremities

Drug-Induced Serum Sickness/Serum Sickness-Like Reaction

Drugs may also cause a "serum sickness-like reaction" (SSLR), characterized by the development of cutaneous eruption, arthralgia/arthritis, and often fever [73]. Cutaneous eruption may be variable such as palpable purpura with/without hemorrhagic vesicles, urticarial lesions, or EM-like lesions in SSLR. Leukocytoclastic vasculitis is usually seen in the histopathology of cutaneous lesions. Urticarial lesions seen in drug-induced SSLR commonly represent urticarial vasculitis. Unlike the true serum sickness, a type III hypersensitivity reaction, however, vasculitis and fever are not consistent findings in the reported cases of SSLR. Besides, gastrointestinal disturbances, lymphadenopathy, low complement levels, circulating immune complexes, and proteinuria associated with renal involvement are usually absent or rarely reported in drug-induced SSLR [4, 73]. Cases with detected circulating immune complexes to drugs are better termed as "drug-induced serum sickness." Penicillins, cephalosporins, sulfonamides, and many other drugs have been implicated to cause drug-induced serum sickness or SSLR. Cardiovascular drugs such as beta-blockers are also among the inducers of this type of reaction.

Other Skin Reactions

Pruritus and *flushing* are other frequently reported adverse reactions of drug therapy. Cardiovascular drugs including statins have been reported among the main inducers of drug-induced pruritus [74]. Flushing may occur with vasodilators and CCBs.

Xerosis is a common side effect of lipid-lowering drugs.

Peripheral edema is frequently associated with the use of adrenergic neuron blockers (reserpine), CCBs, and vasodilators.

Some drugs may cause *ulceration of the skin and mucosa.* There are increasing reports on perianal, peristomal, oral, or skin ulcerations with nicorandil, a vasodilatory drug used to treat angina [75].

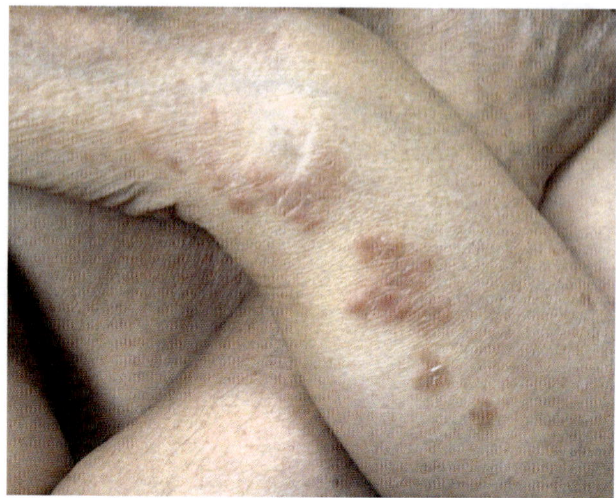

Fig. 1.66 Indurated, reddish, confluent papules on the extensor surface of the forearm in a patient with interstitial granulomatous drug reaction from thalidomide

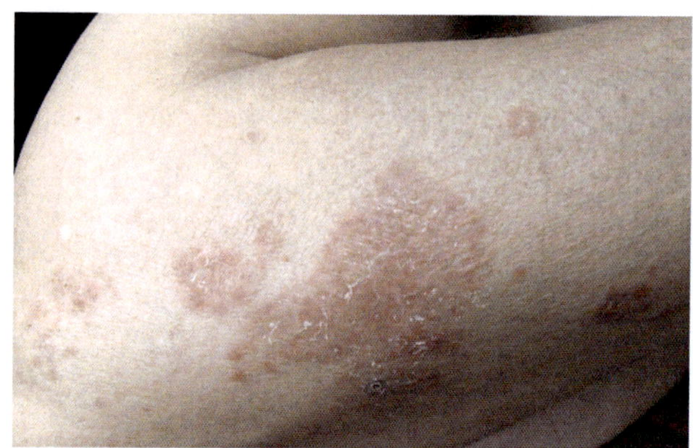

Fig. 1.67 Erythemato-squamous plaque and indurated, reddish papules on the extensor surface of the forearm in a patient with interstitial granulomatous drug reaction from thalidomide

Drugs including thiazides and ACEIs (captopril) may induce a *pityriasis rosea-like eruption* [76].

Drug-induced papuloerythroderma of Ofuji [77] has been reported in association with cardiovascular drugs as well, such as furosemide and aspirin in single cases [78, 79].

Drug-induced Sweet syndrome is a rare condition, reported to occur with granulocyte colony-stimulating factor, all-trans-retinoic acid, and miscellaneous drugs [80]. The upper extremities are more frequently involved, and peripheral neutrophilia is usually absent in drug-induced Sweet syndrome [81].

Interstitial granulomatous drug reaction (IGDR) resembles interstitial granulomatous dermatitis, which is mostly a histopathological entity describing any condition characterized by the arrangement of histiocytes when they are splayed singly or in groups between collagen bundles [82]. The clinical presentation of IGDR

(Figs. 1.66 and 1.67) is variable such as plaques, generalized erythematous macular and/or papular lesions, and erythema nodosum [83–87].

Among the cardiovascular drugs, ACEIs, CCBs, beta-blockers, lipid-lowering drugs, anticoagulants, and diuretics, i.e., furosemide, were implicated in the evolution of IGDR [83].

Drug-Induced Hyperhidrosis/Hypohidrosis

Drugs may also alter the human sweating response. Cholinesterase inhibitors, selective serotonin reuptake inhibitors, opioids, and tricyclic antidepressants may cause hyperhidrosis, whereas antimuscarinic anticholinergic agents, carbonic anhydrase inhibitors, and tricyclic antidepressants may cause hypohidrosis [88]. Various cardiovascular drugs were found to be associated with hyperhidrosis.

Drug-Induced Mucosal Lesions

Drug eruptions may also present with mucosal lesions, mainly oral or genital, showing lichenoid, bullous/erosive, aphthous, or erythematous pattern. Burning mouth/tongue, scalded mouth syndrome, xerostomia, taste disturbances/dysgeusia, and gingival hyperplasia may also occur [89]. In a study on 531 patients taking cardiovascular drugs, oral symptoms and/or signs were reported in 14.1 % with xerostomia being the most common (7.5 %), followed by lichenoid lesions (3.6 %) and dysgeusia (1.9 %) [90]. Xerostomia was less frequent in patients receiving therapy with ACEIs [90]. It may frequently occur with alpha-adrenergic receptor blockers, adrenergic neuron blockers, alpha-2 adrenergic receptor agonists, class I antiarrhythmics, CCBs, beta-blockers, and diuretics. Phenytoin and CCBs (mainly nifedipine) are well-known inducers of gingival hyperplasia.

Drug-Induced Hair Changes

Drugs may induce hair changes. Alopecia with anticoagulants, beta-blockers, and statins; hypertrichosis with phenytoin, minoxidil, acetazolamide, and diazoxide are well-known hair problems in patients taking cardiovascular drugs [3]. Drug-induced alopecia is nonscarring and usually reversible following withdrawal of the drug [91, 92]. Cytostatics, carbamazepine, valproate, cimetidine, acitretin, ketoconazole, and carbimazole are other drugs which may cause alopecia [4, 91, 92]. Other causative drugs of hypertrichosis include cyclosporine, interferon, danazol, penicillamine, and zidovudine [84, 92].

Drug-Induced Nail Changes

Drugs may cause various nail changes that are often dose-related and disappear after stopping the causative agent [93]. Some changes are usually asymptomatic and only cause cosmetic problems, but there might be painful onycholysis and subungual abscesses or ingrown nails, paronychia, and pyogenic granuloma, the latter mainly associated with the use of tyrosine kinase inhibitors of the epidermal growth factor receptor (e.g., erlotinib, gefitinib) [93]. Symptoms vary according to the affected site of the nail such as the matrix, nail bed, nail folds, or vessels.

Among the cardiovascular drugs, indapamide may induce photo-onycholysis, whereas warfarin and other anticoagulants can cause bleeding of the nail bed [93]. Digital gangrene can be seen with beta-blockers as a serious side effect [94].

Difficulties in Analyzing the Published Reports on Drug Eruptions

Unfortunately, a considerable amount of the published reports fail to describe the cutaneous lesions properly, i.e., a "rash" or "exanthema" does not say much about the type of the reaction, the latter often used for erythema or maculopapular/morbilliform eruption. It is also not clear whether several reported variations of "edema" such as facial edema, periorbital edema, lid edema, or genital edema represent angioedema or not. Even reaction types lack a systematic classification; some reactions are named according to the elementary lesion of the eruption (maculopapular, bullous, pustular), some according to clinicohistopathologic picture (lichenoid, eczematous), some according to dermatosis (FDE, exfoliative dermatitis, EM, SJS, TEN), or some according to the name of the activated dermatosis or disease (psoriasiform, SLE-like).

Pathogenesis

The pathogenesis of ACDR may be either non-immunologic such as overdose, cumulative toxicity, or drug interactions, which are known as dose-dependent and predictable type A (augmented) reactions, or less commonly type B (bizarre) reactions which are unpredictable and not dose-dependent. Type B reactions include mainly immunologic reactions whereas all of the four immune mechanisms according to Coombs and Gell [95] may be involved. Non-immunologic reactions such as "intolerance" occurring with normal doses of a drug and "idiosyncrasy" due to deficiency of drug-metabolizing enzymes in genetic susceptible patients are also covered under type B reactions. Pseudoallergic reactions mimicking true immunologically mediated immediate-type allergic reactions, such as anaphylactoid reactions, are induced by "intolerance" to the drug resulting in mast cell degranulation and liberation of mediators like histamine and leukotrienes which lead to the development of clinical symptoms [96].

Immunologic reactions may be against the active ingredients or their metabolites or the inactive ingredients such as preservatives, emulgators, or dyes in a drug. Angioedema/urticaria is the typical example for IgE-mediated type I (anaphylactic/immediate) hypersensitivity reaction. Among the cardiovascular drugs, ACEIs are the most common inducers of angioedema/urticaria. Some drugs like acetylsalicylic acid, morphine, codeine, muscle relaxants, and radiological contrast materials may cause anaphylactoid reactions that are clinically similar to anaphylactic reactions, but they are non-immunologically mediated. These drugs are able to degranulate mast cells directly as described above. Thrombocytopenia and related purpuric eruptions are the typical examples for IgM- or IgG-mediated type II (cytotoxic/complement-mediated) hypersensitivity reaction such as in quinidine-induced thrombocytopenia. Leukocytoclastic vasculitis is the typical example for IgG- or IgM-mediated type III (immune complex mediated) hypersensitivity reaction, a known side effect of thrombolytic drugs. Diuretic-induced vasculitis is also well known. Finally, generalized eczematous eruption is the typical example for T cell-mediated type IV (cell-mediated/delayed) hypersensitivity reaction, occurring most commonly after systemic intake of a drug or cross-reacting agent with a preexisting contact sensitization. However, a type IV hypersensitivity reaction was also suggested for many other drug eruptions such as maculopapular, lichenoid, or pustular drug eruptions, based on a recent subclassification of type IV hypersensitivity reactions.

Type IV Drug Hypersensitivity Reactions

Delayed-type (type IV) drug hypersensitivity reactions have been divided into four subtypes (type IVa, b, c, d) depending on the predominant type of drug-specific memory T cells and the released cytokines that would determine the clinical phenotype of the drug eruption (Table 1.1) [97–99]. It was recently shown that granulysin (a cationic cytolytic protein released primarily by T lymphocytes and natural killer cells) is responsible for keratinocyte apoptosis in SJS/TEN rather than perforin, granzyme B, and Fas–Fas ligand interaction [100, 101]. Granulysin was expressed in very high concentrations in the blister fluids of patients with SJS/TEN; moreover, reduction in granulysin levels resulted in reduced cytotoxicity [4, 101].

In most reactions, different type IV reactions may occur together, and cytotoxic functions by CD4+ or CD8+ T cells (type IVc) seem to participate in all type IV reactions [97]. It has been suggested that a combination of type IVa and IVc reactions is involved in eczematous eruptions [97] and type IVc reaction in FDE [19]. Moreover, it would not be surprising to see many examples with overlapping features of different drug eruptions, such as with maculopapular and lichenoid morphology in the same patient, because the cytokine pathways often overlap [10, 102].

Table 1.1 The proposed subtypes of type IV hypersensitivity reactions in the immunopathogenesis of drug eruptions

Type IV reactions	T lymphocyte	Cytokines/inflammatory mediators	Examples of drug eruptions
Type IVa	CD4+ Th1	IFN-γ, TNF-α	Eczematous[a]
			BS/SDRIFE
Type IVb	CD4+ Th2	IL-5, IL-4, IL-13, eotaxin	DHS/DRESS
			Maculopapular (with eosinophilia)
			Type I reactions
Type IVc[b]	Cytotoxic T cells (CD4+ and CD8+)	Perforin, granzyme B, FasL Granulysin[c]	EM
			SJS/TEN[c]
			Eczematous/BS/SDRIFE[a]
			Maculopapular
			FDE
			Lichenoid
Type IVd	CD4+ and CD8+ T cells	IL-8, GM-CSF	Pustular/AGEP

Modified from Refs. [97–99, 102]

IFN interferon, *TNF* tumor necrosis factor, *BS* Baboon syndrome, *SDRIFE* symmetrical drug-related intertriginous and flexural exanthema, *IL* interleukin, *DRESS* drug rash with eosinophilia and systemic symptoms, *FasL* Fas ligand, *EM* erythema multiforme, *SJS* Stevens–Johnson syndrome, *TEN* toxic epidermal necrolysis, *FDE* fixed drug eruption, *GM-CSF* granulocyte-macrophage colony-stimulating factor, *AGEP* acute generalized exanthematous pustulosis

[a]A combination of type IVa and IVc reactions was suggested to be involved in eczematous eruptions

[b]Type IVc is the major type in most drug-induced delayed hypersensitivity reactions

[c]It was recently shown that granulysin (a cationic cytolytic protein released primarily by T lymphocytes and natural killer cells) is the key molecule responsible for keratinocyte apoptosis in SJS/TEN [100, 101]

On the other hand, some drugs, e.g., beta-lactam antibiotics such as amoxicillin and ampicillin, are capable to induce different drug eruptions. The mystery why amoxicillin elicits a typical maculopapular eruption in a given patient, and pustular or BS/SDRIFE in others, or even in the same patient in different occasions, might also be explained by the new subclassification of type IV hypersensitivity reactions [10]: the predominant type of specific memory T cells and related effector mechanism via the released cytokines would determine the type of the eruption in a given occasion [98].

p-i Concept

Certain drugs or their metabolites are capable to induce primary sensitization of T cells by direct systemic exposure [103], without known previous topical exposure and demonstrable cutaneous sensitization. This may be explained by a novel pathomechanism, the so-called p-i concept (pharmacologic interaction with immune receptors) [8].

Different from the hapten and prohapten concepts, certain drugs are able to bind directly and non-covalently to a fitting T cell receptor without first being presented by major histocompatibility complex (MHC) molecules and without prior metabolism [10, 97]. When a chemically inert drug is bound to the fitting T cell receptor, it would already exert sufficient T cell activation, even though the binding is labile. An additional interaction of the T cell receptor with the MHC molecule would lead to full activation of T cells [97]. This type of T cell stimulation has been shown in different forms of drug eruptions such as ciprofloxacin-induced maculopapular eruption, sulfamethoxazole-induced maculopapular eruption, lamotrigine- or carbamazepine-induced DRESS, lidocaine-induced EM, and celecoxib-induced AGEP [8].

Genetic Background

Some drug eruptions were found to be associated with HLA class I alleles. HLA-B 5701 was identified as an important risk factor for abacavir-induced severe drug eruption in Caucasians [104], HLA-B 1502 for carbamazepine-induced SJS in Han-Chinese [105], and HLA-B 5801 for severe drug eruption such as SJS from allopurinol [106]. Moreover, statistical correlations were highly significant between HLA-B22 and feprazone-induced FDE and [107, 108] between HLA-A30 or HLA-A30 B13 Cw6 haplotype and co-trimoxazole-induced FDE [109].

Apart from the HLA alleles, the genetic basis of ACDR may also be related with drug-metabolizing enzymes, mainly the cytochrome P-450 enzyme system, and drug transporters [110]. The related genes would influence the pharmacokinetics and pharmacodynamics of drugs [4].

Other Predisposing Factors

Certain patients may be predisposed to the development of ACDR. A concomitant viral infection may alter the immune status, thus increasing the risk for a drug reaction. Viral infections may increase the incidence of morbilliform drug eruptions. The well-documented examples are the increased risk of ampicillin hypersensitivity in patients with Epstein–Barr virus-induced infectious mononucleosis, and the increased risk of co-trimoxazole hypersensitivity in HIV patients. Altered drug metabolism from organ impairment or genetic factors, e.g., slow acetylating of drugs, might be another predisposing factor. Another important point is that some patients reacting to one drug might have a propensity to react against other chemically unrelated drugs probably due to a deficient ability to develop a tolerogenic immune response. Multiple drug allergy (MDA) is a recently proposed term to describe this condition. It was estimated that up to 10 % of patients with severe drug hypersensitivity have a tendency for developing MDA [111].

Multiple Drug Allergy

MDA is characterized by hypersensitivity to two or more chemically unrelated drugs simultaneously or sequentially [111–113]. The reported cases of MDA were mainly presented with immediate type of drug eruptions such as urticaria, angioedema, or anaphylaxis [112, 113]. Delayed type of drug eruptions have been rarely reported in MDA as maculopapular eruption, FDE, AGEP, DHS, EM, SJS, TEN, and undefined rashes [111, 113, 114]. Generalized eczematous eruption seems to be an extremely rare clinical variant of delayed- type MDA [115, 116].

Diagnosis of Adverse Cutaneous Drug Reactions

The diagnosis of a drug eruption is usually difficult to establish. The first step for the diagnosis is to determine the type of the reaction; dermatologic examination often accompanied by histopathological evaluation is essential for this. The second step is to designate a certain drug as the cause of this certain type of reaction. Skin tests, although not reliable in most of the cases, might be performed such as prick or scratch tests for type I immunologic reactions; intradermal tests for type I, III, or IV immunologic reactions; or patch tests for type IV immunologic reactions. Determination of drug-specific IgE in the serum for type I immunologic reactions could be performed for a limited number of drugs and is also not helpful in most of the cases. Systemic provocation with the suspected drug might be performed in selected cases of localized drug eruptions, especially in localized FDE where systemic challenge is still the gold standard in the diagnosis. Otherwise, it is usually contraindicated especially in severe drug reactions, in patients with documented anaphylaxis, or for drugs with potential risk of developing anaphylactic/anaphylactoid reactions.

History and Clinical Investigation

A chronological history of drugs that were used in the last weeks or months before the onset of the drug eruption is essential. The time between drug intake and the onset of the eruption is a major clue for identifying the culprit drug. However, one should be aware that the latency period between the initiation of therapy and onset of the drug eruption might be variable. For the common maculopapular eruptions, the reaction typically starts after 5–10 days, whereas in FDE, it usually starts within 10–30 minutes to hours [19], and in antiepileptic-induced DHS up to 8 weeks following therapy [4]. SJS/TEN usually begins within 4 weeks of exposure to the causative drug [4]. In drug-induced lupus, symptoms may first occur after 1 year of drug therapy [4].

Table 1.2 The Naranjo adverse drug reaction probability scale

Criteria	Yes	No	?	Total score
Presence of previous conclusive reports on this ADR	+1	0	0	
Appearance of ADR after administration of the suspected drug	+2	−1	0	
Improvement of ADR after discontinuation of the drug	+1	0	0	
Reappearance of ADR following readministration of the drug	+2	−1	0	
Reappearance of ADR following a placebo	−1	+1	0	
Alternative causes (other than drug)	−1	+2	0	
Dose-dependent severity of ADR	+1	0	0	
Toxic concentration of the drug in blood (or other fluids)	+1	0	0	
History of any similar reaction to the same or similar drugs	+1	0	0	
Confirmation of ADR by any objective evidence	+1	0	0	

Adapted from Naranjo et al. [117] and modified from Özkaya and Babuna [102]
Probability categories according to total score [117]: definite if ≥9, probable if 5–8, possible if 1–4, doubtful if ≤0
ADR adverse drug reaction

History of similar eruptions in the past, the morphology of the eruption, coexisting fever, and lymphadenopathy should be identified. Alternative causes of the eruption, such as infection, should also be excluded. Drug imputability scores such as the Naranjo adverse drug reaction probability score (Table 1.2) or other causality assessment criteria would help find out a causal relationship between drugs and the eruption [102, 117–119].

A positive withdrawal test, i.e., improvement of the eruption after drug withdrawal, and a positive rechallenge test, i.e., reappearance of ACDR following readministration of the drug, would suggest a causal relationship between the drug and the eruption.

Histopathology

Histopathology is not diagnostic, but it may help identify the type of the eruption and exclude the differential diagnostic conditions. However, the widespread belief that blood and tissue eosinophilia is helpful in identifying drug-induced eruptions and their differentiation from viral exanthemas could not be verified in a recent study on patients with morbilliform eruption [120].

Immunofluorescence Microscopy

Immunofluorescence microscopy would be helpful in diagnosing bullous eruptions, e.g., pemphigus, pemphigoid, linear IgA dermatosis, and other reactions such as lupus erythematosus, and vasculitis, e.g., HSP. However, there is lack of strong positivity rates in direct immunofluorescence (DIF) in drug-induced pemphigus [4, 25].

In Vivo Diagnostic Tests

In vivo tests for identifying the culprit drug in drug eruptions include skin prick/scratch/intradermal tests and systemic provocation tests for type I hypersensitivity reactions; and patch test, skin prick/intradermal tests with late readings up to 1 week, and systemic provocation tests for type IV hypersensitivity reactions.

It might be recommended to start with open skin tests first, in order to exclude immediate reactions. If open tests are negative after 20–60 minutes, skin prick/scratch/intradermal tests with the suspected drugs might be performed for the diagnosis of type I hypersensitivity reactions, however, with a high rate of false-positive reactions.

Patch test is an important diagnostic step for most of the drug eruptions. In case of a negative patch test reaction with the suspected drug, it was suggested to perform late readings of skin prick/intradermal tests which would be useful [121]. Phototest and photopatch tests may be performed if there is suspicion of drug-induced photosensitivity. A positive phototest, showing a decrease in the minimal dose of the UVA and UVB radiation required to induce an erythema in a patient while taking the suspected drug, would suggest a drug-induced phototoxic eruption. A positive photopatch test with the suspected drug, on the other hand, would contribute to the diagnosis of photoallergic drug eruption.

Patch testing and photopatch testing in drug eruptions and examples of patch/photopatch testing with cardiovascular drugs are detailed in Chap. 16.

In Vitro Diagnostic Tests

In vitro tests include the determination of drug-specific IgE, basophil activation test and mast cell degranulation test for type I hypersensitivity reactions; and lymphocyte transformation/activation tests for type IV hypersensitivity reactions [122].

Serum-Specific IgE Testing

In case of suspicion of ACDR related with type I hypersensitivity reaction, i.e., drug-induced angioedema/urticaria, drug-specific IgE levels may be determined; however, only a limited number of drugs can be investigated by this method. Specific IgE to penicillin G, penicillin V, amoxicillin, and ampicillin are most frequently studied. The results suggest, however, that skin testing offers greater reliability and sensitivity than beta-lactam-specific IgE determination [123].

Basophil Activation Test

In patients with type I hypersensitivity reactions, a flow cytometric basophil activation test has been shown to contribute to the diagnosis of drug-induced anaphylactic reaction with several drugs such as beta-lactams, NSAIDs, and muscle relaxants [122].

Lymphocyte Transformation Test/Lymphocyte Activation Test/Other Tests

As an adjunct to skin testing in delayed-type hypersensitivity reactions, drug-specific T cell activity may be assessed in vitro by the lymphocyte transformation test (LTT; synonyms: lymphocyte proliferation test, lymphocyte stimulation test) or the lymphocyte activation test (LAT) [124]. LTT was found to be positive especially in maculopapular drug eruption, SJS, BS, bullous EM, AGEP, and DRESS [122, 124, 125]. In contrast, it was mainly negative in FDE and TEN [122, 124]. In LAT, activation of T lymphocytes can be measured by means of upregulation of the activation marker CD69 or by means of cell-cycle analysis through DNA content [122, 126]. Positive LTT and LAT responses to the drugs in vitro would suggest involvement of T cells in the pathogenesis of drug eruptions. However, clinical relevance of positive LTT and LAT responses might sometimes be lacking, so further confirmatory studies are needed.

The in vitro interferon-gamma release test from lymphocytes may also be a helpful clue for the diagnosis of ACDR [127].

Systemic Challenge with Drugs

In case of a negative patch test result with the suspected drug, systemic challenge, usually oral provocation test, is considered to be the only reliable method to find out the responsible drug. It is generally considered safe to perform a drug challenge in most of the delayed-type immune reactions [128]. The clinical relevance of cross-reactive drugs might also be investigated by this method. Systemic challenge is the gold standard in the diagnosis of FDE; however, it should not be performed in severe drug eruptions, e.g., DRESS, SJS, and TEN.

Apart from finding the culprit drug, systemic challenge would also allow to find out an alternative drug that would be safe for the patient. For this purpose, it would be best to perform systemic challenge with a drug with a negative patch test finding.

Systemic challenge with drugs is also not well standardized. Regarding FDE, it might be recommended to perform a systemic provocation test at least 4 weeks after resolution of the eruption to avoid false-negative results due to a refractory period [19]. It would be best to perform a systemic challenge test with the least implicated drug first, followed by more likely drugs [129]. In delayed hypersensitivity reactions, it is usually started with a subtherapeutic initial dose, e.g., with 1/8 of a tablet, that is increased every 12–24 hours up to a whole tablet [130]. In case of immediate hypersensitivity reactions, doses are much lower, e.g., 1/100 of the therapeutic dose, and are usually increased every 30–60 minutes by approximately 10-fold up to the full therapeutic dose.

False-negative reactions might be seen due to the lack of cofactors like viral infection that would alter the immune response.

Subcutaneous provocation testing was found superior to patch testing with low molecular weight heparins (LMWHs) for finding out the culprit drug as low doses of LMWH may inhibit the elicitation of allergic contact dermatitis [131].

Management of Adverse Cutaneous Drug Reactions

The suspected drug must be stopped immediately or changed to a non-cross-reacting alternative agent. Indeed, it was reported that rapid withdrawal of the suspected drugs may decrease mortality in SJS/TEN [55]. However, this is especially difficult in elderly and those on multiple hard-to-replace drugs with vital indications. For mild ACDR, a symptomatic therapy with systemic antihistamines and topical corticosteroids would help in many types of reactions, but systemic corticosteroids (usually 1 mg/kg/day prednisolone or its equivalent) are usually necessary for severe ACDR although their use is still controversial in TEN.

Patients should be warned not to use the causative drug and its cross-reactants in the future. Avoidance is the best treatment for ACDR.

The most commonly reported adverse cutaneous reactions of cardiovascular drugs are summarized according to the drug class and to the type of the reaction in Tables 1.3 and 1.4, respectively. Possible cross-reactions are shown in Table 1.5.

Table 1.3 Overview of the main adverse cutaneous reactions to specific class of cardiovascular drugs

Cardiovascular drug	Type of the adverse drug reaction
Angiotensin-converting enzyme inhibitors (mainly captopril, enalapril)	Angioedema, bullous eruption-mainly pemphigus, lichenoid eruption, lymphomatoid eruption, psoriasiform eruption, eczematous eruption, drug-induced lupus erythematosus, photosensitivity, scalded mouth syndrome
Angiotensin II receptor blockers	Angioedema, psoriasiform eruption, eczematous eruption, lymphomatoid eruption, vasculitis, bullous eruptions, lichenoid eruption
Alpha-2 adrenergic receptor agonists	Drug-induced lupus erythematosus (methyldopa), photosensitivity, lichenoid eruption (methyldopa), eczematous eruption (methyldopa), local side effects (transdermal clonidine), psoriasiform eruption (clonidine), xerostomia
Class I antiarrhythmics	Drug-induced lupus erythematosus (mainly procainamide), photosensitivity (quinidine), maculopapular eruption, drug rash with eosinophilia and systemic symptoms (phenytoin, mexiletine), hyperpigmentation (quinidine, phenytoin), acneiform/pustular eruption, purpura (quinidine), injection site reactions, angioedema/urticaria, xerostomia, gingival hyperplasia (phenytoin)
Beta-blockers	Psoriasiform eruption, oculomucocutaneous syndrome (practolol), lichenoid eruption, angioedema/urticaria, drug-induced lupus erythematosus, Peyronie's disease, vasculitis, peripheral vascular disease, alopecia
Class III antiarrhythmics	Photosensitivity (amiodarone), hyperpigmentation (amiodarone), drug-induced lupus erythematosus (amiodarone)

Table 1.3 (continued)

Cardiovascular drug	Type of the adverse drug reaction
Calcium channel blockers	Peripheral edema, flushing, gingival hyperplasia (nifedipine), gynecomastia, maculopapular eruption, photosensitivity, hyperpigmentation (diltiazem), nonvasculitic eruptive telangiectasia, drug-induced lupus erythematosus-mainly subacute type, psoriasiform reactions, angioedema/urticaria, AGEP (diltiazem), pemphigus and bullous eruptions, purpura (amlodipine), erythema multiforme, SJS/TEN
Diuretics	Photosensitivity (thiazide), drug-induced lupus erythematosus-mainly subacute type, bullous eruptions-mainly pemphigoid, AGEP, erythema multiforme, SJS/TEN, vasculitis, lichenoid eruption, angioedema/urticaria, hypertrichosis (acetazolamide)
Vasodilators	Flushing, peripheral edema, hypertrichosis (diazoxide, minoxidil), drug-induced lupus erythematosus (hydralazine), vasculitis (hydralazine), contact dermatitis (transdermal nitroglycerin), erythema multiforme, SJS/TEN, mucocutaneous ulcers (nicorandil), erythroderma (epoprostenol, pentaerythritol tetranitrate, glyceryl trinitrate)
Lipid-lowering drugs	Lichenoid eruption (statins), dermatomyositis (statins), drug-induced lupus erythematosus (statins), eczematous eruption (statins), alopecia (statins), xerosis/ichthyosis, photosensitivity (fibrates), angioedema/urticaria (fibrates), flushing (niacin), acanthosis nigricans (niacin)
Platelet inhibitors	Angioedema/urticaria, anaphylactoid reaction (aspirin), maculopapular eruption, bleeding/purpura, thrombotic thrombocytopenic purpura, lichenoid eruption, drug-induced lupus erythematosus (ticlopidine), drug rash with eosinophilia and systemic symptoms, AGEP
Thrombolytics	Purpura, angioedema/urticaria, vasculitis, cholesterol embolism, serum sickness-like reaction (streptokinase)
Anticoagulants	Bleeding/purpura, skin necrosis (heparin, LMWHs, warfarin), eczematous eruption (enoxaparin), angioedema/urticaria, bullous hemorrhagic dermatosis, maculopapular eruption, vasculitis, alopecia, calcinosis cutis (nadroparin), purple toe syndrome (warfarin), drug rash with eosinophilia and systemic symptoms
Sympathomimetics (mainly dopamine, epinephrine/norepinephrine)	Injection site reactions including skin necrosis, peripheral gangrene

The most frequently implicated drugs are indicated in parentheses
AGEP acute generalized exanthematous pustulosis, *LMWH* low molecular weight heparin, *SJS* Stevens–Johnson syndrome, *TEN* toxic epidermal necrolysis

Table 1.4 Overview of the main adverse cutaneous reactions to cardiovascular drugs according to the type of the reaction (in alphabetical order)

Type of the adverse drug reaction	Main causative cardiovascular drug
AGEP	Diltiazem, diuretics, platelet inhibitors
Alopecia	Anticoagulants, beta-blockers, statins
Angioedema/urticaria	ACEIs, ARBs, aspirin and other platelet inhibitors, beta-blockers, thrombolytics, anticoagulants, class I antiarrhythmics, CCBs, fibrates
Bullous eruptions	
Drug-induced pemphigus	Captopril, enalapril, nifedipine
Drug-induced pemphigoid	Furosemide, spironolactone, clonidine, nifedipine, ARBs
Pseudoporphyria	Furosemide, thiazides
DHS/DRESS	Phenytoin, mexiletine, platelet inhibitors, anticoagulants
Eczematous eruption	Anticoagulants (heparin, LMWHs), methyldopa, statins, nitroglycerin (transdermal patch), clonidine (transdermal patch), CCBs, ACEIs, ARBs
Erythema multiforme/SJS/TEN	Phenytoin, diuretics, CCBs
Erythroderma/exfoliative dermatitis	Captopril, CCBs, class I antiarrhythmics, vasodilatory drugs (epoprostenol, pentaerythritol tetranitrate, glyceryl trinitrate)
Fixed drug eruption	Platelet inhibitors, class I antiarrhythmics, beta-blockers
Flushing	Vasodilators, CCBs, niacin
Gingival hyperplasia	Phenytoin, CCBs (nifedipine)
Hyperpigmentation	Amiodarone (blue gray), phenytoin (brown), quinidine (blue gray), diltiazem
Hypertrichosis	Phenytoin, minoxidil, diazoxide, acetazolamide
Lichenoid eruption	ACEIs, ARBs, beta-blockers, diuretics, methyldopa, statins, platelet inhibitors
Lupus erythematosus	
Systemic	Hydralazine, class I antiarrhythmics (mainly procainamide), methyldopa, statins, beta-blockers, ACEIs, amiodarone, ticlopidine
Subacute cutaneous	CCBs, thiazides, statins, ACEIs
Lymphomatoid eruption	ACEIs, ARBs, phenytoin
Maculopapular eruption	ACEIs (captopril), ARBs, CCBs, class I antiarrhythmics, diuretics, platelet inhibitors, aminocaproic acid
Nail changes	
Photo-onycholysis	Indapamide
Bleeding of the nail bed	Anticoagulants
Digital gangrene	Beta-blockers
Pincer nail	Beta-blockers
Necrosis	Anticoagulants (warfarin, heparin, LMWHs, acenocumarol, fluindione), beta-blockers, sympathomimetics, thrombolytics (via cholesterol embolism)
Peripheral edema	CCBs, vasodilators, adrenergic neuron blockers (reserpine)
Photosensitivity	Amiodarone, thiazides, quinidine, CCBs, ACEIs, fibrates (fenofibrate)

Table 1.4 (continued)

Type of the adverse drug reaction	Main causative cardiovascular drug
Pruritus	Almost every cardiovascular drug
Psoriasis/psoriasiform eruption	ACEIs, beta-blockers, ARBs, CCBs
Purpura	Quinidine, diuretics, anticoagulants, platelet inhibitors, thrombolytics, CCBs
Vasculitis	ACEIs, ARBs, hydralazine (ANCA positive), diuretics, quinidine, beta-blockers, thrombolytics, anticoagulants
Xerosis/acquired ichthyosis	Lipid-lowering drugs
Xerostomia	Alpha-adrenergic receptor blockers, alpha-2 adrenergic receptor agonists, class I antiarrhythmics, beta-blockers, CCBs, diuretics, adrenergic neuron blockers

Note: Adverse cutaneous drug reaction to phenytoin mainly occurs from using the drug as an anticonvulsant

AGEP acute generalized exanthematous pustulosis, *ACEIs* angiotensin-converting enzyme inhibitors, *ARBs* angiotensin II receptor blockers, *CCBs* calcium channel blockers, *DHS* drug hypersensitivity syndrome, *DRESS* drug rash with eosinophilia and systemic symptoms, *SJS* Stevens–Johnson syndrome, *TEN* toxic epidermal necrolysis, *LMWH* low molecular weight heparin, *ANCA* antineutrophil cytoplasmic autoantibody

Table 1.5 Cross-reactivity of cardiovascular drugs (cross-reactions usually occur between drugs within the same group or between drugs sharing the same chemical group)

Cardiovascular drug groups	Cross-reactivity
Angiotensin-converting enzyme inhibitors (ACEIs)	Not expected between captopril and other ACEIs, because of the lack of sulfhydryl group in ACEIs other than captopril
	Possible with angiotensin II receptor blockers
Angiotensin II receptor blockers	Possible with ACEIs
Class I antiarrhythmics (sodium channel blockers)	Controversial within class Ib (demonstrated between tocainide and lidocaine, but not with mexiletine)
	Between phenytoin and other aromatic antiepileptics
Beta-blockers (class II antiarrhythmics)	Suggested between cardioselective and noncardioselective beta-blockers
Class III antiarrhythmics	Possible between amiodarone and iodinated radiocontrast agents
Calcium channel blockers (class IV antiarrhythmics)	Controversial among the same subgroup
	Possible between different subgroups (shown between diltiazem and nifedipine, diltiazem and verapamil, diltiazem and amlodipine)
Diuretics	Controversial between sulfonamide diuretics and sulfonamide antibiotics containing arylamine group, and paraphenylenediamine
Vasodilators	Possible among nitrates (shown between topically applied glyceryl trinitrate and isosorbide dinitrate)
Lipid-lowering drugs	Possible among statins (shown between fluvastatin and lovastatin)
	Possible between fenofibrate and topically applied ketoprofen
Platelet inhibitors	Between clopidogrel, ticlopidine, and prasugrel
Anticoagulants	Between heparin, low molecular weight heparins, and danaparoid
	Between fondaparinux and dalteparin
	Note: recombinant hirudins are not shown to cross-react with heparin or low molecular weight heparins and heparinoids

References

1. Lee A, Thomson J. Drug-induced skin reactions. In: Adverse drug reactions. 2nd ed. London: Pharmaceutical Press; 2006. p. 125–56.
2. Turk BG, Gunaydin A, Ertam I, Ozturk G. Adverse cutaneous drug reactions among hospitalized patients: five year surveillance. Cutan Ocul Toxicol. 2013;32:41–5. doi:10.3109/15569527.2012.702837.
3. Valeyrie-Allanore L, Sassolas B, Roujeau JC. Drug-induced skin, nail and hair disorders. Drug Saf. 2007;30:1011–30.
4. Al-Niaimi F. Drug eruptions in dermatology. Expert Rev Dermatol. 2011;6:273–86.
5. Andersen WK, Feingold DS. Adverse drug interactions clinically important for the dermatologist. Arch Dermatol. 1995;131:468–73.
6. Roujeau JC. Clinical heterogeneity of drug hypersensitivity. Toxicology. 2005;209:123–9.
7. Haymore BR, Yoon J, Mikita CP, Klote MM, DeZee KJ. Risk of angioedema with angiotensin receptor blockers in patients with prior angioedema associated with angiotensin-converting enzyme inhibitors: a meta-analysis. Ann Allergy Asthma Immunol. 2008;101:495–9. doi:10.1016/S1081-1206(10)60288-8.
8. Pichler WJ, Beeler A, Keller M, Lerch M, Posadas S, Schmid D, et al. Pharmacological interaction of drugs with immune receptors: the p-I concept. Allergol Int. 2006;55:17–25.
9. Andersen KE, Hjorth N, Menné T. The baboon syndrome: systemically-induced allergic contact dermatitis. Contact Dermatitis. 1984;10:97–100.
10. Özkaya E. Current understanding of Baboon syndrome. Exp Rev Dermatol. 2009;4:163–75.
11. Lerch M, Bircher AJ. Systemically induced allergic exanthem from mercury. Contact Dermatitis. 2004;50:349–53.
12. Häusermann P, Harr T, Bircher AJ. Baboon syndrome resulting from systemic drugs: is there strife between SDRIFE and allergic contact dermatitis syndrome? Contact Dermatitis. 2004;51:297–310.
13. Summers EM, Bingham CS, Dahle KW, Sweeney C, Ying J, Sontheimer RD. Chronic eczematous eruptions in the aging: further support for an association with exposure to calcium channel blockers. JAMA Dermatol. 2013;149:814–8. doi:10.1001/jamadermatol.2013.511.
14. Pfeiff B, Pullmann H. Baboon-artiges Arzneiexanthem auf heparin. Dermatologe. 1991;39:559–60.
15. Tan SC, Tan JW. Symmetrical drug-related intertriginous and flexural exanthema. Curr Opin Allergy Clin Immunol. 2011;11:313–8. doi:10.1097/ACI.0b013e3283489d5f.
16. Almeida J, Levantine A. Lichenoid drugs eruptions. Br J Dermatol. 1971;85:604–7.
17. Woo V, Bonks J, Borukhova L, Zegarelli D. Oral lichenoid drug eruption: a report of a pediatric case and review of the literature. Pediatr Dermatol. 2009;26:458–64. doi:10.1111/j.1525-1470.2009.00953.x.
18. Fessa C, Lim P, Kossard S, Richards S, Peñas PF. Lichen planus-like drug eruptions due to β-blockers: a case report and literature review. Am J Clin Dermatol. 2012;13:417–21. doi:10.2165/11634590-000000000-00000.
19. Özkaya E. Fixed drug eruption: state of the art. J Dtsch Dermatol Ges. 2008;6:181–8.
20. Özkaya E. Oral mucosal fixed drug eruption: characteristics and differential diagnosis. J Am Acad Dermatol. 2013;69:e51–8. doi:10.1016/j.jaad.2012.08.019.
21. Ahmed I, Reichenberg J, Lucas A, Shehan JM. Erythema multiforme associated with phenytoin and cranial radiation therapy: a report of three patients and review of the literature. Int J Dermatol. 2004;43:67–73.
22. Wöhrl S, Loewe R, Pickl WF, Stingl G, Wagner SN. EMPACT syndrome. J Dtsch Dermatol Ges. 2005;3:39–43.
23. Fabbrocini G, Panariello L, Pensabene M, Lauria R, Matano E, Martellotta D, et al. EMPACT syndrome associated with phenobarbital. Dermatitis. 2013;24:37–9. doi:10.1097/DER.0b013e31827ede32.

24. Stavropoulos PG, Soura E, Antoniou C. Drug-induced pemphigoid: a review of the literature. J Eur Acad Dermatol Venereol. 2014;28:1133–40. doi:10.1111/jdv.12366.
25. Brenner S, Goldberg I. Drug-induced pemphigus. Clin Dermatol. 2011;29:455–7. doi:10.1016/j.clindermatol.2011.01.016.
26. Ramsay CA. Drug induced pseudoporphyria. J Rheumatol. 1991;18:799–800.
27. Maruani A, Machet MC, Carlotti A, Giraudeau B, Vaillant L, Machet L. Immunostaining with antibodies to desmoglein provides the diagnosis of drug-induced pemphigus and allows prediction of outcome. Am J Clin Pathol. 2008;130:369–74.
28. Chanal J, Ingen-Housz-Oro S, Ortonne N, Duong TA, Thomas M, Valeyrie-Allanore L, et al. Linear IgA bullous dermatosis: comparison between the drug-induced and spontaneous forms. Br J Dermatol. 2013;169:1041–8. doi:10.1111/bjd.12488.
29. Newby CS, Barr RM, Greaves MW, Mallet AI. Cytokine release and cytotoxicity in human keratinocytes and fibroblasts induce d by phenols and sodium dodecyl sulfate. J Invest Dermatol. 2000;115:292–8.
30. Feliciani C, Toto P, Amerio P, Pour SM, Coscione G, Shivji G, et al. In vitro and in vivo expression of interleukin-1α and tumor necrosis factor-α mRNA in pemphigus vulgaris: interleukin-1α and tumor necrosis factor-α are involved in acantholysis. J Invest Dermatol. 2000;114:71–7.
31. Ruocco V, De Angelis E, Lombardi ML. Drug-induced pemphigus. II. Pathomechanisms and experimental investigations. Clin Dermatol. 1993;11:507–13.
32. Fernando SL. Acute generalised exanthematous pustulosis. Australas J Dermatol. 2012;53:87–92. doi:10.1111/j.1440-0960.2011.00845.x.
33. Roujeau JC, Bioulac-Sage P, Bourseau C, Guillaume JC, Bernard P, Lok C, et al. Acute generalized exanthematous pustulosis. Analysis of 63 cases. Arch Dermatol. 1991;127:1333–8.
34. Sidoroff A, Halevy S, Bavinck JN, Vaillant L, Roujeau JC. Acute generalized exanthematous pustulosis (AGEP)–a clinical reaction pattern. J Cutan Pathol. 2001;28:113–9.
35. Momin SB, Peterson A, Del Rosso JQ. A status report on drug-associated acne and acneiform eruptions. J Drugs Dermatol. 2010;9:627–36.
36. Scheinfeld NS, Chernoff K, Derek Ho MK, Liu YC. Drug-induced photoallergic and phototoxic reactions – an update. Expert Opin Drug Saf. 2014;13:321–40. doi:10.1517/14740338.2014.885948.
37. Badri T, Ben Tekaya N, Cherif F, Ben Osman Dhahri A. Photo-onycholysis: two cases induced by doxycycline. Acta Dermatovenerol Alp Panonica Adriat. 2004;13:135–6.
38. Drucker AM, Rosen CF. Drug-induced photosensitivity: culprit drugs, management and prevention. Drug Saf. 2011;34:821–37. doi:10.2165/11592780-000000000-00000.
39. Dereure O. Drug-induced skin pigmentation. Epidemiology, diagnosis and treatment. Am J Clin Dermatol. 2001;2:253–62.
40. Conroy EA, Liranzo MO, McMahon J, Steck WD, Tuthill RJ. Quinidine-induced pigmentation. Cutis. 1996;57:425–7.
41. Gonzalez-Arriagada WA, Silva AR, Vargas PA, de Almeida OP, Lopes MA. Facial pigmentation associated with amiodarone. Gen Dent. 2013;61:e15–7.
42. Cox NH, Walsh ML, Robson RH. Purpura and bleeding due to calcium-channel blockers: an underestimated problem? Case reports and a pilot study. Clin Exp Dermatol. 2009;34:487–91. doi:10.1111/j.1365-2230.2008.03048.x.
43. Dootson G, Byatt C. Amiodarone-induced vasculitis and a review of the cutaneous side-effects of amiodarone. Clin Exp Dermatol. 1994;19:422–4.
44. Veloso HH, De Paola AA. Thrombophlebitis: a common complication of amiodarone. Am Fam Physician. 2004;70:1448.
45. Al-Niaimi F, Lyon C. Felodipine-induced eruptive telangiectasia following mastectomy and radiotherapy. Br J Dermatol. 2010;162:210–1. doi:10.1111/j.1365-2133.2009.09497.x.
46. Pendergraft WF, Niles JL. Trojan horses: drug culprits associated with antineutrophil cytoplasmic autoantibody (ANCA) vasculitis. Curr Opin Rheumatol. 2014;26:42–9. doi:10.1097/BOR.0000000000000014.

47. Papagrigoraki A, Gisondi P, Rosina P, Cannone M, Girolomoni G. Erythema nodosum: etiological factors and relapses in a retrospective cohort study. Eur J Dermatol. 2010;20:773–7. doi:10.1684/ejd.2010.1116.
48. Sharma G, Govil DC. Allopurinol induced erythroderma. Indian J Pharmacol. 2013;45:627–8. doi:10.4103/0253-7613.121381.
49. Finkelstein Y, Soon GS, Acuna P, George M, Pope E, Ito S, et al. Recurrence and outcomes of Stevens-Johnson syndrome and toxic epidermal necrolysis in children. Pediatrics. 2011;128:723–8. doi:10.1542/peds.2010-3322.
50. Pereira FA, Mudgil AV, Rosmarin DM. Toxic epidermal necrolysis. J Am Acad Dermatol. 2007;56:181–200.
51. Castelain F, Humbert P. Toxic epidermal necrolysis. Curr Drug Saf. 2012;7:332–8.
52. Bastuji-Garin S, Fouchard N, Bertocchi M, Roujeau JC, Revuz J, Wolkenstein P. SCORTEN: a severity-of-illness score for toxic epidermal necrolysis. J Invest Dermatol. 2000;115:149–53.
53. Schwartz RA, McDonough PH, Lee BW. Toxic epidermal necrolysis: part II. Prognosis, sequelae, diagnosis, differential diagnosis, prevention, and treatment. J Am Acad Dermatol. 2013;69:187.e1–16. doi:10.1016/j.jaad.2013.05.002; quiz 203–4.
54. Verma R, Vasudevan B, Pragasam V. Severe cutaneous adverse drug reactions. Med J Armed Forces India. 2013;69:375–83.
55. Garcia-Doval I, LeCleach L, Bocquet H, Otero XL, Roujeau JC. Toxic epidermal necrolysis and Stevens-Johnson syndrome: does early withdrawal of causative drugs decrease the risk of death? Arch Dermatol. 2000;136:323–7.
56. Ständer S, Metze D, Luger T, Schwarz T. Drug reaction with eosinophilia and systemic symptoms (DRESS): a review. Hautarzt. 2013;64:611–22. doi:10.1007/s00105-013-2615-0; quiz 623–4.
57. Kardaun SH, Sidoroff A, Valeyrie-Allanore L, Halevy S, Davidovici BB, Mockenhaupt M, et al. Variability in the clinical pattern of cutaneous side-effects of drugs with systemic symptoms: does a DRESS syndrome really exist? Br J Dermatol. 2007;156:609–11.
58. Yazganoglu KD, Özkaya E, Ergin-Özcan P, Çakar N. Vancomycin-induced drug hypersensitivity syndrome. J Eur Acad Dermatol Venereol. 2005;19:648–50.
59. Choi TS, Doh KS, Kim SH, Jang MS, Suh KS, Kim ST. Clinicopathological and genotypic aspects of anticonvulsant-induced pseudolymphoma syndrome. Br J Dermatol. 2003;148:730–6.
60. Mutasim DF. Lymphomatoid drug eruption mimicking digitate dermatosis: cross reactivity between two drugs that suppress angiotensin II function. Am J Dermatopathol. 2003; 25:331–4.
61. Pulitzer MP, Nolan KA, Oshman RG, Phelps RG. CD30+ lymphomatoid drug reactions. Am J Dermatopathol. 2013;35:343–50. doi:10.1097/DAD.0b013e31826bc1e5.
62. Nazarian RM, Van Cott EM, Zembowicz A, Duncan LM. Warfarin-induced skin necrosis. J Am Acad Dermatol. 2009;61:325–32. doi:10.1016/j.jaad.2008.12.039.
63. Katz U, Zandman-Goddard G. Drug-induced lupus: an update. Autoimmun Rev. 2010;10:46–50. doi:10.1016/j.autrev.2010.07.005.
64. Levine D, Switlyk SA, Gottlieb A. Cutaneous lupus erythematosus and anti-TNF-alpha therapy: a case report with review of the literature. J Drugs Dermatol. 2010;9:1283–7.
65. Marzano AV, Vezzoli P, Crosti C. Drug-induced lupus: an update on its dermatologic aspects. Lupus. 2009;18:935–40. doi:10.1177/0961203309106176.
66. Callen JP. Drug-induced subacute cutaneous lupus erythematosus. Lupus. 2010;19:1107–11. doi:10.1177/0961203310370349.
67. Sontheimer RD, Henderson CL, Grau RH. Drug-induced subacute cutaneous lupus erythematosus: a paradigm for bedside-to-bench patient-oriented translational clinical investigation. Arch Dermatol Res. 2009;301:65–70. doi:10.1007/s00403-008-0890-x.
68. Srivastava M, Rencic A, Diglio G, Santana H, Bonitz P, Watson R, et al. Drug-induced, Ro/SSA-positive cutaneous lupus erythematosus. Arch Dermatol. 2003;139:45–9.

69. Bulut M, Yazganoglu KD, Buyukbabani N, Özkaya E. Subacute cutaneous lupus erythematosus-like eruption possibly induced by filgrastim, a granulocyte colony-stimulating factor. EADV 22nd Congress, İstanbul, 2–6 October 2013, Programme book. p. 152 (P 109).
70. Milavec-Puretić V, Mance M, Ceović R, Lipozenčić J. Drug induced psoriasis. Acta Dermatovenerol Croat. 2011;19:39–42.
71. Tsankov N, Angelova I, Kazandjieva J. Drug-induced psoriasis. Recognition and management. Am J Clin Dermatol. 2000;1:159–65.
72. Wolf R, Ruocco V. Triggered psoriasis. Adv Exp Med Biol. 1999;455:221–5.
73. Yerushalmi J, Zvulunov A, Halevy S. Serum sickness-like reactions. Cutis. 2002;69:395–7.
74. Ständer S, Darsow U, Mettang T, Gieler U, Maurer M, Ständer H, et al. S2k guideline–Chronic Pruritus. J Dtsch Dermatol Ges. 2012;10 Suppl 4:S1–27. doi:10.1111/j.1610-0387.2012.08005.x.
75. Claeys A, Weber-Muller F, Trechot P, Cuny JF, Georges MY, Barbaud A, et al. Cutaneous, perivulvar and perianal ulcerations induced by nicorandil. Br J Dermatol. 2006;155: 494–6.
76. Ghersetich I, Rindi L, Teofoli P, Tsampau D, Palleschi GM, Lotti T. Pityriasis rosea-like skin eruptions caused by captopril. G Ital Dermatol Venereol. 1990;125:457–9.
77. Sugita K, Kabashima K, Nakamura M, Tokura Y. Drug-induced papuloerythroderma: analysis of T-cell populations and a literature review. Acta Derm Venereol. 2009;89:618–22.
78. Sugita K, Kabashima K, Nakashima D, Tokura Y. Papuloerythroderma of Ofuji induced by furosemide. J Am Acad Dermatol. 2008;58(2 Suppl):S54–5. doi:10.1016/j.jaad.2006.05.046.
79. Sugita K, Koga C, Yoshiki R, Izu K, Tokura Y. Papuloerythroderma caused by aspirin. Arch Dermatol. 2006;142:792–3.
80. Thompson DF, Montarella KE. Drug-induced Sweet's syndrome. Ann Pharmacother. 2007;41:802–11.
81. Roujeau JC. Neutrophilic drug eruptions. Clin Dermatol. 2000;18:331–7.
82. Bremner R, Simpson E, White CR, Morrison L, Deodhar A. Palisaded neutrophilic and granulomatous dermatitis: an unusual cutaneous manifestation of immune-mediated disorders. Semin Arthritis Rheum. 2004;34:610–6.
83. Magro CM, Crowson AN, Schapiro BL. The interstitial granulomatous drug reaction: a distinctive clinical and pathological entity. J Cutan Pathol. 1998;25:72–8.
84. Magro CM, Cruz-Inigo AE, Votava H, Jacobs M, Wolfe D, Crowson AN. Drug-associated reversible granulomatous T cell dyscrasia: a distinct subset of the interstitial granulomatous drug reaction. J Cutan Pathol. 2010;37 Suppl 1:96–111.
85. Perrin C, Lacour JP, Castanet J, Michiels JF. Interstitial granulomatous drug reaction with a histological pattern of interstitial granulomatous dermatitis. Am J Dermatopathol. 2001;23:295–8.
86. Lee MW, Choi JH, Sung KJ, Moon KC, Koh JK. Interstitial and granulomatous drug reaction presenting as erythema nodosum-like lesions. Acta Derm Venereol. 2002;82:473–4.
87. Yazganoğlu KD, Tambay E, Mete Ö, Özkaya E. Interstitial granulomatous drug reaction due to thalidomide. J Eur Acad Dermatol Venereol. 2009;23:490–3. doi:10.1111/j.1468-3083.2008.02953.x.
88. Cheshire WP, Fealey RD. Drug-induced hyperhidrosis and hypohidrosis: incidence, prevention and management. Drug Saf. 2008;31:109–26.
89. Torpet LA, Kragelund C, Reibel J, Nauntofte B. Oral adverse drug reactions to cardiovascular drugs. Crit Rev Oral Biol Med. 2004;15:28–46.
90. Habbab KM, Moles DR, Porter SR. Potential oral manifestations of cardiovascular drugs. Oral Dis. 2010;16:769–73. doi:10.1111/j.1601-0825.2010.01686.x.
91. Pillans PI, Woods DJ. Drug-associated alopecia. Int J Dermatol. 1995;34:149–58.
92. Piraccini BM, Iorizzo M, Rech G, Tosti A. Drug-induced hair disorders. Curr Drug Saf. 2006;1:301–5.
93. Piraccini BM, Alessandrini A. Drug-related nail disease. Clin Dermatol. 2013;31:618–26. doi:10.1016/j.clindermatol.2013.06.013.

94. Kynaston HG, Roberts DH, Davies WT. Peripheral gangrene associated with beta-blockade. Br J Surg. 1987;74:760.
95. Coombs PR, Gell PG. Classification of allergic reactions responsible for clinical hypersensitivity and disease. In: Gell RR, editor. Clinical aspects of immunology. Oxford: Oxford University Press; 1968. p. 575–96.
96. Friedmann PS, Ardern-Jones M. Patch testing in drug allergy. Curr Opin Allergy Clin Immunol. 2010;10:291–6. doi:10.1097/ACI.0b013e32833aa54d.
97. Posadas SJ, Pichler WJ. Delayed drug hypersensitivity reactions – new concepts. Clin Exp Allergy. 2007;37:989–99.
98. Yawalkar N, Pichler WJ. Mechanisms of cutaneous drug reactions. J Dtsch Dermatol Ges. 2004;2:1013–23.
99. Pichler WJ. Delayed drug hypersensitivity reactions. Ann Intern Med. 2003;139:683–93.
100. Lee HY, Chung WH. Toxic epidermal necrolysis: the year in review. Curr Opin Allergy Clin Immunol. 2013;13:330–6. doi:10.1097/ACI.0b013e3283630cc2.
101. Chung WH, Hung SI, Yang JY, Su SC, Huang SP, Wei CY, et al. Granulysin is a key mediator for disseminated keratinocyte death in Stevens-Johnson syndrome and toxic epidermal necrolysis. Nat Med. 2008;14:1343–50. doi:10.1038/nm.1884.
102. Özkaya E, Babuna G. A challenging case: symmetrical drug related intertriginous and flexural exanthem, fixed drug eruption, or both? Pediatr Dermatol. 2011;28:711–4. doi:10.1111/j.1525-1470.2011.01656.x.
103. Schnyder B, Burkhart C, Schnyder-Frutig K, von Greyerz S, Naisbitt DJ, Pirmohamed M, et al. Recognition of sulfamethoxazole and its reactive metabolites by drug-specific CD4+ T cells from allergic individuals. J Immunol. 2000;164:6647–54.
104. Mallal S, Nolan D, Witt C, Masel G, Martin AM, Moore C, et al. Association between presence of HLA-B*5701, HLA-DR7, and HLA-DQ3 and hypersensitivity to HIV-1 reverse-transcriptase inhibitor abacavir. Lancet. 2002;359:727–32.
105. Chung WH, Hung SI, Hong HS, Hsih MS, Yang LC, Ho HC, et al. Medical genetics: a marker for Stevens-Johnson syndrome. Nature. 2004;428:486.
106. Hung SI, Chung WH, Liou LB, Chu CC, Lin M, Huang HP, et al. HLA-B*5801 allele as a genetic marker for severe cutaneous adverse reactions caused by allopurinol. Proc Natl Acad Sci U S A. 2005;102:4134–9.
107. Pellicano R, Ciavarella G, Lomuto M, Di Giorgio G. Genetic susceptibility to fixed drug eruptions: evidence for a link with HLA-B22. J Am Acad Dermatol. 1994;30:52–4.
108. Pellicano R, Lomuto M, Ciavarella G, Di Giorgio G, Gasparini P. Fixed drug eruptions with feprazone are linked to HLA-B22. J Am Acad Dermatol. 1997;36:782–4.
109. Ozkaya E, Akar U. Fixed drug eruption induced by trimethoprim-sulfamethoxazole: evidence for a link to HLA-A30 B13 Cw6 haplotype. J Am Acad Dermatol. 2001;45:712–7.
110. Shapiro LE, Shear NH. Drug interactions: proteins, pumps, and P-450 s. J Am Acad Dermatol. 2002;47:467–84.
111. Gex-Collet C, Helbling A, Pichler WJ. Multiple drug hypersensitivity-proof of multiple drug hypersensitivity by patch and lymphocyte transformation tests. J Investig Allergol Clin Immunol. 2005;15:293–6.
112. Asero R. Multiple drug allergy syndrome: a distinct clinical entity. Curr Allergy Rep. 2001;1:18–22.
113. Halevy S, Grossman N. Multiple drug allergy in patients with cutaneous adverse drug reactions diagnosed by in vitro drug-induced interferon-gamma release. Isr Med Assoc J. 2008;10:865–8.
114. Voltolini S, Bignardi D, Minale P, Pellegrini S, Troise C. Phenobarbital- induced DiHS and ceftriaxone hypersensitivity reaction: a case of multiple drug allergy. Eur Ann Allergy Clin Immunol. 2009;41:62–3.
115. Özkaya E. Eczematous type multiple drug allergy from isoniazid and ethambutol with positive patch test results. Cutis. 2013;92:121–4.
116. Özkaya E, Yazganoglu KD. Sequential development of eczematous type "multiple drug allergy" to unrelated drugs. J Am Acad Dermatol. 2011;65:e26–9. doi:10.1016/j.jaad.2010.12.028.

117. Naranjo CA, Busto U, Sellers EM, Sandor P, Ruiz I, Roberts EA, et al. A method for estimating the probability of adverse drug reactions. Clin Pharmacol Ther. 1981;30:239–45.
118. Moore N, Biour M, Paux G, Loupi E, Begaud B, Boismare F, et al. Adverse drug reaction monitoring: doing it the French way. Lancet. 1985;2(8463):1056–8.
119. The Uppsala Monitoring Centre. The use of the WHO-UMC system for standardised case causality assessment. http://who-umc.org/Graphics/24734.pdf. Accessed 31 Mar 2014.
120. Seitz CS, Rose C, Kerstan A, Trautmann A. Drug-induced exanthems: correlation of allergy testing with histologic diagnosis. J Am Acad Dermatol. 2013;69:721–8. doi:10.1016/j.jaad.2013.06.022.
121. Barbaud A, Reichert-Penetrat S, Tréchot P, Jacquin-Petit MA, Ehlinger A, Noirez V, et al. The use of skin testing in the investigation of cutaneous adverse drug reactions. Br J Dermatol. 1998;139:49–58.
122. Romano A, Demoly P. Recent advances in the diagnosis of drug allergy. Curr Opin Allergy Clin Immunol. 2007;7:299–303.
123. Sanz ML, García BE, Prieto I, Tabar A, Oehling A. Specific IgE determination in the diagnosis of beta-lactam allergy. J Investig Allergol Clin Immunol. 1996;6:89–93.
124. Pichler WJ, Tilch J. The lymphocyte transformation test in the diagnosis of drug hypersensitivity. Allergy. 2004;59:809–20.
125. Goossens C, Sass U, Song M. Baboon syndrome. Dermatology. 1997;194:421–2.
126. Kanny G, Pichler W, Morisset M, Franck P, Marie B, Kohler C, et al. T cell-mediated reactions to iodinated contrast media: evaluation by skin and lymphocyte activation tests. J Allergy Clin Immunol. 2005;115:179–85.
127. Halevy S, Cohen AD, Grossman N. Clinical implications of in vitro drug-induced interferon gamma release from peripheral blood lymphocytes in cutaneous adverse drug reactions. J Am Acad Dermatol. 2005;52:254–61.
128. Aberer W, Bircher A, Romano A, Blanca M, Campi P, Fernandez J, et al. Drug provocation testing in the diagnosis of drug hypersensitivity reactions: general considerations. Allergy. 2003;58:854–63.
129. Mahajan VK, Handa S. Patch testing in cutaneous adverse drug reactions: methodology, interpretation, and clinical relevance. Indian J Dermatol Venereol Leprol. 2013;79:836–41. doi:10.4103/0378-6323.120751.
130. Ozkaya E, Bayazit H, Ozarmagan G. Drug related clinical pattern in fixed drug eruption. Eur J Dermatol. 2000;10:288–91.
131. Méndez J, Sanchís ME, de la Fuente R, Stolle R, Vega JM, Martínez C, et al. Delayed-type hypersensitivity to subcutaneous enoxaparin. Allergy. 1998;53:999–1003.

Part II
Adverse Cutaneous Drug Reactions to Specific Class of Cardiovascular Drugs

Chapter 2
Angiotensin-Converting Enzyme Inhibitors

Keywords Angiotensin-converting enzyme inhibitor • Captopril • Enalapril • Angioedema • Pemphigus • Lupus erythematosus • Photosensitivity • Psoriasis/psoriasiform • Kaposi sarcoma • Lymphomatoid • Lichenoid • Scalded mouth syndrome

Angiotensin-converting enzyme inhibitors (ACEIs) can be classified into two subgroups according to their chemical structure: the one containing a thiol (or sulfhydryl [SH]) group such as captopril and zofenopril, and the other lacking a thiol group such as enalapril, ramipril, cilazapril, fosinopril, quinapril, trandolapril, lisinopril, perindopril, moexipril, benazepril, imidapril, delapril, alacepril, and spirapril.

ACEIs inhibit angiotensin-converting enzyme (ACE) activity that leads to the inhibition of conversion of angiotensin I to angiotensin II which is a vasoconstrictive agent. Additionally, inhibition of ACE prevents the degradation of bradykinin, substance P, enkephalins, and some of the reproductive peptide hormones [1, 2]. The mechanisms for the pathogenesis of adverse cutaneous drug reactions associated with ACEIs were proposed to be an allergic, immune-mediated reaction on one side and on the other side a pharmacologic, dose-dependent reaction mainly as a result of potentiation of kinin activity [3, 4]. Half of the adverse reactions to ACEIs are suggested to occur in the skin [1].

The adverse cutaneous drug reactions described below are meant to be sorted by starting from the well-known reactions of ACEIs to the lesser known ones. The major ones are summarized in Table 2.1.

Angioedema/Urticaria

Angioedema is the most well-documented adverse cutaneous drug reaction of ACEIs. It was stated to be a class effect of ACEIs [5]. It is a potentially fatal adverse effect. The incidence was reported to be between 0.2 and 2.5 % [6]. It was indicated to occur more in African-Americans [6–8]. Seasonal allergies and a history of drug rash were found to be independent risk factors for angioedema in a large prospective study of enalapril-treated patients [8]. Another study revealed that ACEI-associated

E. Özkaya, K.D. Yazganoğlu, *Adverse Cutaneous Drug Reactions to Cardiovascular Drugs*, DOI 10.1007/978-1-4471-6536-1_2

Table 2.1 Major adverse cutaneous drug reactions with angiotensin-converting enzyme inhibitors (ACEIs)

Adverse cutaneous drug reaction	Main inducers
Angioedema	Class effect of ACEIs
Bullous reactions	
Pemphigus	Captopril, enalapril, lisinopril, fosinopril, ramipril, cilazapril, quinapril
Linear IgA dermatosis	Captopril, benazepril
Bullous pemphigoid	Captopril, enalapril, lisinopril
Lichen planus pemphigoides	Captopril, ramipril
Lichen planus/lichenoid eruptions	Captopril, enalapril, lisinopril
Lymphomatoid drug eruption	Captopril, enalapril, lisinopril
Psoriasis/psoriasiform eruption	Captopril, enalapril[a], lisinopril, ramipril, perindopril[b]
Pityriasis rosea-like eruption	Captopril, enalapril, lisinopril
Kaposi sarcoma	Captopril, lisinopril, cilazapril
Drug-induced lupus erythematosus	Captopril, lisinopril, enalapril, cilazapril
Photosensitivity	Captopril, enalapril, ramipril, quinapril
Vasculitis	Captopril, enalapril, lisinopril, ramipril
Maculopapular eruption	Captopril
Eczematous eruption	Captopril, enalapril, ramipril, fosinopril, benazepril, quinapril
Erythroderma	Captopril
Stevens–Johnson syndrome/ toxic epidermal necrolysis	Captopril, ramipril
DRESS	Captopril, ramipril
Alopecia	Captopril, enalapril
Scalded mouth syndrome	Captopril, enalapril, lisinopril

DRESS drug rash with eosinophilia and systemic symptoms
[a]Probable cross-reaction to atenolol
[b]Probable cross-reaction to captopril

angioedema was more likely to occur during the months when pollen counts were increased [9]. Tongue, lip, facial, and supraglottic edema were the common reported clinical manifestations of the reaction [7].

The underlying mechanisms of ACEI-associated angioedema have not been clearly defined. The pathogenesis is suggested to be related with several different factors including immunological reactions, accumulation of mediators like bradykinin and substance P, a decrease in aminopeptidase P and dipeptidyl peptidase IV activity (the main enzymes degrading bradykinin and substance P when ACE is inhibited), and genetic factors [1, 6]. The main causative factor seems to be the increased levels and prolonged activity of bradykinin, due to ACE activity inhibition. This vasodilating agent is indicated to cause an increase in vascular permeability that results in fluid leakage, leading to edema of the deep dermis, hypodermis, or submucosal areas, consequently causing angioedema [2, 6]. Moreover, it was also stated that similar to hereditary angioedema patients, some patients using ACEIs could develop angioedema after localized tissue trauma like dental and surgical procedures and local anesthetic injections [6].

Most of the patients experienced the reaction within a few weeks after the onset of treatment [10–12]. However, angioedema might occur in several hours after the initial administration of ACEI [2, 13] or after long-term therapy for months or years [10, 14–18]. A patient was reported who developed angioedema after 7 years of captopril therapy [15], and another one after 11 years of lisinopril use [17]. Enalapril was even suggested to be the reason of the angioedema developing in a patient after 23 years of therapy [19]. It was indicated that the actual incidence of ACEI-related angioedema could be higher [1, 7] due to its underdiagnosis, especially in cases presenting with angioedema after long-term treatment with ACEIs [7].

The ACEI-associated angioedema is generally regarded as not dose dependent [5]. However, Pillans et al. reported 3 patients with angioedema/urticaria after an increase in dose in their large review of 116 patients with ACEI-associated angioedema and/or urticaria [10] and concluded that the relationship was not clear between angioedema and ACEI dosage [10]. They also reported that patients could have more than one episode of angioedema and the interval between these episodes could be long [10].

The management of ACEI-related angioedema strictly necessitates withdrawal of the ACEI. The patient should not be given another type of ACEI; instead, other classes of drugs should be considered for the treatment of the hypertension or the underlying disease [6, 14]. Apart from the severe cases necessitating intubation, close observation is recommended until one is certain that angioedema does not progress especially in patients with angioedema limited to the lips or face [5]. On the other hand, it is not clear whether the classic treatment regimen of angioedema with antihistamines, corticosteroids, and epinephrine is effective in ACEI-related angioedema [5]. In relation with the pathogenesis of ACEI-associated angioedema, bradykinin is indicated to be targeted in the therapy [20]. Icatibant, which is used in hereditary angioedema, is a bradykinin receptor antagonist that is stated to be useful in severe cases of ACEI-associated angioedema, too [6]. Other suggested therapeutic options include concentrate of C1 inhibitor and fresh frozen plasma [20]. Similar to icatibant, ecallantide, a kallikrein inhibitor, is also an emerging therapy that is tried in ACEI-related angioedema [20].

It was stated that ACEIs are contraindicated in patients with a history of idiopathic angioedema [13] or hereditary angioedema [6]. Moreover, it was also pointed out that patients using ACEI should not be concomitantly treated with dipeptidyl-peptidase IV inhibitors (a new class of antidiabetic agents) as the risk of angioedema will be highly increased. Dipeptidyl-peptidase IV is another enzyme degrading substance P, and inhibition of this enzyme will also lead to the accumulation of substance P [6].

Regarding angioedema, cross-reactivity may occur between ACEIs and angiotensin II receptor blockers, with a risk of 9.4 % according to a meta-analysis [21], so the use of the angiotensin II receptor blockers in patients with ACEI-associated angioedema is not always safe. Interestingly, angioedema might continue to occur chronically in some cases after the withdrawal of the causative drug [6].

The concomitant occurrence of urticaria is usually not expected in patients with angioedema triggered by ACEIs [6], although urticaria might also be induced by ACEIs [10]. Captopril was stated to be more likely to cause urticaria than other ACEIs [1].

Bullous Eruptions

Pemphigus

Drug-related pemphigus is suggested to be classified into two subgroups: drug-induced and drug-triggered pemphigus [22]. The former is implicated to be mainly associated with drugs containing a thiol (–SH) group, such as captopril, or a sulfur-containing group that can form a thiol group. Withdrawal of the drug usually results in resolution of the drug-induced pemphigus. In contrast, in drug-triggered pemphigus, the triggers do not contain a sulfur group, such as enalapril, ramipril, cilazapril, fosinopril, and quinapril, and withdrawal of the drug may not result in the resolution of the symptoms. It was indicated that immunofluorescence, histopathological, and clinical findings in drug-related pemphigus are usually not distinguishable from idiopathic pemphigus [23]. The time of the development of pemphigus after the use of ACEIs is variable and can be as long as years [23]. The cases with a long latency period are further challenging to differentiate from idiopathic pemphigus.

On the other hand, it was also stated that while direct immunofluorescence (DIF) findings were more frequently positive, indirect immunofluorescence (IIF) findings could be rather different as not all the patients with drug-related pemphigus had circulating antibodies, and because the titers of circulating antibodies were not in correlation with the severity of the disease [23, 24]. A case of lisinopril-associated oral bullous eruption was reported with negative DIF and IIF findings. The authors questioned whether this could be a case of drug-related pemphigus in the absence of immunofluorescence findings [24]. Some in vitro studies showed that ACEIs might also cause direct acantholysis in the absence of autoantibody formation, which may explain the negative DIF findings in some patients with drug-induced pemphigus [25, 26].

Different pemphigus types including pemphigus vulgaris, pemphigus foliaceus, and pemphigus vegetans can be seen with ACEIs like captopril, enalapril, lisinopril, fosinopril, ramipril, quinapril, and cilazapril [23, 27–38].

In the management of drug-related pemphigus, withdrawal of the drug and treatment of the condition as idiopathic pemphigus are recommended. It is suggested to change the suspected drug by another class of antihypertensives [23], as another ACEI may cause the recurrence of the lesions [37]. However, a case of captopril-induced pemphigus with no recurrence after treatment with enalapril was also reported [38].

Linear IgA Dermatosis

Benazepril and captopril have been reported to be associated with linear IgA dermatosis. The reaction started within 1 week after starting treatment in the benazepril-induced case and resolved completely within 10 days after discontinuation of the therapy [39]. In the captopril-induced case, the reaction began 2 weeks after the administration of therapy, and new lesions continued to occur even after cessation of the therapy. Therefore, dapsone and prednisone were added to the regimen. It was reported that the patient continued to take dapsone, and blistering still occurred occasionally after one year [40].

Lichen Planus Pemphigoides

Captopril [41, 42] and ramipril [43, 44] have been reported to be associated with lichen planus pemphigoides. The reaction was seen within 2–4 weeks after the administration of the ACEI and mostly resolved after discontinuation of the drug [42–44] except in a case that continued for 10 months after withdrawal of the drug [41]. The reaction resolved with solely discontinuation of the drug, that is, without necessitating topical or systemic corticosteroid therapy in one case [44].

Bullous Pemphigoid

Bullous pemphigoid has been reported with captopril [45, 46], enalapril [47], and lisinopril [48].

Lichen Planus/Lichenoid Eruptions

Both lichen planus and lichenoid eruptions have been reported to occur with captopril [49–55], enalapril [56–58], and lisinopril [59]. The eruption was reported to begin within 1–6 months [52, 54, 56] following treatment with these drugs. Withdrawal of the drug led to clinical improvement within 2–3 months [49, 51], although additional therapy might have been necessary [56]. The lesions healed with residual hyperpigmentation [51, 56].

Pityriasis rosea-like eruption evolving into lichenoid drug eruption has also been reported with captopril [52, 53]. In one report, the lichenoid eruption due to captopril was stated to be dose related [54]. In another, alopecia was associated with the lichenoid eruption [55].

Lisinopril was also implicated to be the cause of lichenoid drug reaction in a patient. This case had white reticulated lesions on the lips in addition to cutaneous lichenoid eruption [59].

Lymphomatoid Drug Eruption

Captopril, enalapril, and lisinopril may induce lymphomatoid drug eruption [60, 61]. Eight patients (six receiving captopril, two receiving enalapril) have been observed to develop erythematous eruption, some of which evolved into lichenified and hyperkeratotic lesions on an erythrodermic background in the chronic stage [60]. Patients were being treated with ACEIs for 2–6 weeks before the eruption developed except in two patients who received only single doses of captopril. The histopathological examination revealed mainly perivascular infiltration of histiocytic cells and lymphocytes in the upper dermis showing numerous mitoses. The lymphocytes had large nuclei with cerebriform contours. These features mostly resembled the early stages of cutaneous T cell lymphoma (CTCL) with the exception of the observed perivascular mononuclear infiltration instead of a band-like infiltration that is commonly seen in CTCL, and less atypical lymphoid cells. Moreover, immunohistochemical studies showed similarities between CTCL and the rash [60]. The reaction was even diagnosed as mycosis fungoides in one of the cases receiving enalapril. Rechallenge was performed with the same drug in two patients which resulted in the recurrence of the reaction following a single dose of captopril within 3 days [60]. An immunological pathogenesis was suggested in that the accumulation of the ACEI in the skin and their persistence might cause an abnormal stimulation of the Langerhans cells and T-helper cells. The reaction was reported to be non-dose related with slow resolution after the withdrawal of the drug [60].

Another case was reported with generalized pustular eruption and fever with repeated staphylococcal bacteremia, axillary lymphadenopathy, and splenomegaly [62]. Skin and lymph node biopsies revealed the diagnosis of mycosis fungoides. Withdrawal of captopril led to resolution of the reaction. Positive macrophage inhibiting factor response was observed for both captopril and enalapril [62].

A case of lymphomatoid drug eruption with clinical findings resembling digitate dermatosis was also reported with lisinopril. The eruption resolved within a few months after discontinuation of the drug but started a few weeks later with initiation of valsartan, an angiotensin receptor blocker [61].

Psoriasis/Psoriasiform Eruption

Although rare, new-onset psoriasis or exacerbations of preexisting psoriasis were reported with ACEIs like captopril, enalapril, lisinopril, and ramipril [3, 63–67].

The reaction occurred within 1 week to 4 months of therapy with ACEIs, and resolved within 10 days to 3 months after withdrawal of the drug [3, 65]. Palmoplantar pustulosis associated with captopril and showing recurrence after replacement with perindopril has been reported in a patient [68]. On the other hand, generalized pustular psoriasis has been reported due to ramipril in a patient with psoriatic arthritis [69].

In three patients using enalapril, captopril, or captopril + hydrochlorothiazide, psoriasis-like lesions were observed clinically and histopathologically in addition to eczematous eruption [67].

An immunological pathogenesis was proposed in a patient with new-onset psoriasis which was resistant to therapy [3]. Mast cell degranulation (MCD) test and macrophage migration inhibition (MIF) test performed with the suspected drugs revealed positive results only for captopril in the MCD test. The lesions cleared completely within 3 months after withdrawal of captopril, without systemic therapy [3].

Another patient with a probable atenolol-induced psoriasis experienced an exacerbation of psoriasis 2 weeks after substitution of atenolol by enalapril [3]. MCD and MIF tests were negative with enalapril, but the MIF test was positive with atenolol. Enalapril was discontinued and topical corticosteroids were applied which led to clearance within 10 days. It was supposed that the reaction occurred as a result of cutaneous increase in kinin levels due to enalapril [3].

On the contrary, it was pointed out that due to inhibition of leukotriene A4 (LTA4) hydrolase by captopril, LTA4 will not be converted to LTB4, and as the latter is responsible for leukocyte chemotaxis and keratinocyte proliferation, reduction of its level would theoretically alleviate psoriatic lesions [70].

Pityriasis Rosea-Like Eruption

This type of reaction has been reported with captopril [71–73], lisinopril [71, 74], and enalapril [71].

In a study, eight cases (2 %) were recorded to have pityriasis rosea-like eruption among 380 patients with adverse cutaneous drug reactions occurring during a 3-year period [71]. The suspected inducer drugs were ACEIs in four cases: captopril and hydrochlorothiazide in one case, lisinopril and hydrochlorothiazide in another case, and lisinopril and enalapril in each one case. The reaction occurred between 9 and 14 days after starting therapy with ACEI. The clinical manifestations were reported to be very similar to pityriasis rosea. However, different from the idiopathic disease, the authors noticed the absence of an "herald" patch, bright violet-red color of the lesions, severe itching unresponsive to antihistamines, and an increase of blood and skin eosinophils. The relatively older ages of the patients were also different from those with the idiopathic form of pityriasis rosea. The clinical manifestations improved soon after the suspected drugs were discontinued.

Kaposi Sarcoma

Captopril [75, 76], lisinopril [77], and cilazapril [78] have been reported to be associated with Kaposi sarcoma. The lesions appeared 6–8 months after the start of ACEI therapy [76–78] and disappeared within 3–8 months upon withdrawal of the suspected drugs [75, 77, 78].

The lesions were limited to the skin or associated with visceral and nodal involvement [77, 78]. Development of Kaposi sarcoma was attributed to the possible immunosuppressive activity of ACEIs including the inhibition of IL-12 which plays an important role in cellular immunity [77, 78].

It was further suggested that the immunosuppressive activity of the drugs could cause opportunistic herpetic infections including HHV-8 infection that is supposed to be associated with Kaposi sarcoma [79].

On the contrary, captopril has been shown to be related with the regression of Kaposi sarcoma in an immunosuppressive patient [80].

Drug-Induced Lupus Erythematosus

Systemic lupus erythematosus (SLE) or subacute cutaneous lupus erythematosus (SCLE) were reported with ACEIs such as captopril [81–84], lisinopril [85, 86], cilazapril [87], and enalapril [86].

SLE was reported to occur even after 2.5 years of therapy [84]. Antinuclear antibody (ANA) and/or antihistone antibodies were positive [81, 84]. The cessation of the drug led to both clinical and laboratory improvement [81, 84].

Captopril was also reported to induce the formation of ANA without any clinical findings [88].

While some SCLE patients manifested with annular scaly plaques typical of SCLE, some presented with cutaneous eruption like photodistributed erythema. Systemic findings were absent. Moreover, patients had positive anti-Ro/SSA [86]. Lisinopril, enalapril, and cilazapril have been implicated to be causes of this reaction [86, 87]. The cessation of the drug with or without topical corticosteroid therapy led to clinical resolution, but laboratory improvement was not seen in all cases [86, 87].

Photosensitivity

Photosensitivity was reported to be caused by captopril [89], enalapril [58], quinapril [90], and ramipril [91]. Photopatch tests were performed showing positive results with captopril, ramipril, and quinapril [89–91]. Interestingly, histopathological changes suggestive of follicular mucinosis were found on the photoexposed sites in the captopril-induced case [89].

Vasculitis

Cutaneous vasculitis including Henoch–Schönlein purpura and necrotizing vasculitis has been reported with captopril [92–96], enalapril [97–100], lisinopril [101, 102], and ramipril [103].

Vasculitis was reported to start after several days, weeks, or even months after commencing ACEI therapy [93, 94, 98, 101, 103]. While the reaction might be dose related [92, 97], withdrawal of the drug [92, 93, 101] and therapy with corticosteroids [94, 98] might be necessary. Even systemic vasculitic involvement has been reported [98]. Rechallenge confirmed the causative agent in some cases [93, 101].

In a study, adverse cutaneous drug reactions were reported in 15 of 89 patients (17 %) treated with captopril [92]. The reaction was dose dependent as the decrease of the drug dosage helped in the improvement of the eruption. However, recurrences were observed in six patients, and the drug had to be stopped in four patients. Histopathological examination of the skin biopsies revealed lymphocytic vasculitis. Positive epicutaneous skin tests were observed in 1/3 of the patients, and positive intracutaneous skin tests in 2/3. The in vitro lymphocyte transformation test was also positive in most patients [92]. It was concluded that a positive epicutaneous skin test with captopril was a good indicator for the necessity of captopril withdrawal.

A patient who had tolerated lisinopril previously was reported to present with vasculitis after 3 days of ramipril therapy [103].

Maculopapular Eruption

ACEIs are commonly reported to cause maculopapular eruption and erythema, usually described as exanthematous eruptions in the literature.

Patch testing in cases of captopril-induced maculopapular or eczematous eruptions revealed positive reactions to captopril but negative to several other ACEIs such as enalapril, lisinopril, fosinopril, ramipril, quinapril, and benazepril [104–106]. The reaction was confirmed with positive rechallenge with captopril [104, 106]. However, as the oral provocation tests with enalapril and lisinopril were negative, it was concluded that there was no cross-reactivity between captopril and other ACEIs [106]. The sulfhydryl group of captopril was regarded as the cause of positive patch test reactions [105, 106].

One of the patients with maculopapular rash from captopril had systemic signs and symptoms like mild renal insufficiency, eosinophilia, and diarrhea that resolved after withdrawal of the drug, suggesting drug hypersensitivity syndrome [104].

Eczematous Eruption

Eczematous eruption has been reported to occur with ACEIs [67, 105, 107]. In a recent article documenting eczematous eruption due to ACEIs or angiotensin receptor blockers, diffuse or localized eczematous lesions were seen in a total of 16 patients using ACEIs (enalapril, captopril, ramipril, fosinopril, benazepril, quinapril), 7 of whom were also using another antihypertensive, namely, hydrochlorothiazide [67]. Apart from the spongiotic dermatitis found in some cases, associated psoriasiform lesions were also observed [67]. The reaction was reported to disappear with the cessation of the suspected drug and treatment with topical or systemic corticosteroids in all of the patients. Furthermore, rechallenge test could be performed in 8 patients with the suspected drug (ACEI alone in 6 patients, ACEI + hydrochlorothiazide in 2 patients) and caused reaction in 5 of them (3 with ACEI alone, 2 with ACEI + hydrochlorothiazide) in an average period of 12–16 weeks. As the latency period after rechallenge was long and the remaining 3 patients who did not experience any recurrence of the lesions used a lower dose than the initial one, the authors suggested that the reaction could be regarded as non-immunologic and dose dependent. Moreover, they have stated that old age, polytherapy, poor water intake, and decreased renal efficiency could be potential risk factors of this type of reaction [67].

Regarding eczematous eruption, cross-reactivity may occur between ACEIs and angiotensin II receptor blockers [107], but it is usually not expected between captopril and other ACEIs. Indeed, in one case with captopril-induced systemic contact dermatitis, there was no cross-sensitivity to other ACEIs including fosinopril, quinapril, and benazepril [105].

Erythroderma

Erythroderma or exfoliative dermatitis has been reported with captopril [108–110]. Four patients were reported to develop an erythematous eruption with some eczematous features which evolved to erythroderma. The reaction occurred within 3–6 weeks after captopril was started. It resolved within 2–6 weeks after discontinuation of the drug. Rechallenge, performed in two cases, showed positive results. One of these cases has tolerated enalapril well. The reaction was considered to be an allergic response due to the sulfhydryl group of the captopril molecule [110].

Stevens–Johnson Syndrome/Toxic Epidermal Necrolysis

Severe reactions such as Stevens–Johnson syndrome or toxic epidermal necrolysis have been reported during treatment with captopril [111–113] and ramipril [114].

Drug Rash with Eosinophilia and Systemic Symptoms

Drug rash with eosinophilia and systemic symptoms has been reported with captopril [104, 115] and ramipril [116]. The rash was maculopapular in captopril-induced reactions, and patch test to captopril was positive [104, 115].

Alopecia

Alopecia was suggested to occur as a result of therapy with captopril and enalapril [117–119]. It was reported to start after 1 month of therapy and was reversible upon withdrawal of the drug [117–119]. Rechallenge was positive in the enalapril-induced case [119]. Some other ACEIs were also reported to induce alopecia [120].

Pruritus

Pruritus is a nonspecific cutaneous adverse reaction of drugs. It was reported in patients receiving ACEI therapy [1, 121, 122]. It usually accompanies different types of drug eruptions [56, 97, 105, 106, 110].

Oral Mucosal Reactions

Various types of oral mucosal reactions have been described to be induced by ACEIs. Burning mouth/tongue, scalded mouth syndrome, xerostomia, taste disturbances/dysgeusia, oral lichenoid eruption, and oral ulceration have been defined [12, 120, 123–127]. Xerostomia which was implicated as the most common oral symptom of cardiovascular drugs in a study, was found to be less frequently related with ACEIs [127]. Taste disturbances or dysgeusia are among the general adverse effects of ACEIs [1, 123]. Captopril-induced taste disturbance was found to be more frequent in females, mostly appearing within 3 months of therapy, and could be severe enough leading to withdrawal of the drug [12].

Burning mouth, burning tongue, stomatodynia, stomatopyrosis, glossopyrosis, or glossodynia suggest the same disorder presenting with burning sensation of the tongue or other oral structures. ACEIs were also reported to be associated with scalded mouth syndrome [124, 125]. It seems to be similar to burning mouth, and was described as the burning sensation of the oral mucosa like the tongue, throat, lips, and palate with no apparent clinical findings but more similar to the oral sensation that is seen after consuming hot coffee or pizza due to scalding [124]. Enalapril, captopril, and lisinopril have been implicated to cause scalded mouth syndrome

[124, 125]. The discontinuation of the drug led to the resolution of the symptoms [124, 125]. Interestingly, in one case, the medication was changed from enalapril, which was the offending drug, to lisinopril, another ACEI, and the patient did not experience the same disorder [124]. Another interesting point was the occurrence of the symptoms after long-term use of the drugs [124]. It was further suggested that the scalded mouth syndrome could be a subclinical presentation of drug-induced oral lichen planus [124].

A retrospective study investigating an association between mucosal lichen planus and drugs like beta-blockers, ACEIs, and nonsteroidal antiinflammatory drugs demonstrated an inverse association between ACEI usage and lichen planus, suggesting that ACEIs may have a protective effective against mucosal lichen planus [128].

Other Reported Adverse Cutaneous Drug Reactions to Angiotensin-Converting Enzyme Inhibitors

The other reported skin side effects to ACEIs were *lymphocytic infiltration of Jessner–Kanof* due to enalapril (with probable cross-reaction to valsartan) [129], *onycholysis* with captopril [130, 131], *scleroderma* due to fosinopril [132], *eosinophilic fasciitis* due to fosinopril [132], *follicular mucinosis* with captopril [89], and *hyperpigmentation* due to captopril [133]. *Interstitial granulomatous drug reaction* has been reported due to enalapril alone or in combination with different drugs [134, 135].

Edema/facial edema/peripheral edema and *diaphoresis* were linked to most of the ACEIs [120].

References

1. Steckelings UM, Artuc M, Wollschlager T, Wiehstutz S, Henz BM. Angiotensin-converting enzyme inhibitors as inducers of adverse cutaneous reactions. Acta Derm Venereol. 2001;81:321–5.
2. Kyrmizakis DE, Papadakis CE, Liolios AD, Karatzanis AD, Malandrakis S, Skoulakis CE, et al. Angiotensin-converting enzyme inhibitors and angiotensin II receptor antagonists. Arch Otolaryngol Head Neck Surg. 2004;130:1416–9.
3. Wolf R, Tamir A, Brenner S. Psoriasis related to angiotensin-converting enzyme inhibitors. Dermatologica. 1990;181:51–3.
4. Wilkin JK, Hammond JJ, Kirkendall WM. The captopril-induced eruption. A possible mechanism: cutaneous kinin potentiation. Arch Dermatol. 1980;116:902–5.
5. Winters ME, Rosenbaum S, Vilke GM, Almazroua FY. Emergency department management of patients with ACE-inhibitor angioedema. J Emerg Med. 2013;45:775–80.
6. Rasmussen ER, Mey K, Bygum A. Angiotensin-converting Enzyme Inhibitor-induced Angioedema – A Dangerous New Epidemic. Acta Derm Venereol. 2014;94:260–4. doi:10.2340/00015555-1760.
7. Cohen EG, Soliman AM. Changing trends in angioedema. Ann Otol Rhinol Laryngol. 2001;110:701–6.

8. Kostis JB, Kim HJ, Rusnak J, Casale T, Kaplan A, Corren J, Levy E. Incidence and characteristics of angioedema associated with enalapril. Arch Intern Med. 2005;165:1637–42.
9. Straka B, Nian H, Sloan C, Byrd JB, Woodard-Grice A, Yu C, Stone E, et al. Pollen count and presentation of Angiotensin-converting enzyme inhibitor-associated angioedema. J Allergy Clin Immunol Pract. 2013;1:468–73.
10. Pillans PI, Coulter DM, Black P. Angiooedema and urticaria with angiotensin converting enzyme inhibitors. Eur J Clin Pharmacol. 1996;51:123–6.
11. Hedner T, Samuelsson O, Lunde H, Lindholm L, Andren L, Wiholm BE. Angio-oedema in relation to treatment with angiotensin converting enzyme inhibitors. BMJ. 1992;304:941–6.
12. Chalmers D, Whitehead A, Lawson DH. Postmarketing surveillance of captopril for hypertension. Br J Clin Pharmacol. 1992;34:215–23.
13. Lee A, Thomson J. Drug-induced skin reactions. In: Adverse drug reactions. 2nd ed. London: Pharmaceutical Press; 2006. p. 125–56.
14. Vleeming W, van Amsterdam JG, Stricker BH, de Wildt DJ. ACE inhibitor-induced angioedema. Incidence, prevention and management. Drug Saf. 1998;18:171–88.
15. Chu TJ, Chow N. Adverse effects of ACE inhibitors. Ann Intern Med. 1993;118:314.
16. Garcia-Pavia P, Tomas JM, Alonso-Pulpón L. Late-onset angioedema due to an angiotensin-converting enzyme inhibitor. Can J Cardiol. 2007;23:315–6.
17. Norman JL, Holmes WL, Bell WA, Finks SW. Life-threatening ACE inhibitor-induced angioedema after eleven years on lisinopril. J Pharm Pract. 2013;26:382–8.
18. Amey G, Waidyasekara P, Kollengode R. Delayed presentation of ACE inhibitor-induced angio-oedema. BMJ Case Rep. 2013;2013. doi: 10.1136/bcr-2013-010453.
19. Howarth D. ACE inhibitor angioedema – a very late presentation. Aust Fam Physician. 2013;42:860–2.
20. Lewis LM. Angioedema: etiology, pathophysiology, current and emerging therapies. J Emerg Med. 2013;45:789–96.
21. Haymore BR, Yoon J, Mikita CP, Klote MM, DeZee KJ. Risk of angioedema with angiotensin receptor blockers in patients with prior angioedema associated with angiotensin-converting enzyme inhibitors: a meta-analysis. Ann Allergy Asthma Immunol. 2008;101:495–9.
22. Wolf R, Tamir A, Brenner S. Drug-induced versus drug-triggered pemphigus. Dermatologica. 1991;182:207–10.
23. Ong CS, Cook N, Lee S. Drug-related pemphigus and angiotensin converting enzyme inhibitors. Australas J Dermatol. 2000;41:242–6.
24. Baričević M, Mravak Stipetić M, Situm M, Marinović B, Seiwerth S, Baričević D, et al. Oral bullous eruption after taking lisinopril–case report and literature review. Wien Klin Wochenschr. 2013;125:408–11. doi:10.1007/s00508-013-0382-7.
25. Al-Niaimi F. Drug eruptions in dermatology. Expert Rev Dermatol. 2011;6:273–86.
26. Ruocco V, de Angelis E, Lombardi ML, Pisani M. In vitro acantholysis by captopril and thiopronine. Dermatologica. 1988;176:115–23.
27. Butt A, Burge SM. Pemphigus vulgaris induced by captopril. Br J Dermatol. 1995;132:315–6.
28. Thami GP, Kaur S, Kanwar AJ. Severe childhood pemphigus vulgaris aggravated by enalapril. Dermatology. 2001;202:341.
29. Parodi A, Cozzani E, Milesi G, Drosera M, Rebora A. Fosinopril as a possible pemphigus-inducing drug. Dermatology. 2002;204:139–41.
30. Shelton RM. Pemphigus foliaceus associated with enalapril. J Am Acad Dermatol. 1991;24:503–4.
31. Vignes S, Paul C, Flageul B, Dubertret L. Ramipril-induced superficial pemphigus. Br J Dermatol. 1996;135:657–8.
32. Buzon E, Perez-Bernal AM, de la Pena F, Rios JJ, Camacho F. Pemphigus foliaceus associated with cilazapril. Acta Derm Venereol. 1998;78:227.
33. Patterson CR, Davies MG. Pemphigus foliaceus: an adverse reaction to lisinopril. J Dermatolog Treat. 2004;15:60–2.

34. Pinto GM, Lamarao P, Vale T. Captopril-induced pemphigus vegetans with Charcot-Leyden crystals. J Am Acad Dermatol. 1992;27:281–4.
35. Bastiaens MT, Zwan NV, Verschueren GL, Stoof TJ, Nieboer C. Three cases of pemphigus vegetans: induction by enalapril–association with internal malignancy. Int J Dermatol. 1994;33:168–71.
36. Adriano AR, Gomes Neto A, Hamester GR, Nunes DH, Di Giunta G. Pemphigus vegetans induced by use of enalapril. An Bras Dermatol. 2011;86:1197–200.
37. Ruocco V, Satriano RA, Guerrera V. "Two-step" pemphigus induction by ACE-inhibitors. Int J Dermatol. 1992;31:33–6.
38. Kaplan RP, Potter TS, Fox JN. Drug-induced pemphigus related to angiotensin-converting enzyme inhibitors. J Am Acad Dermatol. 1992;26:364–6.
39. Femiano F, Scully C, Gombos F. Linear IgA dermatosis induced by a new angiotensin-converting enzyme inhibitor. Oral Surg Oral Med Oral Pathol Oral Radiol Endod. 2003;95:169–73.
40. Friedman IS, Rudikoff D, Phelps RG, Sapadin AN. Captopril-triggered linear IgA bullous dermatosis. Int J Dermatol. 1998;37:608–12.
41. Flageul B, Foldes C, Wallach D, Vignon-Pennamen MD, Cottenot F. Captopril-induced lichen planus pemphigoides with pemphigus-like features. A case report. Dermatologica. 1986;173:248–55.
42. Ben Salem C, Chenguel L, Ghariani N, Denguezli M, Hmouda H, Bouraoui K. Captopril-induced lichen planus pemphigoides. Pharmacoepidemiol Drug Saf. 2008;17:722–4.
43. Ogg GS, Bhogal BS, Hashimoto T, Coleman R, Barker JN. Ramipril-associated lichen planus pemphigoides. Br J Dermatol. 1997;136:412–4.
44. Zhu YI, Fitzpatrick JE, Kornfeld BW. Lichen planus pemphigoides associated with ramipril. Int J Dermatol. 2006;45:1453–5.
45. Mallet L, Cooper JW, Thomas J. Bullous pemphigoid associated with captopril. DICP. 1989;23:63.
46. Fitzgerald DA. Subepidermal bullous eruption induced by captopril. Clin Exp Dermatol. 1993;18:196–7.
47. Smith EP, Taylor TB, Meyer LJ, Zone JJ. Antigen identification in drug-induced bullous pemphigoid. J Am Acad Dermatol. 1993;29(5 Pt 2):879–82.
48. Kalińska-Bienias A, Rogoziński TT, Woźniak K, Kowalewski C. Can pemphigoid be provoked by lisinopril? Br J Dermatol. 2006;155:854–5.
49. Wong SS, Long CC, Holt PJ. Lichenoid eruption induced by low dose captopril. Acta Derm Venereol. 1992;72:358–9.
50. Revenga Arranz F, Gonzalo Garijo MA. Lichenioid reaction induced by captopril. Rev Clin Esp. 1996;196:412.
51. Cox NH, Tapson JS, Farr PM. Lichen planus associated with captopril: a further disorder demonstrating the 'tin-tack' sign. Br J Dermatol. 1989;120:319–21.
52. Rotstein E, Rotstein H. Drug eruptions with lichenoid histology produced by captopril. Australas J Dermatol. 1989;30:9–14.
53. Reinhardt LA, Wilkin JK, Kirkendall WM. Lichenoid eruption produced by captopril. Cutis. 1983;31:98–9.
54. Bravard P, Barbet M, Eich D, Weber M, Daniel F, Lauret P. Captopril induced lichenoid eruption. Ann Dermatol Venereol. 1983;110:433–8.
55. Wolf R, Tamir A, Srebrnik A, Brenner S. Lichenoid eruption and alopecia associated with captopril treatment. J Dermatolog Treat. 1990;1:155–7.
56. Ruiz Villaverde R, Blasco Melguizo J, Linares Solano J, Serrano Ortega S. Lichen planus-like eruption due to enalapril. J Eur Acad Dermatol Venereol. 2003;17:612–4.
57. Roten SV, Mainetti C, Donath R, Saurat JH. Enalapril-induced lichen planus-like eruption. J Am Acad Dermatol. 1995;32:293–5.
58. Kanwar AJ, Dhar S, Ghosh S. Photosensitive lichenoid eruption due to enalapril. Dermatology. 1993;187:80.
59. Shackelton JB, English 3rd JC. Acute-onset reticulated white lip. JAMA. 2011;306:2267–8.

60. Furness PN, Goodfield MJ, MacLennan KA, Stevens A, Millard LG. Severe cutaneous reactions to captopril and enalapril; histological study and comparison with early mycosis fungoides. J Clin Pathol. 1986;39:902–7.
61. Mutasim DF. Lymphomatoid drug eruption mimicking digitate dermatosis: cross reactivity between two drugs that suppress angiotensin II function. Am J Dermatopathol. 2003;25: 331–4.
62. Carroll J, Thaler M, Grossman E, Alder A, Trau H, Rosenthal T. Generalized pustular eruption associated with converting enzyme inhibitor therapy. Cutis. 1995;56:276–8.
63. Wolf R, Dorfman B, Krakowski A. Psoriasiform eruption induced by captopril and chlorthalidone. Cutis. 1987;40:162–4.
64. Coulter DM, Pillans PI. Angiotensin-converting enzyme inhibitors and psoriasis. N Z Med J. 1993;106:392–3.
65. Gilleaudeau P, Vallat VP, Carter DM, Gottlieb AB. Angiotensin-converting enzyme inhibitors as possible exacerbating drugs in psoriasis. J Am Acad Dermatol. 1993;28:490–2.
66. Antonov D, Grozdev I, Pehlivanov G, Tsankov N. Psoriatic erythroderma associated with enalapril. Skinmed. 2006;5:90–2.
67. Vena GA, Cassano N, Coco V, De Simone C. Eczematous reactions due to angiotensin-converting enzyme inhibitors or angiotensin II receptor blockers. Immunopharmacol Immunotoxicol. 2013;35:447–50.
68. Eriksen JG, Christiansen JJ, Asmussen I. Postulosis palmoplantaris caused by angiotensin-converting enzyme inhibitors. Ugeskr Laeger. 1995;157:3335–6.
69. Thakor P, Padmanabhan M, Johnson A, Pararajasingam T, Thakor S, Jorgensen W. Ramipril-induced generalized pustular psoriasis: case report and literature review. Am J Ther. 2010;17:92–5.
70. Ikai K. Exacerbation and induction of psoriasis by angiotensin-converting enzyme inhibitors. J Am Acad Dermatol. 1995;32:819.
71. Atzori L, Pinna AL, Ferreli C, Aste N. Pityriasis rosea-like adverse reaction: review of the literature and experience of an Italian drug-surveillance center. Dermatol Online J. 2006;12:1.
72. Ghersetich I, Rindi L, Teofoli P, Tsampau D, Palleschi GM, Lotti T. Pityriasis rosea-like skin eruptions caused by captopril. G Ital Dermatol Venereol. 1990;125:457–9.
73. Wilkin JK, Kirkendall WM. Pityriasis rosea-like rash from captopril. Arch Dermatol. 1982;118:186–7.
74. Atzori L, Ferreli C, Pinna AL, Aste N. 'Pityriasis rosea-like' adverse reaction to lisinopril. J Eur Acad Dermatol Venereol. 2004;18:743–5.
75. Puppin Jr D, Rybojad M, de la Chapelle C, Morel P. Kaposi's sarcoma associated with captopril. Lancet. 1990;336:1251–2.
76. Larbre JP, Nicolas JF, Collet P, Larbre B, Llorca G. Kaposi's sarcoma in a patient with rheumatoid arthritis possible responsibility of captopril in the development of lesions. J Rheumatol. 1991;18:476–7.
77. Bilen N, Bayramgurler D, Aydeniz B, Apaydin R, Ozkara SK. Possible causal role of lisinopril in a case of Kaposi's sarcoma. Br J Dermatol. 2002;147:1042–4.
78. Dervis E, Demirkesen C. Kaposi's sarcoma in a patient with psoriasis vulgaris. Acta Dermatovenerol Alp Panonica Adriat. 2010;19:31–4.
79. Di Carlo A. Lisinopril and Kaposi's sarcoma. Br J Dermatol. 2004;150:158–9.
80. Vogt B, Frey FJ. Inhibition of angiogenesis in Kaposi's sarcoma by captopril. Lancet. 1997;349:1148.
81. Ratliff 3rd NB. Captopril induced lupus. J Rheumatol. 2002;29:1807–8.
82. Patri P, Nigro A, Rebora A. Lupus erythematosus-like eruption from captopril. Acta Derm Venereol. 1985;65:447–8.
83. Sieber C, Grimm E, Follath F. Captopril and systemic lupus erythematosus syndrome. BMJ. 1990;301:669.
84. Bertin P, Kamdem J, Bonnet C, Arnaud M, Treves R. Captopril-induced lupus. Clin Exp Rheumatol. 1993;11:695.

85. Carter JD, Valeriano-Marcet J, Kanik KS, Vasey FB. Antinuclear antibody-negative, drug-induced lupus caused by lisinopril. South Med J. 2001;94:1122–3.
86. Srivastava M, Rencic A, Diglio G, Santana H, Bonitz P, Watson R, et al. Drug-induced, Ro/SSA-positive cutaneous lupus erythematosus. Arch Dermatol. 2003;139:45–9.
87. Fernandez-Diaz ML, Herranz P, Suarez-Marrero MC, Borbujo J, Manzano R, Casado M. Subacute cutaneous lupus erythematosus associated with cilazapril. Lancet. 1995;345:398.
88. Reidenberg MM, Case DB, Drayer DE, Reis S, Lorenzo B. Development of antinuclear antibody in patients treated with high doses of captopril. Arthritis Rheum. 1984;27:579–81.
89. Pérez-Ferriols A, Martínez-Menchón T, Fortea JM. Follicular mucinosis secondary to captopril-induced photoallergy. Actas Dermosifiliogr. 2005;96:167–70.
90. Rodríguez Granados MT, Abalde T, García Doval I, De la Torre C. Systemic photosensitivity to quinapril. J Eur Acad Dermatol Venereol. 2004;18:389–90.
91. Wagner SN, Welke F, Goos M. Occupational UVA-induced allergic photodermatitis in a welder due to hydrochlorothiazide and ramipril. Contact Dermatitis. 2000;43:245–6.
92. Smit AJ, Van der Laan S, De Monchy J, Kallenberg CG, Donker AJ. Cutaneous reactions to captopril. Predictive value of skin tests. Clin Allergy. 1984;14:413–9.
93. Miralles R, Pedro-Botet J, Farre M, Rubies-Prat J. Captopril and vasculitis. Ann Intern Med. 1988;109:514.
94. Laaban J, Marie JP, Wallach D, Blanchard D, Lafay M, Gruffaz F. Necrotising vasculitis associated with captopril therapy. Eur Heart J. 1987;8:319.
95. Guillevin L, Le Roux G, Breau JL. Leukocytoclasic vasculitis during treatment with low-dose captopril. Ann Med Interne (Paris). 1987;138:658–9.
96. Jensen ON, Ahlquist P. Schoenlein-Henoch purpura in a geriatric patient after captopril therapy. Ugeskr Laeger. 1996;158:4926–7.
97. Carrington PR, Sanusi ID, Zahradka S, Winder PR. Enalapril-associated erythema and vasculitis. Cutis. 1993;51:121–3.
98. Goncalves R, Cortez Pinto H, Serejo F, Ramalho F. Adult Schonlein-Henoch purpura after enalapril. J Intern Med. 1998;244:356–7.
99. Moots RJ, Keeling PJ, Morgan SH. Adult Schonlein-Henoch purpura after enalapril. Lancet. 1992;340:304–5.
100. Ayani I, Martinez MJ, Lekuona I, Manrique P. Enalapril-induced vasculitis. Med Clin (Barc). 1991;96:596.
101. Barlow RJ, Schulz EJ. Lisinopril-induced vasculitis. Clin Exp Dermatol. 1988;13:117–20.
102. Disdier P, Harle JR, Verrot D, Jouglard J, Weiller PJ. Adult Schonlein-Henoch purpura after lisinopril. Lancet. 1992;340:985.
103. Gupta S, Gandhi NM, Ferguson J. Cutaneous vasculitis secondary to ramipril. J Drugs Dermatol. 2004;3:81–2.
104. Cnudde F, Leynadier F, Dry J. Cutaneous reaction to captopril: value of patch tests. Contact Dermatitis. 1990;23:375–6.
105. Pfützner W, Rueff F, Przybilla B. Systemic contact dermatitis due to captopril without cross-sensitivity to fosinopril, quinapril and benazepril. Acta Derm Venereol. 2004;84:91–2.
106. Martinez JC, Fuentes MJ, Armentia A, Vega JM, Fernandez A. Dermatitis to captopril. Allergol Immunopathol (Madr). 2001;29:279–80.
107. Touraud JP, Collet E, Louguet C, Sgro C, Dalac S, Dutronc Y, Lambert D. Cross-sensitivity between angiotensin-converting enzyme inhibitors and angiotensin II receptor antagonist. Ann Dermatol Venereol. 2002;129:1033–6.
108. Solinger AM. Exfoliative dermatitis from captopril. Cutis. 1982;29:473–4.
109. O'Neill PG, Rajan N, Charlat ML, Bolli R. Captopril-related exfoliative dermatitis. Tex Med. 1989;85:40–1.
110. Goodfield MJ, Millard LG. Severe cutaneous reactions to captopril. Br Med J (Clin Res Ed). 1985;290:1111.
111. Pennell DJ, Nunan TO, O'Doherty MJ, Croft DN. Fatal Stevens-Johnson syndrome in a patient on captopril and allopurinol. Lancet. 1984;1:463.

112. Alkurtass DA, Al-Jazairi AS. Possible captopril-induced toxic epidermal necrolysis. Ann Pharmacother. 2003;37:380–3.
113. Winfred RI, Nanda S, Horvath G, Elnicki M. Captopril-induced toxic epidermal necrolysis and agranulocytosis successfully treated with granulocyte colony-stimulating factor. South Med J. 1999;92:918–20.
114. Oskay T, Ozcelik T, Kutluay L. Stevens-Johnson Syndrome associated with ramipril. Int J Dermatol. 2003;42:580–1.
115. Chaabane A, Fadhl NB, Chadly Z, Fredj NB, Boughattas NA, Aouam K. Captopril-induced DRESS: first reported case confirmed by patch test. Dermatitis. 2013;24:255–7.
116. Pileri A, Brunasso AM, Tilz H, Wolf P, Massone C. Ramipril-induced drug reaction with eosinophilia and systemic symptoms (DRESS). Eur J Dermatol. 2011;21:624–5.
117. Motel PJ. Captopril and alopecia: a case report and review of known cutaneous reactions in captopril use. J Am Acad Dermatol. 1990;23:124–5.
118. Leaker B, Whitworth JA. Alopecia associated with captopril treatment. Aust N Z J Med. 1984;14:866.
119. Ahmad S. Enalapril and reversible alopecia. Arch Intern Med. 1991;151:404.
120. Litt JZ. Drug eruption reference manual. 19th ed. Boca Raton: CRC Press (Taylor and Francis Group); 2013.
121. Frishman WH, Brosnan BD, Grossman M, Dasgupta D, Sun DK. Adverse dermatologic effects of cardiovascular drug therapy: part II. Cardiol Rev. 2002;10:285–300.
122. Thestrup-Pedersen K. Adverse reactions in the skin from anti-hypertensive drugs. Dan Med Bull. 1987;34 Suppl 1:3–5.
123. Torpet LA, Kragelund C, Reibel J, Nauntofte B. Oral adverse drug reactions to cardiovascular drugs. Crit Rev Oral Biol Med. 2004;15:28–46.
124. Brown RS, Krakow AM, Douglas T. Choksi SK."Scalded mouth syndrome" caused by angiotensin converting enzyme inhibitors: two case reports. Oral Surg Oral Med Oral Pathol Oral Radiol Endod. 1997;83:665–7.
125. Savino LB, Haushalter NM. Lisinopril-induced "scalded mouth syndrome". Ann Pharmacother. 1992;26:1381–2.
126. Triantos D, Kanakis P. Stomatodynia (burning mouth) as a complication of enalapril therapy. Oral Dis. 2004;10:244–5.
127. Habbab KM, Moles DR, Porter SR. Potential oral manifestations of cardiovascular drugs. Oral Dis. 2010;16:769–73.
128. Clayton R, Chaudhry S, Ali I, Cooper S, Hodgson T, Wojnarowska F. Mucosal (oral and vulval) lichen planus in women: are angiotensin-converting enzyme inhibitors protective, and beta-blockers and non-steroidal anti-inflammatory drugs associated with the condition? Clin Exp Dermatol. 2010;35:384–7. doi:10.1111/j.1365-2230.2009.03581.x.
129. Schepis C, Lentini M, Siragusa M, Batolo D. ACE-inhibitor-induced drug eruption resembling lymphocytic infiltration (of Jessner-Kanof) and Lupus erythematosus tumidus. Dermatology. 2004;208:354–5.
130. Borders JV. Captopril and onycholysis. Ann Intern Med. 1986;105:305–6.
131. Brueggemeyer CD, Ramirez G. Onycholysis associated with captopril. Lancet. 1984;1:1352–3.
132. Biasi D, Caramaschi P, Carletto A, Bambara LM. Scleroderma and eosinophilic fasciitis in patients taking fosinopril. J Rheumatol. 1997;24:1242.
133. O'Neil MB, Balfe JW, Geary DF. Captopril related hyperpigmentation. Br Med J. 1987;295:333.
134. Magro CM, Crowson AN, Schapiro BL. The interstitial granulomatous drug reaction: a distinctive clinical and pathological entity. J Cutan Pathol. 1998;25:72–8.
135. Perrin C, Lacour JP, Castanet J, Michiels JF. Interstitial granulomatous drug reaction with a histological pattern of interstitial granulomatous dermatitis. Am J Dermatopathol. 2001;23:295–8.

Chapter 3
Angiotensin II Receptor Blockers

Keywords Angiotensin II receptor blocker • Losartan • Candesartan • Valsartan • Angioedema • Lymphomatoid • Psoriasis • Eczema • Lichenoid • Maculopapular • Bullous

The angiotensin II receptor blockers (ARBs) inhibit the activity of angiotensin II at the angiotensin II receptor level (AT-1, AT-2 receptors). Losartan potassium is the prototype of the ARBs. Others are candesartan, irbesartan, valsartan, telmisartan, olmesartan, eprosartan, and azilsartan.

The adverse cutaneous drug reactions described below are meant to be sorted by starting from the well-known reactions of ARBs to the lesser known ones. The major ones are summarized in Table 3.1.

Angioedema/Urticaria

Angioedema that is a well-known bradykinin-mediated side effect of angiotensin-converting enzyme inhibitors (ACEIs) is also reported with ARBs, although theoretically ARBs do not affect ACE and the degradation of bradykinin. The underlying mechanism of this adverse effect is not clear [1, 2]. However, it is stated that selective effects of ARBs on the AT-1 subtype of angiotensin II receptor may cause increase of bradykinin in tissue levels causing angioedema [3].

Losartan, candesartan, valsartan, telmisartan, olmesartan, and irbesartan are the reported ARBs to be associated with angioedema that may be severe in some cases [1–10]. The reaction was reported to develop within a wide range of lag time, occurring within 24 hours to 16 months [2], or even approximately 3 years [8] after the initiation of therapy. It was reported to be dose dependent in a valsartan-induced case [4].

It is a matter of debate whether ARBs can be used in patients with a previous history of ACEI-related angioedema. There are patients with previous history of angioedema from ACEIs who safely used ARBs such as losartan, candesartan, irbesartan, or telmisartan [11]. On the other hand, it is also known that angioedema may occur with ARBs in patients with a previous history of ACEI-associated

E. Özkaya, K.D. Yazganoğlu, *Adverse Cutaneous Drug Reactions to Cardiovascular Drugs*, DOI 10.1007/978-1-4471-6536-1_3

Table 3.1 Major adverse cutaneous drug reactions with angiotensin II receptor blockers

Adverse cutaneous drug reaction	Main inducers
Angioedema	Losartan, valsartan, candesartan, telmisartan, olmesartan, irbesartan
Psoriasis/psoriasiform eruption	Losartan, candesartan, irbesartan, valsartan, valsartan + hydrochlorothiazide
Eczematous eruption	Losartan, valsartan, irbesartan, olmesartan, valsartan + hydrochlorothiazide, irbesartan + hydrochlorothiazide
Lymphomatoid drug eruption	Losartan, valsartan, irbesartan
Vasculitis	Losartan, candesartan
Bullous eruptions	
Linear IgA dermatosis	Candesartan (eprosartan[a])
Bullous pemphigoid	Losartan, valsartan
Pemphigus foliaceus	Candesartan (telmisartan[a])
Lichenoid eruption	Valsartan, irbesartan + hydrochlorothiazide
Maculopapular eruption	Valsartan, irbesartan
Erythema multiforme	Candesartan, irbesartan
Stevens–Johnson syndrome	Losartan
Oral mucosal reactions	Losartan, valsartan, candesartan, eprosartan
SDRIFE	Telmisartan + hydrochlorothiazide

SDRIFE symmetrical drug-related intertriginous and flexural exanthema
[a]Probable cross-reaction to candesartan

angioedema [1, 2, 5]. According to a meta-analysis, this risk was found as 9.4 % [12]. It was suggested that in patients with a history of angioedema, especially ACEI-associated angioedema, ARBs may be avoided or used very cautiously although a strict contraindication was not stated [1, 2, 13, 14].

ARBs were also reported to cause angioedema in the setting of type III hereditary angioedema [15], which is a newly described type of angioedema seen in women with normal C1 inhibitor level and function [16].

Although rare, urticaria may accompany ARB-induced angioedema in some cases [10].

Psoriasis

New-onset psoriasis or exacerbation of preexisting psoriasis was reported in patients using ARBs like losartan, candesartan, irbesartan, and valsartan [17–20]. New-onset psoriasis started within 1 week to 9 months after the initiation of treatment with ARBs; exacerbation of psoriasis occurred within several days to 9 months after the onset of the drug [17, 19, 20]. The clinical manifestation of some of the cases were interesting as psoriasis lesions were reported to occur on sun-exposed areas such as on the back of the hands and forearms [19]. Accompanying nail involvement was also reported in some cases [19].

In one patient with valsartan-induced psoriasis, lesions resolved following withdrawal of the drug but relapsed after initiation of therapy with candesartan [19]. Apart from the suggested direct pharmacological action of ARBs, the keratinocyte proliferating effect of angiotensin II that is increased with ARBs was also suggested as an important factor that could be related with psoriasis from ARBs [19].

Psoriasis-like lesions were observed clinically and histopathologically in a patient using valsartan + hydrochlorothiazide [21].

Eczematous Eruption

Eczematous eruption has been reported with ARBs like losartan, valsartan, irbesartan, olmesartan, and eprosartan [21–23].

In a recent report, diffuse or localized eczematous eruption was seen in a total of seven patients using ARBs, five of whom were also using another antihypertensive, namely, hydrochlorothiazide [21]. In one of the patients, who was using valsartan + hydrochlorothiazide, psoriasis-like lesions were observed clinically and histopathologically. The reaction was reported to disappear with the cessation of the suspected drug and with the use of topical or systemic corticosteroids in all patients. Furthermore, rechallenge test performed in three patients with the suspected drug (irbesartan + hydrochlorothiazide in two patients, olmesartan in one patient) led to recurrence of eczematous lesions in two patients taking irbesartan + hydrochlorothiazide [21].

The possibility of a cross-sensitivity reaction between ACEIs and ARBs was mentioned in an article reporting two cases who developed eczematous eruption first while taking an ACEI and then after switching it to an ARB [22].

Lymphomatoid Drug Eruption

Different clinical patterns of lymphomatoid drug eruptions have been reported in association with ARBs, namely, valsartan, losartan, and irbesartan.

A lisinopril-associated lymphomatoid drug eruption with clinical findings resembling digitate dermatosis resolving after discontinuation of lisinopril, but recurring after therapy with valsartan, was reported [24].

Another case with valsartan-induced maculopapular eruption was reported to develop CD30+ pseudolymphomatous eruption appearing as generalized papules after a 4-month discontinuation of valsartan [25]. The maculopapular eruption has been completely resolved at that time. In spite of the long latency period after the discontinuation of the drug, the authors attributed the lymphomatoid drug eruption to valsartan due to the positive lymphocyte stimulation test, and suggested that overstimulation of valsartan-reactive T cells might have caused the eruption [25].

A case of irbesartan-induced maculopapular eruption with some histopathological features resembling early stage of mycosis fungoides has also been reported [26].

Two cases of atypical cutaneous lymphoid hyperplasia were attributed to losartan therapy. The papular eruption developed approximately 3 weeks after the onset of losartan in one patient and resolved after discontinuation of the drug [27]. The other case developed plaques over the trunk and groin 2 months after the onset of losartan that regressed after withdrawal of the drug. According to the histopathological and immunohistochemical findings, and polymerase chain reaction analysis, the authors considered the first condition as cutaneous T cell pseudolymphoma and the latter one as regressive true cutaneous T cell lymphoma [27].

Vasculitis

Vasculitis was defined during therapy with losartan and candesartan [28–31].

Two patients have been reported with Henoch–Schönlein purpura occurring 1 and 4 weeks, respectively, after starting losartan therapy [28, 29]. Both of them showed increased levels of IgA. Discontinuation of the drugs led to clinical improvement within 8 days and 3 weeks, respectively. In one of the cases, rechallenge with losartan resulted in reappearance of the lesions within 2 days [28]. In the other one, antineutrophilic cytoplasmic antibodies (ANCA) were positive, and still detected positive after discontinuation of losartan [29].

One case of Henoch–Schönlein purpura associated with acute nephritic syndrome occurring after 2 years of therapy with candesartan was reported. The lesions resolved within 1 week after withdrawal of the therapy [30].

One case of severe leukocytoclastic vasculitis with the presence of ANCA was reported from losartan [31]. Interestingly, ANCA were still positive after discontinuation of losartan therapy.

Bullous Eruption

Linear IgA Dermatosis

A case of candesartan-induced linear IgA dermatosis was reported [32]. The reaction started 2 weeks after the initiation of candesartan therapy. One month after discontinuation of therapy, the lesions fully disappeared. However, 10 months later, eprosartan, another ARB, was given to the patient, which led to the recurrence of the lesions. Discontinuation of the drug and therapy with low-dose systemic corticosteroids resulted in clearance of the lesions [32].

Bullous Pemphigoid

Two cases of bullous pemphigoid were suggested to occur in association with ARBs, namely, losartan and valsartan [33, 34]. In the case with bullous pemphigoid triggered by losartan, the patient had coexisting psoriasis, and the blistering showed recurrence even after cessation of losartan [33].

Pemphigus Foliaceus

A case of candesartan-induced pemphigus foliaceus was reported [35]. The reaction started 2 months after initiation of therapy with candesartan. After discontinuation of candesartan and additional immunosuppressive treatment, the lesions resolved. However, they recurred with another ARB, telmisartan, after 2 months of administration [35].

Lichenoid Drug Eruption

Lichenoid drug eruption has been reported in patients taking valsartan and irbesartan + hydrochlorothiazide [36, 37].

Two cases of valsartan-induced linear lichenoid eruption have been reported, but one had a history of prior lichen planus [36]. In the case of irbesartan + hydrochlorothiazide-induced lichenoid eruption, patch testing with irbesartan and hydrochlorothiazide as single substances revealed negative results, but it was positive for the combination drug suggesting that the reaction was a "compound allergy" [37].

Maculopapular Eruption

Valsartan has been reported to induce maculopapular eruption in several cases [25, 26, 38]. In one of the valsartan-induced cases, CD30+ pseudolymphomatous eruption developed after resolution of the maculopapular eruption and a 4-month discontinuation of valsartan [25]. Another patient with irbesartan-induced maculopapular eruption showed some targetoid lesions and mucosal involvement suggesting an overlap with "erythema multiforme major" [26]. This case had additionally some histopathological features resembling early mycosis fungoides [26].

Erythema Multiforme/Stevens–Johnson Syndrome

ARBs have also been reported to induce erythema multiforme. A patient with an isolated ulcer on the lip, which was interpreted as erythema multiforme, has been reported during the use of candesartan [39]. Targetoid lesions and mucosal involvement accompanied in a patient with irbesartan-induced maculopapular eruption suggesting an overlap of maculopapular eruption with erythema multiforme major [26]. This case showed some histopathological features resembling early mycosis fungoides [26].

Stevens–Johnson syndrome from losartan has been reported [40].

Oral Mucosal Reactions

Oral mucosal reactions like xerostomia, dysgeusia/ageusia, burning mouth, or aphthous ulcers have been described to be induced by ARBs including losartan, valsartan, eprosartan, and candesartan [41–46].

Pruritus

Pruritus is a nonspecific cutaneous adverse reaction of drugs. It was reported to accompany different types of drug eruptions in patients receiving ARBs [6, 26, 36–38, 47].

Other Reported Adverse Cutaneous Drug Reactions to Angiotensin II Receptor Blockers

Symmetrical drug-related intertriginous and flexural exanthema from telmisartan + hydrochlorothiazide [48], *nail clubbing* and *nail pigmentation* with losartan (with a probable cross-reaction to valsartan) [49], and *photosensitivity* with valsartan [6] have been reported.

Other skin side effects linked to ARBs include *facial edema/peripheral edema/edema* with valsartan, losartan, olmesartan, telmisartan, candesartan, irbesartan, and eprosartan; *diaphoresis/hyperhidrosis* due to losartan, candesartan, telmisartan, and eprosartan; *xerosis* with losartan, and *alopecia* with losartan and olmesartan [23].

References

1. Kyrmizakis DE, Papadakis CE, Liolios AD, Karatzanis AD, Malandrakis S, Skoulakis CE, et al. Angiotensin-converting enzyme inhibitors and angiotensin II receptor antagonists. Arch Otolaryngol Head Neck Surg. 2004;130:1416–9.

2. van Rijnsoever EW, Kwee-Zuiderwijk WJ, Feenstra J. Angioneurotic edema attributed to the use of losartan. Arch Intern Med. 1998;158:2063–5.
3. Nykamp D, Winter EE. Olmesartan medoxomil-induced angioedema. Ann Pharmacother. 2007;41:518–20.
4. Irons BK, Kumar A. Valsartan-induced angioedema. Ann Pharmacother. 2003;37:1024–7.
5. Abdi R, Dong VM, Lee CJ, Ntoso KA. Angiotensin II receptor blocker-associated angioedema: on the heels of ACE inhibitor angioedema. Pharmacotherapy. 2002;22:1173–5.
6. Frye CB, Pettigrew TJ. Angioedema and photosensitive rash induced by valsartan. Pharmacotherapy. 1998;18:866–8.
7. Borazan A, Ustün H, Yilmaz A. Angioedema induced by angiotensin II blocker telmisartan. Allergy. 2003;58:454.
8. Chiu AG, Krowiak EJ, Deeb ZE. Angioedema associated with angiotensin II receptor antagonists: challenging our knowledge of angioedema and its etiology. Laryngoscope. 2001;111:1729–31.
9. Nielsen EW. Hypotensive shock and angio-oedema from angiotensin II receptor blocker: a class effect in spite of tripled tryptase values. J Intern Med. 2005;258:385–7.
10. Kazim SF, Shahid M. Losartan associated anaphylaxis and angioneurotic oedema. J Pak Med Assoc. 2010;60:685–6.
11. Gavras I, Gavras H. Are patients who develop angioedema with ACE inhibition at risk of the same problem with AT1 receptor blockers? Arch Intern Med. 2003;163:240–1.
12. Haymore BR, Yoon J, Mikita CP, Klote MM, DeZee KJ. Risk of angioedema with angiotensin receptor blockers in patients with prior angioedema associated with angiotensin-converting enzyme inhibitors: a meta-analysis. Ann Allergy Asthma Immunol. 2008;101:495–9.
13. MacLean JA, Hannaway PJ. Angioedema and AT1 receptor blockers: proceed with caution. Arch Intern Med. 2003;163:1488–9.
14. Rasmussen ER, Mey K, Bygum A. Angiotensin-converting enzyme inhibitor-induced angioedema – a dangerous new epidemic. Acta Derm Venereol. 2014;94:260–4. doi:10.2340/00015555-1760.
15. Bork K, Dewald G. Hereditary angioedema type III, angioedema associated with angiotensin II receptor antagonists, and female sex. Am J Med. 2004;116:644–5.
16. Bork K, Barnstedt SE, Koch P, Traupe H. Hereditary angioedema with normal C1-inhibitor activity in women. Lancet. 2000;356:213–7.
17. Lamba G, Palaniswamy C, Singh T, Shah D, Lal S, Vinnakota R, et al. Psoriasis induced by losartan therapy: a case report and review of the literature. Am J Ther. 2011;18:e78–80.
18. Kawamura A, Ochiai T. Candesartan cilexetil induced pustular psoriasis. Eur J Dermatol. 2003;13:406–7.
19. Marquart-Elbaz C, Grosshans E, Lipsker D, Lipsker D. Sartans, angiotensin II receptor antagonists, can induce psoriasis. Br J Dermatol. 2002;147:617–8.
20. AT1-receptor antagonists and psoriasis. http://www.lareb.nl/LarebCorporateWebsite/media/publicaties/kwb_2006_1_angio.pdf. Accessed 14 May 2014.
21. Vena GA, Cassano N, Coco V, De Simone C. Eczematous reactions due to angiotensin-converting enzyme inhibitors or angiotensin II receptor blockers. Immunopharmacol Immunotoxicol. 2013;35:447–50.
22. Touraud JP, Collet E, Louguet C, Sgro C, Dalac S, Dutronc Y, Lambert D. Cross-sensitivity between angiotensin-converting enzyme inhibitors and angiotensin II receptor antagonist. Ann Dermatol Venereol. 2002;129:1033–6.
23. Litt JZ. Drug eruption reference manual. 19th ed. Boca Raton: CRC Press (Taylor and Francis Group); 2013.
24. Mutasim DF. Lymphomatoid drug eruption mimicking digitate dermatosis: cross reactivity between two drugs that suppress angiotensin II function. Am J Dermatopathol. 2003;25:331–4.
25. Sawada Y, Yoshiki R, Kawakami C, Fukamachi S, Sugita K, Nakamura M, Tokura Y. Valsartan-induced drug eruption followed by CD30+ pseudolymphomatous eruption. Acta Derm Venereol. 2010;90:521–2.

26. Gambini D, Sala F, Gianotti R, Cusini M. Exanthematous reaction to irbesartan. J Eur Acad Dermatol Venereol. 2003;17:472–3.
27. Viraben R, Lamant L, Brousset P. Losartan-associated atypical cutaneous lymphoid hyperplasia. Lancet. 1997;350:1366.
28. Bosch X. Henoch-Schonlein purpura induced by losartan therapy. Arch Intern Med. 1998;158:191–2.
29. Brouard M, Piguet V, Chavaz P, Borradori L. Schonlein-Henoch purpura associated with losartan treatment and presence of antineutrophil cytoplasmic antibodies of x specificity. Br J Dermatol. 2001;145:362–3.
30. Morton A, Muir J, Lim D. Rash and acute nephritic syndrome due to candesartan. BMJ. 2004;328:25.
31. Piérard Franchimont C, Henry F, Piérard GE. Severe pustular and polymorphous vasculitis caused by losartan. Ann Dermatol Venereol. 2001;128(10 Pt 1):1040–2.
32. Pena-Penabad C, Rodriguez-Lozano J, del Pozo J, Garcia-Silva J, Fonseca E. Linear IgA bullous dermatosis induced by angiotensin receptor antagonists. Am J Med. 2003;114:163–4.
33. Saraceno R, Citarella L, Spallone G, Chimenti S. A biological approach in a patient with psoriasis and bullous pemphigoid associated with losartan therapy. Clin Exp Dermatol. 2008; 33:154–5.
34. Femiano F. Mucocutaneous bullous pemphigoid induced by valsartan. A clinical case. Minerva Stomatol. 2003;52:187–90.
35. Bae YI, Yun SJ, Lee SC, Park GT, Lee JB. Pemphigus foliaceus induced by an angiotensin II receptor blocker. Clin Exp Dermatol. 2008;33:721–3.
36. Gencoglan G, Ceylan C, Kazandi AC. Linear lichenoid drug eruption induced by valsartan. Clin Exp Dermatol. 2009;34:e334–5.
37. Pfab F, Athanasiadis GI, Kollmar A, Ring J, Ollert M. Lichenoid drug eruption due to an antihypertonic drug containing irbesartan and hydrochlorothiazide. Allergy. 2006;61:786–7.
38. Ozturk G, Turk BG, Senturk B, Turkmen M, Kandiloglu G. Exanthematous drug eruption due to valsartan. Cutan Ocul Toxicol. 2012;31:335–7.
39. Ejaz AA, Walsh JS, Wasiluk A. Erythema multiforme associated with candesartan cilexetil. South Med J. 2004;97:614–5.
40. Bonnici H, Bygum A. Losartan-induced Stevens-Johnson syndrome in a geriatric patient. Ugeskr Laeger. 2007;169:1233–4.
41. Habbab KM, Moles DR, Porter SR. Potential oral manifestations of cardiovascular drugs. Oral Dis. 2010;16:769–73.
42. Chen C, Chevrot D, Contamin C, Romanet T, Allenet B, Mallaret M. Stomatitis and ageusia induced by candesartan. Nephrologie. 2004;25:97–9.
43. Goffin E, Pochet JM, Lejuste P, De Plaen JF. Aphthous ulcers of the mouth associated with losartan. Clin Nephrol. 1998;50:197.
44. Castells X, Rodoreda I, Pedrós C, Cereza G, Laporte JR. Drug points: dysgeusia and burning mouth syndrome by eprosartan. BMJ. 2002;325:1277.
45. Heeringa M, van Puijenbroek EP. Reversible dysgeusia attributed to losartan. Ann Intern Med. 1998;129:72.
46. Schlienger RG, Saxer M, Haefeli WE. Reversible ageusia associated with losartan. Lancet. 1996;347:471–2.
47. Frishman WH, Brosnan BD, Grossman M, Dasgupta D, Sun DK. Adverse dermatologic effects of cardiovascular drug therapy: part II. Cardiol Rev. 2002;10:285–300.
48. Ferreira O, Mota A, Morais P, Cunha AP, Azevedo F. Symmetrical drug-related intertriginous and flexural exanthema (SDRIFE) induced by telmisartan-hydrochlorothiazide. Cutan Ocul Toxicol. 2010;29:293–5.
49. Packard KA, Arouni AJ, Hilleman DE, Gannon JM. Fingernail clubbing and chromonychia associated with the use of angiotensin II receptor blockers. Pharmacotherapy. 2004;24: 546–50.

Chapter 4
Alpha-2 Adrenergic Receptor Agonists

Keywords Alpha-2 adrenergic receptor agonist • Methyldopa • Clonidine • Photosensitivity • Lupus • Lichenoid • Eczema • Psoriasis/Psoriasiform • Xerostomia

Alpha-2 adrenergic receptor agonists include clonidine, guanfacine, guanabenz, methyldopa, rilmenidine, and moxonidine. These are centrally active antihypertensive drugs.

The adverse cutaneous drug reactions described below are meant to be sorted by starting from the well-known reactions of alpha-2 adrenergic receptor agonists to the lesser known ones. The major ones are summarized in Table 4.1.

Drug-Induced Lupus Erythematosus

Methyldopa has been shown to induce the formation of antinuclear antibodies (ANA) and/or systemic lupus erythematosus, but a photosensitive eruption or cutaneous features of lupus were rarely reported [1–5]. The reaction started within several months to over a year of therapy with methyldopa [2–5]. Antihistone antibodies, which are frequently associated with drug-induced lupus erythematosus, were found positive [2, 4]. The reaction resolved and the level of ANA declined or returned to normal upon discontinuation of methyldopa and/or with treatment of lupus syndrome [2–4]. Clonidine has also been implicated as a cause of lupus-like syndrome [6].

Photosensitivity

Photosensitivity has been reported to occur during the use of rilmenidine [7] and methyldopa [8]. Photosensitivity to methyldopa can be a part of the systemic lupus erythematosus induced by this drug [2]. In a recent study, it was found that the risk of the development of basal cell carcinoma was increased in patients with a long-term use of methyldopa [9].

E. Özkaya, K.D. Yazganoğlu, *Adverse Cutaneous Drug Reactions to Cardiovascular Drugs*, DOI 10.1007/978-1-4471-6536-1_4

Table 4.1 Major adverse cutaneous drug reactions with alpha-2 adrenergic receptor agonists

Adverse cutaneous drug reaction	Main inducers
Drug-induced lupus erythematosus (systemic lupus erythematosus)	Methyldopa
Photosensitivity	Methyldopa, rilmenidine
Lichenoid eruption	Methyldopa
Eczematous eruption	Methyldopa
Cicatricial pemphigoid	Clonidine
Psoriasis/psoriasiform eruption	Clonidine
Local side effects from topical use	Clonidine
Xerostomia	Methyldopa, clonidine, rilmenidine, moxonidine, guanabenz
Drug rash with eosinophilia and systemic symptoms	Methyldopa

Lichenoid Eruption

Both oral and cutaneous lichenoid eruptions were reported from the use of methyldopa [10–14]. The reaction may start after several months to years of therapy. In some cases, the reaction was confirmed by rechallenge with the suspected drug [11, 12]. Complete resolution of the reaction can take several months after stopping the drug. Unusual clinical and histopathological manifestations of lichenoid drug eruptions were also reported in patients using methyldopa [11, 15]. One of these cases had an ulcerative lichenoid eruption on the feet and toes, accompanied by generalized eczema that occurred after approximately 1 year of treatment with methyldopa [11]. Discontinuation of methyldopa led to clearance of the eczema within 3 weeks, while the ulceration on the feet healed in 5 months. Rechallenge with methyldopa for only 1 day caused recurrence of the eczema and burning symptom of the soles of the feet [11].

Eczematous Eruption

Eczematous eruptions have also been reported during treatment with methyldopa [16, 17]. A report of 16 cases with methyldopa-associated eczema included seborrheic dermatitis mainly involving the scalp and face as well as nummular or generalized eczema [17]. Both new-onset eczema and exacerbation of healed eczema were reported. Five of these 16 patients had a history of previous eczema like atopic dermatitis, seborrheic dermatitis, and hair dye dermatitis, and one had a history of ichthyosis. The reaction has started within a few weeks to 60 months of therapy and, in some cases, following a dose increase [17]. The eruption healed within 1–12 weeks after stopping the drug. Eight of the patients were rechallenged with methyldopa; the reaction recurred within a 2-day period in all patients except one who used a smaller dose. In another patient, after a 6-month period of clearance, methyldopa was started again, but the reaction did not recur. Patch testing with 1 % aqueous solution of methyldopa performed in six patients was negative. The occurrence of eczema after an increase in drug dosage in some cases, immediate relapse of the eczema on full doses, and relatively late relapses on smaller doses led the authors to suggest that the reaction was rather dose related [17].

Bullous Eruption

Cicatricial Pemphigoid

A case of cicatricial pemphigoid involving perianal skin and anal/vulvar mucosa was reported with long-term clonidine therapy [18].

Psoriasis/Psoriasiform Eruption

Exacerbation of psoriasis after 3 days of therapy with clonidine was reported that was supposed to be related to clonidine-induced inhibition of adenylate cyclase which might lead to a decrease in intracellular level of cyclic adenosine monophosphate (cAMP) with subsequent promotion of epidermal cell proliferation [19].

Local Side Effects from Topical Use

The clonidine transdermal therapeutic system is used in the treatment of hypertension as well, and with fewer systemic adverse effects compared to oral formulation [20]. However, dermatitis to topical clonidine was reported to be frequent (in up to 38 % of the patients) [20]. The reaction can be irritant or allergic in nature which includes pruritus, erythema, scaling, vesiculation, excoriation, and induration at the transdermal application site [6, 20, 21]. The drug itself is thought to be the cause of the allergic reactions rather than the excipients of transdermal systems [20, 21]. Hyperpigmentation and depigmentation are other local side effects occurring at the site of the clonidine patch [20, 22, 23]. Generalized maculopapular eruption following the use of systemic clonidine in a patient with previous eczematous skin reaction from topical clonidine use was reported, suggesting systemic allergic (contact) dermatitis [21].

Pruritus

Pruritus is a nonspecific cutaneous adverse reaction of drugs. It was reported in patients receiving alpha-2 adrenergic receptor agonists including clonidine, guanfacine, guanabenz, and methyldopa [6, 24].

Oral Mucosal Reactions

Oral mucosal reactions like *oral lichenoid eruption* have been described to be induced by methyldopa [10, 13] and *xerostomia* by methyldopa, clonidine, rilmenidine, moxonidine, and guanabenz [6, 25]. Clonidine has been reported to cause xerostomia by central and peripheral mechanisms [25].

Other Reported Adverse Cutaneous Drug Reactions to Alpha-2 Adrenergic Receptor Agonists

The other reported adverse cutaneous drug reactions were *drug rash with eosinophilia and systemic symptoms* [26], *black tongue* [27], and *cutaneous nodules* with methyldopa revealing granulomatous infiltration with multinucleated giant cells containing birefringent crystalline material [28].

Angioedema/urticaria induced by clonidine, guanfacine, methyldopa, and moxonidine; *alopecia* due to clonidine, guanfacine, and methyldopa; *diaphoresis* with clonidine, guanfacine, and guanabenz; *gynecomastia* due to guanabenz and methyldopa; *peripheral edema/edema* induced by clonidine, guanfacine, and methyldopa; and *purpura* from guanfacine and methyldopa were also reported [6, 24].

References

1. Breckenridge A, Dollery CT, Worlledge SM, Holborow EJ, Johnson GD. Positive direct Coombs tests and antinuclear factor in patients treated with methyldopa. Lancet. 1967;2: 1265–7.
2. Nordstrom DM, West SG, Rubin RL. Methyldopa-induced systemic lupus erythematosus. Arthritis Rheum. 1989;32:205–8.
3. Dupont A, Six R. Lupus-like syndrome induced by methyldopa. Br Med J (Clin Res Ed). 1982;285:693–4.
4. Harrington TM, Davis DE. Systemic lupus-like syndrome induced by methyldopa therapy. Chest. 1981;79:696–7.
5. Sherman JD, Love DE, Harrington JF. Anemia, positive lupus and rheumatoid factors with methyldopa. A report of three cases. Arch Intern Med. 1967;120:321–6.
6. Frishman WH, Brosnan BD, Grossman M, Dasgupta D, Sun DK. Adverse dermatologic effects of cardiovascular drug therapy: part III. Cardiol Rev. 2002;10:337–48.
7. Mota AV, Vasconcelos C, Correia TM, Barros MA, Mesquita-Guimaraes J. Rilmenidine-induced photosensitivity reaction. Photodermatol Photoimmunol Photomed. 1998;14:132–3.
8. Vaillant L, Le Marchand D, Grognard C, Hocine R, Lorette G. Photosensitivity to methyldopa. Arch Dermatol. 1988;124:326–7.
9. Kaae J, Boyd HA, Hansen AV, Wulf HC, Wohlfahrt J, Melbye M. Photosensitizing medication use and risk of skin cancer. Cancer Epidemiol Biomarkers Prev. 2010;19:2942–9.
10. Burry JN, Kirk J. Letter: Lichenoid drug reaction from methyldopa. Br J Dermatol. 1974;91:475–6.
11. Burry JN. Ulcerative lichenoid eruption from methyldopa. Arch Dermatol. 1976;112:880.

12. Holt PJ, Navaratnam A. Lichenoid eruption due to methyldopa. Br Med J. 1974;3:234.
13. Stevenson CJ. Lichenoid eruptions due to methyldopa. Br J Dermatol. 1971;85:600.
14. Hay KD, Reade PC. Methyldopa as a cause of oral mucous membrane reactions. Br Dent J. 1978;145:195–203.
15. Gonzalez JG, Marcus MD, Cruz DJ. Giant cell lichenoid dermatitis. J Am Acad Dermatol. 1986;15:87–92.
16. Heid E, Samsoen M, Juillard J, Eberst E, Foussereau J. Papulo-vesicular endogenous eruptions induced by methyldopa and clofibrate. Ann Dermatol Venereol. 1977;104:494–6.
17. Church R. Eczema provoked by methyl dopa. Br J Dermatol. 1974;91:373–8.
18. van Joost T, Faber WR, Manuel HR. Drug-induced anogenital cicatricial pemphigoid. Br J Dermatol. 1980;102:715–8.
19. Wilkin J. Exacerbation of psoriasis during clonidine therapy. Arch Dermatol. 1981;117:4.
20. Prisant LM. Transdermal clonidine skin reactions. J Clin Hypertens (Greenwich). 2002;4: 136–8.
21. Crivellaro MA, Bonadonna P, Dama A, Senna G, Passalacqua G. Skin reactions to clonidine: not just a local problem. Case report. Allergol Immunopathol (Madr). 1999;27:318–9.
22. Doe N, Seth S, Hebert LA. Skin depigmentation related to transdermal clonidine therapy. Arch Intern Med. 1995;155:2129.
23. Wiser TH, Kazakis AM, LaCivita CL. Transdermal clonidine: an association with recurrent herpes simplex and hyperpigmentation. J Am Acad Dermatol. 1987;17:143–4.
24. Litt JZ. Drug eruption reference manual. 19th ed. Boca Raton: CRC Press (Taylor and Francis Group); 2013.
25. Torpet LA, Kragelund C, Reibel J, Nauntofte B. Oral adverse drug reactions to cardiovascular drugs. Crit Rev Oral Biol Med. 2004;15:28–46.
26. Wolf R, Tamir A, Werbin N, Brenner S. Methyldopa hypersensitivity syndrome. Ann Allergy. 1993;71:166–8.
27. Brody HJ, Cohen M. Black tongue secondary to methyldopa therapy. Cutis. 1986;38:187–8.
28. Wells JD, Kurtay M, Lochner JC, George WL. Letter: Granulomatous skin lesions and alpha-methyldopa. Ann Intern Med. 1974;81:701–2.

Chapter 5
Class I Antiarrhythmic Drugs

Keywords Class I antiarrhythmic • Quinidine • Procainamide • Mexiletine • Phenytoin • Lupus erythematosus • Photosensitivity • Maculopapular • Drug rash with eosinophilia and systemic symptoms • Stevens–Johnson syndrome/toxic epidermal necrolysis • Hyperpigmentation • Purpura

Class I antiarrhythmic drugs, also known as sodium channel blockers, are classified into three subgroups such as class Ia (quinidine, procainamide, disopyramide, acecainide), class Ib (lidocaine, mexiletine, tocainide, phenytoin), and class Ic (propafenone, flecainide, encainide, moricizine).

Acecainide (*N*-acetylprocainamide) is the *N*-acetylated metabolite of procainamide. Mexiletine and tocainide are the oral analogs of parenteral lidocaine. Cutaneous side effects from lidocaine used as a local anesthetic are not detailed in this chapter.

Phenytoin, also known as diphenylhydantoin, is more commonly associated with cutaneous reactions due to its use as an anticonvulsant. It is less frequently used in cardiovascular medicine. Therefore, side effects of phenytoin will be mentioned but not given in detail in this chapter. Cross-reactivity may occur between phenytoin and other aromatic antiepileptics like phenobarbital and carbamazepine.

The adverse cutaneous drug reactions described below are meant to be sorted by starting from the well-known reactions of class I antiarrhythmic drugs to the lesser known ones. The major ones are summarized in Table 5.1.

Drug-Induced Lupus Erythematosus

Systemic lupus erythematosus (SLE) is a well-known adverse effect of procainamide. It is stated to have the highest risk among drugs implicated to cause SLE with an incidence of 15–20 % [1]. On the other hand, administration of the *N*-acetylated metabolite of procainamide, namely, acecainide, is indicated to reduce this risk [2]. There are controversial reports on the importance of acetylator phenotypes, namely, slow and rapid acetylators, in the induction of SLE due to procainamide [2, 3]. Thrombosis may occur due to lupus anticoagulants induced by procainamide [4].

E. Özkaya, K.D. Yazganoğlu, *Adverse Cutaneous Drug Reactions to Cardiovascular Drugs*, DOI 10.1007/978-1-4471-6536-1_5

Table 5.1 Major adverse cutaneous drug reactions with class I antiarrhythmic drugs

Adverse cutaneous drug reaction	Main inducers
Drug-induced lupus erythematosus (mainly systemic lupus erythematous)	Procainamide, quinidine, phenytoin, propafenone, tocainide
Photosensitivity	Quinidine, phenytoin
Maculopapular eruption	Phenytoin, mexiletine, tocainide, lidocaine[a], acecainide, procainamide, quinidine
Drug rash with eosinophilia and systemic symptoms	Phenytoin, mexiletine
Erythema multiforme/Stevens–Johnson syndrome/toxic epidermal necrolysis	Phenytoin, quinidine, tocainide
EMPACT	Phenytoin
Hyperpigmentation	Quinidine, phenytoin
Lymphomatoid drug eruption	Mexiletine, phenytoin
Acute generalized exanthematous pustulosis	Mexiletine, propafenone
Acneiform eruption	Phenytoin, quinidine, propafenone
Fixed drug eruption	Phenytoin, flecainide, lidocaine, quinidine
Vasculitis	Quinidine, procainamide, phenytoin
Purpura	Quinidine, disopyramide, mexiletine, phenytoin, procainamide, propafenone
Injection site reactions	
Nicolau syndrome	Lidocaine
Purple glove syndrome	Phenytoin
Angioedema/urticaria	Lidocaine, quinidine, procainamide, flecainide, propafenone, disopyramide, mexiletine, moricizine, tocainide, phenytoin
Oral mucosal reactions	
Xerostomia	Class effect
Gingival hyperplasia	Phenytoin
Erythroderma	Phenytoin, quinidine, tocainide
Linear IgA dermatosis	Phenytoin
Hirsutism	Phenytoin

EMPACT Erythema Multiforme associated with Phenytoin And Cranial radiation Therapy
[a]Probable cross-reaction with tocainide

Quinidine is an inducer of SLE as well [5–8]. The reaction was reported usually to occur after 1–18 months of treatment, but earlier or later onset is also possible. The frequency of cutaneous involvement was indicated to be higher in quinidine-induced lupus than procainamide-induced lupus. Maculopapular, discoid, malar, photosensitive, or petechial eruptions were described [8].

Other antiarrhythmics like propafenone [9], and tocainide [10, 11] have also been found in association with SLE. On the other hand, propafenone has been recorded as a cause of an eruption that would be compatible with subacute cutaneous lupus erythematosus [12].

Phenytoin was among the implicated drugs which trigger SLE and other collagen vascular diseases including subacute cutaneous lupus erythematosus, dermatomyositis, scleroderma, systemic sclerosis-like disease, and Sjögren-like syndrome [13, 14].

Mexiletine was considered a safe antiarrhythmic alternative without an apparent risk of inducing lupus erythematosus, as no rise in antinuclear factor titer could be shown during a long-term follow-up (mean 47.8 months) of 12 patients [15].

Photosensitivity

Photosensitivity is one of the well-described adverse cutaneous effects of quinidine. It can present as erythematous, lichenoid, eczematous, or livedo reticularis-like eruption on sun-exposed skin [16–24]. While the reaction resolves after withdrawal of quinidine, it can be provoked by photopatch test or by rechallenge in some cases [17, 19, 22] but not in all [16]. The dermatitis was also reproduced after intradermal injection of quinidine sulfate solution that was irradiated with UVA in vitro, but only in the presence of the patient's serum [20, 21]. Therefore, it was suggested that a carrier protein in the serum or skin could have bounded to quinidine sulfate and caused this type of photodermatitis [20, 21].

Phenytoin induced a photodistributed cutaneous eruption in a patient who had additional symptoms suggestive of drug hypersensitivity syndrome [25].

Maculopapular Eruption

Maculopapular eruptions can be seen with various class I antiarrhythmic drugs like phenytoin, lidocaine, tocainide, mexiletine, acecainide, procainamide, and quinidine [13, 26–31]. It may be seen as part of the drug hypersensitivity syndrome [30–32]. Maculopapular eruption seems to be the most common cutaneous reaction induced by phenytoin [13].

Regarding maculopapular eruption, cross-reactivity was shown between tocainide and lidocaine, but not with mexiletine in a patient. Different structures of the drugs, namely, tocainide and lidocaine containing amide moiety and mexiletine containing ether moiety, were suggested to be responsible for the cross-reaction [28].

Drug Rash with Eosinophilia and Systemic Symptoms

Drug rash with eosinophilia and systemic symptoms (DRESS) is a well-known cutaneous adverse reaction induced by phenytoin [13, 33–35].

DRESS was also reported to develop in patients treated with mexiletine [30–32, 36–38], all from Far Eastern countries, mainly Japanese patients, suggesting a genetic predisposition in relation with ethnicity [38]. The eruption was mainly maculopapular or papuloerythematous, while it was pustular in one case described as acute generalized exanthematous pustulosis. The onset of the reaction was approximately 1 month later after the start of mexiletine, but in two patients the lag time was long, i.e., after 5 and 6 months in each case [37, 38]. The reaction was confirmed by positive patch test in some cases [30, 32, 37, 38]. Interestingly, reactivation of human herpesvirus 6 and 7 and cytomegalovirus was found in some cases suggesting a pathogenic role for viruses as cofactors in drug hypersensitivity syndrome [32, 36, 37].

Erythema Multiforme/Stevens–Johnson Syndrome/Toxic Epidermal Necrolysis

Erythema multiforme and severe reactions like Stevens–Johnson syndrome/toxic epidermal necrolysis may develop with phenytoin [35, 39–41]. The risk of developing Stevens–Johnson syndrome/toxic epidermal necrolysis was reported to be highest within the first 8 weeks of phenytoin therapy [39, 40]. It can be part of the drug hypersensitivity syndrome [35, 41].

The development of erythema multiforme confined to the radiation field during or following cranial radiation in patients receiving prophylactic anticonvulsant therapy with phenytoin, was recently defined as EMPACT (Erythema Multiforme associated with Phenytoin And Cranial radiation Therapy) [42, 43].

Quinidine [29, 44] and tocainide [45] have been reported as other inducers of erythema multiforme/Stevens–Johnson syndrome/toxic epidermal necrolysis. According to a report analyzing the serious skin reactions to tocainide, erythema multiforme/Stevens–Johnson syndrome, erythroderma, and rashes (not specified) with or without stomatitis were reported in 21 patients using tocainide. It should be stated that most of these patients were also using other medication, but the great majority of them ($n=17$) improved after withdrawal of tocainide. In 4 patients, however, data were not available. The onset of the reaction was within the first 3 weeks of treatment in most of the patients [45].

Hyperpigmentation

Mucosal pigmentation and blue-gray pigmentation of the skin have been reported with quinidine [46, 47]. The blue-gray pigmentation induced by quinidine was assumed to be similar to the pigmentation induced by antimalarials as pretibial areas, nose, ears, forearms, subungual tissues, and hard palate were involved clinically, and there were pigment granules containing melanin and hemosiderin in the histopathology [47].

Phenytoin may cause a brownish pigmentation resembling chloasma on sun-exposed areas [13, 48], and this effect might be related with its prolonged administration [48]. Acquired acromelanosis has been reported to be induced by phenytoin [49].

Lymphomatoid Drug Eruption

Pseudolymphomatous reaction and lymphadenopathy occurred in a patient 4 weeks after initiation of mexiletine [50]. Clinically, a generalized maculopapular and squamatous eruption was seen, but histopathological investigation showed mycosis fungoides-like features. While discontinuation of the drug led to regression within 2 days, reinstitution of the drug caused recurrence of the lesions resolving completely within 2 weeks [50]. Phenytoin was indicated to cause pseudolymphoma, lymphoid hyperplasia, malignant lymphoma, and mycosis fungoides-like lesions as well [13].

Pustular Eruption

Acute Generalized Exanthematous Pustulosis

Acute generalized exanthematous pustulosis was reported to occur in patients treated with mexiletine that was confirmed by patch testing [51], and with propafenone, after 5 days of treatment [52]. The mexiletine-induced case of acute generalized exanthematous pustulosis rather suggests a drug hypersensitivity syndrome because of the presence of facial edema, liver dysfunction, and hypereosinophilia [51].

Acneiform Eruption

Acneiform eruptions have been related to quinidine, propafenone, and phenytoin in the reported cases [29, 53]. Phenytoin has been attributed to cause acne due to its androgenic effect [54]. Acne keloidalis-like lesions was reported in a patient taking both phenytoin and carbamazepine [55].

Fixed Drug Eruption

Fixed drug eruption (FDE) has been reported to occur with phenytoin [56]. Lidocaine-induced FDE is mainly associated with its use as a local anesthetic [57, 58]. Flecainide has been reported as the probable cause of FDE in a patient, however, without any further confirmatory tests [59]. Quinidine was also linked to FDE [60].

Vasculitis

Leukocytoclastic vasculitis or Henoch–Schönlein purpura has been reported to develop during quinidine therapy [61, 62]. Procainamide may cause urticarial vasculitis and vasculitis as a part of SLE in some cases [63–65]. Phenytoin was also implicated as a cause of vasculitis [13].

Purpura

Quinidine can induce purpura in relation with thrombocytopenia, a well-known side effect of this drug that may be even fatal [66, 67]. Phenytoin, disopyramide, mexiletine, procainamide, and propafenone were also linked to purpura [13, 29, 68].

Injection Site Reactions

Nicolau syndrome (*embolia cutis medicamentosa*) was reported following injection of lidocaine as a local anesthetic [69], while intravenous administration may cause phlebitis [70].

Intravenous administration of phenytoin, usually on the dorsum of the hand, may cause soft tissue damage like "*purple glove syndrome*" [71, 72]. It presents usually with an initial blue-purple discoloration at the injection site with subsequent development of edema that can spread up the extremity causing severe pain that may rarely evolve into necrosis, ischemia, vascular compression, or compartment syndrome necessitating surgical intervention [71, 72].

Angioedema/Urticaria

Urticaria, angioedema, and anaphylactoid reactions are the well-known cutaneous side effects of lidocaine, mainly due to its use as a local anesthetic [29]. Some other class I antiarrhythmic drugs such as quinidine, procainamide, flecainide, propafenone, disopyramide, mexiletine, moricizine, tocainide, and phenytoin may also cause angioedema/urticaria [29, 68, 73, 74].

Pruritus

Pruritus has also been implicated among the adverse effects of class I antiarrhythmic drugs [29]. It may accompany different types of cutaneous eruptions [28, 30, 31].

Oral Mucosal Reactions

Xerostomia is a common reaction with this group of drugs [75]. It was stated to be seen during the use of quinidine, disopyramide, flecainide, and moricizine due to their anticholinergic effects [75]. Propafenone was associated with bitter or metallic taste [75], and flecainide was reported as a cause of bitter taste [76].

Gingival hyperplasia induced by phenytoin is a well-described reaction in the literature. It is associated with long-term use of phenytoin [13]. The prevalence of gingival enlargement in patients with chronic phenytoin use was reported to be about 40 % [77]. It was regarded as a dose-dependent side effect [77, 78]. Phenytoin-induced decrease in folic acid levels may cause oral ulcerations, cheilitis, and glossitis [75].

Mucosal pigmentation has been reported with quinidine [46, 47].

Stomatitis was reported in patients using tocainide, accompanying different kinds of skin eruptions, mostly not specified [45]. Disopyramide was reported to cause oral mucosal ulceration [79].

Other Reported Adverse Cutaneous Drug Reactions to Class I Antiarrhythmic Drugs

Erythroderma can develop during treatment with quinidine [80, 81], tocainide [45], phenytoin [13], flecainide, lidocaine, and mexiletine [29, 68].

Linear IgA dermatosis has been reported with phenytoin therapy [82, 83]. Interestingly, it showed clinical features similar to erythema multiforme and toxic epidermal necrolysis in two different cases [82, 83]. One of the patients received concomitant radiotherapy and developed erythema multiforme-like eruption, but histopathological and immunofluorescence findings were compatible with linear IgA dermatosis [83].

Coarsening of the facies including lip and nose enlargement and thickening of the face and scalp may be induced after long-term phenytoin use [13]. *Thickening of the heel pads* (above 20 mm) was reported to occur in patients receiving long-term phenytoin treatment [84]. *Hirsutism* may also be seen after long-term phenytoin use. It was stated to develop mostly on the extensor parts of the extremities, trunk, and face within 3 months of phenytoin use, usually subsiding within 1 year after stopping the drug, but it may also persist [13].

Psoriasis/psoriasiform eruption with flecainide [85] and quinidine [86, 87], *contact dermatitis* with lidocaine [88, 89], *porphyria* with phenytoin [13], *pseudoporphyria* with quinidine [90], *lichen planus* with quinidine [91], *erythema nodosum* with disopyramide [92], and *allergic granulomatous angiitis* with cutaneous involvement in the form of maculopapular eruption and palpable purpura in a patient using both quinidine and digoxin were also reported [93].

Other adverse cutaneous drug reactions linked to class I antiarrhythmic drugs include *alopecia* with disopyramide, flecainide, mexiletine, propafenone, quinidine, tocainide, and phenytoin; *edema/periorbital edema/facial edema* with disopyramide, flecainide, mexiletine, propafenone, encainide, and moricizine; *flushing* with flecainide, tocainide, procainamide, and quinidine; *hyperhidrosis* with flecainide, mexiletine, moricizine, propafenone, and tocainide; *xerosis* with disopyramide, mexiletine, and moricizine; *granuloma annulare* with quinidine; and *Sneddon–Wilkinson disease* with quinidine [29, 68].

References

1. Vedove CD, Del Giglio M, Schena D, Girolomoni G. Drug-induced lupus erythematosus. Arch Dermatol Res. 2009;301:99–105.
2. Reidenberg MM, Drayer DE. Procainamide, N-acetylprocainamide, antinuclear antibody and systemic lupus erythematosus. Angiology. 1986;37:968–71.
3. Sonnhag C, Karlsson E, Hed J. Procainamide-induced lupus erythematosus-like syndrome in relation to acetylator phenotype and plasma levels of procainamide. Acta Med Scand. 1979;206:245–51.
4. List AF, Doll DC. Thrombosis associated with procainamide-induced lupus anticoagulant. Acta Haematol. 1989;82:50–2.
5. Cohen MG, Kevat S, Prowse MV, Ahern MJ. Two distinct quinidine-induced rheumatic syndromes. Ann Intern Med. 1988;108:369–71.
6. Sukenik S, Horowitz J, Katz A, Henkin J, Buskila D. Quinidine-induced lupus erythematosus-like syndrome: three case reports and a review of the literature. Isr J Med Sci. 1987;23:1232–4.
7. West SG, McMahon M, Portanova JP. Quinidine-induced lupus erythematosus. Ann Intern Med. 1984;100:840–2.
8. Alloway JA, Salata MP. Quinidine-induced rheumatic syndromes. Semin Arthritis Rheum. 1995;24:315–22.
9. Guindo J, Rodriguez de la Serna A, Borja J, Oter R, Jane F, Bayes de Luna A. Propafenone and a syndrome of the lupus erythematosus type. Ann Intern Med. 1986;104:589.
10. Oliphant LD, Goddard M. Tocainide-associated neutropenia and lupus-like syndrome. Chest. 1988;94:427–8.
11. Gelfand MS, Yunus F, White FL. Bone marrow granulomas, fever, pancytopenia, and lupus-like syndrome due to tocainide. South Med J. 1994;87:839–41.
12. Couto N, Ferreira M, Reis E. Neutropenia and cutaneous lesions secondary to propafenone. Eur J Dermatol. 2009;19:365–7.
13. Scheinfeld N. Phenytoin in cutaneous medicine: its uses, mechanisms and side effects. Dermatol Online J. 2003;9:6.
14. Ross S, Ormerod AD, Roberts C, Dwyer C, Herriot R. Subacute cutaneous lupus erythematosus associated with phenytoin. Clin Exp Dermatol. 2002;27:474–6.
15. Johansson BW, Stavenow L, Hanson A. Long-term clinical experience with mexiletine. Am Heart J. 1984;107:1099–102.
16. Armstrong RB, Leach EE, Whitman G, Harber LC, Poh-Fitzpatrick MB. Quinidine photosensitivity. Arch Dermatol. 1985;121:525–8.
17. Wolf R, Dorfman B, Krakowski A. Quinidine-induced lichenoid and eczematous photodermatitis. Dermatologica. 1987;174:285–9.
18. Bonnetblanc JM, Bernard P, Catanzano G, Souyri N. Quinidine-induced lichenoid photodermatitis. Ann Dermatol Venereol. 1987;114:957–61.
19. Gammer S, Gross PR. Photoallergy induced by quinidine. Cutis. 1976;17:72–4.
20. Schurer NY, Holzle E, Plewig G, Lehmann P. Photosensitivity induced by quinidine sulfate: experimental reproduction of skin lesions. Photodermatol Photoimmunol Photomed. 1992;9:78–82.

21. Schurer NY, Lehmann P, Plewig G. Quinidine-induced photoallergy. A clinical and experimental study. Hautarzt. 1991;42:158–61.
22. Marx JL, Eisenstat BA, Gladstein AH. Quinidine photosensitivity. Arch Dermatol. 1983;119:39–43.
23. Manzi S, Kraus VB, St Clair EW. An unusual photoactivated skin eruption. Quinidine-induced livedo reticularis. Arch Dermatol. 1989;125(417–8):421–2.
24. Bruce S, Wolf Jr JE. Quinidine-induced photosensitive livedo reticularis-like eruption. J Am Acad Dermatol. 1985;12:332–6.
25. Bhalla M, Garg G, Thami GP. Photodistribution of rash in phenytoin-induced drug rash with eosinophilia and systemic symptoms. Clin Exp Dermatol. 2011;36:553–4.
26. Habot B, Rabinovitz C, Friedensohn A, Schlesinger Z, Baumel Y. A severe skin reaction following mexiletene. Harefuah. 1992;123:462, 506.
27. Dunn JM, Groth PE, DeSimone A. Tocainide: a severe adverse reaction. Drug Intell Clin Pharm. 1988;22:142–5.
28. Duff HJ, Roden DM, Marney S, Colley DG, Maffucci R, Primm RK, et al. Molecular basis for the antigenicity of lidocaine analogs: tocainide and mexiletine. Am Heart J. 1984;107:585–9.
29. Frishman WH, Brosnan BD, Grossman M, Dasgupta D, Sun AD. Adverse dermatologic effects of cardiovascular drug therapy: part I. Cardiol Rev. 2002;10:230–46.
30. Higa K, Hirata K, Dan K. Mexiletine-induced severe skin eruption, fever, eosinophilia, atypical lymphocytosis, and liver dysfunction. Pain. 1997;73:97–9.
31. Seino Y, Yamauchi M, Hirai C, Okumura A, Kondo K, Yamamoto M, Okazaki Y. A case of fulminant Type 1 diabetes associated with mexiletine hypersensitivity syndrome. Diabet Med. 2004;21:1156–7.
32. Morito H, Ogawa K, Kobayashi N, Fukumoto T, Asada H. Drug-induced hypersensitivity syndrome followed by persistent arthritis. J Dermatol. 2012;39:178–9.
33. Pereira de Silva N, Piquioni P, Kochen S, Saidon P. Risk factors associated with DRESS syndrome produced by aromatic and non-aromatic antipiletic drugs. Eur J Clin Pharmacol. 2011;67:463–70.
34. Oelze LL, Pillow MT. Phenytoin-induced drug reaction with eosinophilia and systemic symptoms (DRESS) syndrome: a case report from the emergency department. J Emerg Med. 2013;44:75–8.
35. Sherertz EF, Jegasothy BV, Lazarus GS. Phenytoin hypersensitivity reaction presenting with toxic epidermal necrolysis and severe hepatitis. Report of a patient treated with corticosteroid "pulse therapy". J Am Acad Dermatol. 1985;12(1 Pt 2):178–81.
36. Sekiguchi A, Kashiwagi T, Ishida-Yamamoto A, Takahashi H, Hashimoto Y, Kimura H, et al. Drug-induced hypersensitivity syndrome due to mexiletine associated with human herpes virus 6 and cytomegalovirus reactivation. J Dermatol. 2005;32:278–81.
37. Yagami A, Yoshikawa T, Asano Y, Koie S, Shiohara T, Matsunaga K. Drug-induced hypersensitivity syndrome due to mexiletine hydrochloride associated with reactivation of human herpesvirus 7. Dermatology. 2006;213:341–4.
38. Lee SP, Kim SH, Kim TH, Sohn JW, Shin DH, Park SS, Yoon HJ. A case of mexiletine-induced hypersensitivity syndrome presenting as eosinophilic pneumonia. J Korean Med Sci. 2010;25:148–51.
39. Rzany B, Correia O, Kelly JP, Naldi L, Auquier A, Stern R. Risk of Stevens-Johnson syndrome and toxic epidermal necrolysis during first weeks of antiepileptic therapy: a case-control study. Study Group of the International Case Control Study on Severe Cutaneous Adverse Reactions. Lancet. 1999;353:2190–4.
40. Roujeau JC, Kelly JP, Naldi L, Rzany B, Stern RS, Anderson T, et al. Medication use and the risk of Stevens-Johnson syndrome or toxic epidermal necrolysis. N Engl J Med. 1995;333:1600–7.
41. Smith DA, Burgdorf WH. Universal cutaneous depigmentation following phenytoin-induced toxic epidermal necrolysis. J Am Acad Dermatol. 1984;10:106–9.
42. Ahmed I, Reichenberg J, Lucas A, Shehan JM. Erythema multiforme associated with phenytoin and cranial radiation therapy: a report of three patients and review of the literature. Int J Dermatol. 2004;43:67–73.

43. Wöhrl S, Loewe R, Pickl WF, Stingl G, Wagner SN. EMPACT syndrome. J Dtsch Dermatol Ges. 2005;3:39–43.
44. Adornato MC. Toxic epidermal necrolysis associated with quinidine administration. N Y State Dent J. 2000;66:38–40.
45. Arrowsmith JB, Creamer JI, Bosco L. Severe dermatologic reactions reported after treatment with tocainide. Ann Intern Med. 1987;107:693–6.
46. Birek C, Main JH. Two cases of oral pigmentation associated with quinidine therapy. Oral Surg Oral Med Oral Pathol. 1988;66:59–61.
47. Mahler R, Sissons W, Watters K. Pigmentation induced by quinidine therapy. Arch Dermatol. 1986;122:1062–4.
48. Lee A, Thomson J. Drug-induced skin reactions. In: Adverse drug reactions. 2nd ed. London: Pharmaceutical Press; 2006. p. 125–56.
49. Kanwar AJ, Jaswal R, Thami GP, Bedi GK. Acquired acromelanosis due to phenytoin. Dermatology. 1997;194:373–4.
50. Kardaun SH, Scheffer E, Vermeer BJ. Drug-induced pseudolymphomatous skin reactions. Br J Dermatol. 1988;118:545–52.
51. Sasaki K, Yamamoto T, Kishi M, Yokozeki H, Nishioka K. Acute exanthematous pustular drug eruption induced by mexiletine. Eur J Dermatol. 2001;11:469–71.
52. Huang YM, Lee WR, Hu CH, Cheng KL. Propafenone-induced acute generalized exanthematous pustulosis. Int J Dermatol. 2005;44:256–7.
53. Burkhart CG. Quinidine-induced acne. Arch Dermatol. 1981;117:603–4.
54. Lolis MS, Bowe WP, Shalita AR. Acne and systemic disease. Med Clin North Am. 2009;93:1161–81.
55. Grunwald MH, Ben-Dor D, Livni E, Halevy S. Acne keloidalis-like lesions on the scalp associated with antiepileptic drugs. Int J Dermatol. 1990;29:559–61.
56. Sharma VK, Dhar S, Gill AN. Drug related involvement of specific sites in fixed eruptions: a statistical evaluation. J Dermatol. 1996;23:530–4.
57. Garcia JC, Torre F, Sanchez M, Martin JA, Canto G. Fixed drug eruption induced by lidocaine and patch testing. J Investig Allergol Clin Immunol. 1997;7:127–8.
58. Kawada A, Noguchi H, Hiruma M, Tajima S, Ishibashi A, Marshall J. Fixed drug eruption induced by lidocaine. Contact Dermatitis. 1996;35:375.
59. Knapp 3rd CF, Cooke ER, Sheehan DJ. Bullous fixed drug eruption caused by flecainide. J Am Acad Dermatol. 2009;60:e3.
60. Almeyda J, Levantine A. Cutaneous reactions to cardiovascular drugs. Br J Dermatol. 1973;88:313–9.
61. Shalit M, Flugelman MY, Harats N, Galun E, Ackerman Z, Kopolovic J, Eliakim M. Quinidine-induced vasculitis. Arch Intern Med. 1985;145:2051–2.
62. Aviram A. Henoch-Schonlein syndrome associated with quinidine. JAMA. 1980;243:432–3.
63. Rosin JM. Vasculitis following procaineamide therapy. Am J Med. 1967;42:625–9.
64. Knox JP, Welykyj SE, Gradini R, Massa MC. Procainamide-induced urticarial vasculitis. Cutis. 1988;42:469–72.
65. Jackson C, Phillips PE. Procainamide-induced lupus with vasculitis. Clin Exp Rheumatol. 1986;4:290–2.
66. Nieminen U, Kekomaki R. Quinidine-induced thrombocytopenic purpura: clinical presentation in relation to drug-dependent and drug-independent platelet antibodies. Br J Haematol. 1992;80:77–82.
67. Brenner WI, Heslov SF, Deosaransingh M. Fatal quinidine-induced thrombocytopenia following open-heart surgery. Tex Heart Inst J. 1990;17:237–9.
68. Litt JZ. Drug eruption reference manual. 19th ed. Boca Raton: CRC Press (Taylor and Francis Group); 2013.
69. García-Vilanova-Comas A, Fuster-Diana C, Cubells-Parrilla M, Pérez-Ferriols MD, Pérez-Valles A, Roig-Vila JV. Nicolau syndrome after lidocaine injection and cold application: a rare complication of breast core needle biopsy. Int J Dermatol. 2011;50:78–80.

70. Bassan MM, Sheikh-Hamad D. Prevention of lidocaine-infusion phlebitis by heparin and hydrocortisone. Chest. 1983;84:439–41.
71. Cadenbach A, Rottger K, Muller MK. Purple glove syndrome. Severe soft tissue reaction following phenytoin infusion. Dtsch Med Wochenschr. 1998;123:318–22.
72. Chokshi R, Openshaw J, Mehta NN, Mohler 3rd E. Purple glove syndrome following intravenous phenytoin administration. Vasc Med. 2007;12:29–31.
73. Ponte CD, Horner P. Suspected procainamide-induced angioedema. Drug Intell Clin Pharm. 1985;19:139–40.
74. Incorvaia C, Pravettoni C, Riario-Sforza GG. Urticaria-angioedema reaction caused by propafenone. Allergy. 2006;61:269.
75. Torpet LA, Kragelund C, Reibel J, Nauntofte B. Oral adverse drug reactions to cardiovascular drugs. Crit Rev Oral Biol Med. 2004;15:28–46.
76. Martinez-Selles M, Castillo I, Montenegro P, Martin ML, Almendral J, Sanjurjo M. Pharmacogenetic study of the response to flecainide and propafenone in patients with atrial fibrillation. Rev Esp Cardiol. 2005;58:745–8.
77. Casetta I, Granieri E, Desidera M, Monetti VC, Tola MR, Paolino E, et al. Phenytoin-induced gingival overgrowth: a community-based cross-sectional study in Ferrara, Italy. Neuroepidemiology. 1997;16:296–303.
78. Perlik F, Kolinova M, Zvarova J, Patzelova V. Phenytoin as a risk factor in gingival hyperplasia. Ther Drug Monit. 1995;17:445–8.
79. Wittkowsky AK, Reddy R, Bardy GH. Oral mucosal ulceration from disopyramide. Ann Pharmacother. 1995;29:1299–300.
80. Bellogini GC, Oneglia C. Exfoliative dermatitis caused by quinidine. Description of a clinical case. Minerva Cardioangiol. 1987;35:457–9.
81. Gouffault J, Pawlotsky Y, Morel H, Bourel M. Erythrodermia of quinidine origin. Sem Hop. 1965;41:1350–3.
82. Tran D, Kossard S, Shumack S. Phenytoin-induced linear IgA dermatosis mimicking toxic epidermal necrolysis. Australas J Dermatol. 2003;44:284–6.
83. Acostamadiedo JM, Perniciaro C, Rogers 3rd RS. Phenytoin-induced linear IgA bullous disease. J Am Acad Dermatol. 1998;38(2 Pt 2):352–6.
84. Kattan KR. Thickening of the heel-pad associated with long-term Dilantin therapy. Am J Roentgenol Radium Ther Nucl Med. 1975;124:52–6.
85. Mancuso G, Tampieri E, Berdondini RM. Psoriasis-like eruption caused by flecainide. G Ital Dermatol Venereol. 1988;123:171–2.
86. Brenner S, Cabili S, Wolf R. Psoriasiform eruption induced by quinidine. Widespread erythematous scaly plaques in an adult. Arch Dermatol. 1993;129(1331–2):1334–5.
87. Harwell WB. Quinidine-induced psoriasis. J Am Acad Dermatol. 1983;9:278.
88. Kaufmann JM, Hale EK, Ashinoff RA, Cohen DE. Cutaneous lidocaine allergy confirmed by patch testing. J Drugs Dermatol. 2002;1:192–4.
89. Mackley CL, Marks Jr JG, Anderson BE. Delayed-type hypersensitivity to lidocaine. Arch Dermatol. 2003;139:343–6.
90. Petersen CS, Thomsen K. Pseudoporphyria. Ugeskr Laeger. 1992;154:1713–5.
91. Sarkany I. Lichen planus following quinidine therapy. Br J Dermatol. 1967;79:123.
92. Niv Y, Shafriri P, Shlonski Z, Harush F. Erythema nodosum due to disopyramide. Harefuah. 1985;108:490.
93. Quin J, Adamski M, Howlin K, Jones W, O'Neill P, Stewart G, Young A. Quinidine-induced allergic granulomatous angiitis: an unusual cause of acute renal failure. Med J Aust. 1988;148:145–6.

Chapter 6
Beta Adrenergic Receptor Blockers (Class II Antiarrhythmics)

Keywords Beta-blockers • Psoriasis/psoriasiform • Oculomucocutaneous syndrome • Lichenoid • Angioedema/urticaria • Lupus erythematosus • Peyronie's disease • Vasculitis • Cold extremity • Gangrene • Alopecia

Beta-blockers are classified into two major subgroups as cardioselective (β_1) (acebutolol, atenolol, metoprolol, betaxolol, bisoprolol, esmolol, nebivolol) and noncardioselective ($\beta_{1+}\beta_2$) blockers (propranolol, nadolol, oxprenolol, pindolol, timolol, sotalol, carteolol, penbutolol). Additionally, there are other ones with both α and β receptor blocking activities such as labetalol and carvedilol. While β_1 receptors are found mostly in the heart muscle, β_2 receptors are located mostly on the vascular and bronchial smooth muscle [1]. β_2 receptors are also found in the skin [2, 3]. Practolol is no longer used because of its various side effects.

The best known adverse cutaneous drug reaction from beta-blockers is psoriasis or psoriasiform eruption. On the other hand, allergic contact dermatitis is a well-described adverse cutaneous drug reaction due to the topical use of beta-blockers in eye drops [4].

The adverse cutaneous drug reactions described below are meant to be sorted by starting from the well-known reactions of beta-blockers to the lesser known ones. The major ones are summarized in Table 6.1.

Psoriasis/Psoriasiform Eruption

Beta-blockers are among the most common drugs that are associated with psoriasis. In fact, they are considered among the drugs with undoubted causal relationship to psoriasis [5, 6]. New-onset psoriasis, therapy-resistant psoriasis, and exacerbation of preexisting psoriasis have been reported with beta-blockers [2, 3, 5, 7–10]. Practolol, atenolol, metoprolol, propranolol, nadolol, pindolol, oxprenolol, cetamolol, and alprenolol were among the culprit drugs.

E. Özkaya, K.D. Yazganoğlu, *Adverse Cutaneous Drug Reactions to Cardiovascular Drugs*, DOI 10.1007/978-1-4471-6536-1_6

Table 6.1 Major adverse cutaneous drug reactions with beta-blockers

Adverse cutaneous drug reaction	Main inducers
Psoriasis/psoriasiform eruption	Practolol, atenolol, metoprolol, propranolol, nadolol, pindolol, oxprenolol, cetamolol, alprenolol
Oculomucocutaneous syndrome	Practolol, oxprenolol, metoprolol, nadolol, pindolol, timolol
Lichen planus/lichenoid eruption	Atenolol, propranolol, labetalol, pindolol, metoprolol, sotalol, oxprenolol, nebivolol, practolol, timolol, levobunolol
Angioedema/urticaria	Propranolol, metoprolol, labetalol and other beta-blockers
Drug-induced lupus erythematosus	Acebutolol, atenolol, betaxolol, metoprolol, pindolol, propranolol, labetalol, practolol
Peyronie's disease	Practolol, propranolol, metoprolol, labetalol
Vasculitis	Atenolol, acebutolol, sotalol, propranolol, carvedilol
Peripheral vascular disease	Propranolol, metoprolol, practolol, alprenolol, atenolol, pindolol, oxprenolol
Alopecia	Propranolol, metoprolol, nadolol
Erythema multiforme/Stevens–Johnson syndrome/toxic epidermal necrolysis	Metoprolol, carvedilol, propranolol
Fixed drug eruption	Atenolol, propranolol, bisoprolol
Pincer nails	Acebutolol, metoprolol
Xerostomia	Class effect
Aphthous ulcer	Beta-blockers (not specified)

In a retrospective analysis of beta-blockers' effects on psoriasis, the rate of exacerbations of psoriasis was found to be 72.4 % among patients using beta-blockers [2].

The eruption may develop in a wide range of time after starting therapy with beta-blockers, even after a year or longer [3, 5]. Some of the cutaneous reactions were stated to be diagnosed solely with clinical findings, without confirmation by histopathological examination. It is further indicated that not all of the clinically diagnosed psoriasiform-type reactions were typical for psoriasis by histopathology [2, 3, 9].

Beta-blockers may also transform plaque-type psoriasis into pustular or erythrodermic type [5], such as reported with propranolol [8].

A patient without a history of psoriasis within a 5-year period of propranolol therapy developed psoriasis after changing the drug to cetamolol. The diagnosis was made by histopathology and was confirmed by rechallenge with cetamolol [7].

The mechanism of beta-blocker-induced psoriasiform reactions is not clear. It was postulated that it could be associated with the blockage of β-adrenergic receptors that are present in the epidermis that might cause a decrease in intraepidermal cyclic adenosine monophosphate (cAMP) resulting in an increase in the epidermal cell turnover [2, 3, 5].

Cross-sensitivity was suggested to occur between beta-blockers, but this remains controversial [3].

Oculomucocutaneous Syndrome

Oculomucocutaneous syndrome affecting the eye, skin, and mucosal sites has been reported mainly with practolol [11] which was therefore withdrawn worldwide. Oxprenolol, metoprolol, nadolol, pindolol, and timolol were the other beta-blockers associated with this reaction [12, 13].

Dry eye (xerophthalmia) due to lacrimal gland fibrosis was the common symptom of ocular manifestations which usually started with conjunctival hyperemia and led to conjunctival scarring, shrinkage, and visual loss. Reduction of tear flow, reduction of lysozyme, and absence of secretory IgA were found [11, 14]. The cutaneous findings were reported as psoriasiform plaques on extensor surfaces of the forearms, or hyperkeratosis of the palms, soles, knees, elbows, knuckles, and fingertips. Ulceration of the oral and nasal mucosa accompanied in some cases. Antinuclear antibodies were shown to be positive, without any symptoms for systemic lupus erythematosus (SLE) [11, 12, 14]. The condition progressed to SLE after the diagnosis of oculomucocutaneous syndrome in one patient [11], so follow-up seemed to be necessary.

The underlying mechanism of this reaction is not known. Circulating antibodies were found in the sera of these patients, but their effect on the reaction was not clear [11, 15]. Practolol therapy has been associated with immunological abnormalities like cutaneous anergy to *Candida albicans* and streptokinase/streptodornase antigens, and in vitro depression of lymphocyte function, and with serologic abnormalities such as positivity of antinuclear antibody and rheumatoid factor [16].

Lichen Planus/Lichenoid Eruption

Both oral and cutaneous lichenoid eruptions have been reported with beta-blockers like atenolol, propranolol, labetalol, pindolol, metoprolol, sotalol, oxprenolol, nebivolol, practolol, timolol, and levobunolol, the latter two associated with topical use as eye drops [13, 17–24]. Atenolol seems to be the most common beta-blocker inducing lichenoid reactions [24].

The latency period between the initial administration of the drug and the onset of the lichenoid lesions may vary in a wide range of time, from a few days to many years of use of the suspected beta-blocker [24]. The extent of the reaction may vary; it may involve different body sites including most commonly the extremities and trunk, and also other sites such as the hands, feet, face, nails, oral mucosa, and genital area [24]. The eruption may be localized or generalized [24]. Ulcerative and bullous forms have been described [18, 19]. Lichenoid reaction activated by beta-blockers seems to be driven by T cell-mediated response. According to the recently proposed subtypes of type IV drug hypersensitivity reactions, a type IVc reaction seems to be involved in the pathogenesis of lichenoid drug eruptions (Table 1.1). Cross-reactivity is stated to be rare among beta-blockers regarding lichenoid eruptions [24].

In a retrospective study investigating an association between mucosal lichen planus and drugs like beta-blockers, angiotensin-converting enzyme inhibitors, and nonsteroidal antiinflammatory drugs, a relation was found between beta-blocker usage and lichen planus, particularly the vulvar type [25].

Angioedema/Urticaria

Angioedema and/or urticaria and even anaphylaxis have been reported to occur due to beta-blockers like propranolol, metoprolol, and labetalol. Severe anaphylaxis triggered by other allergens which is slow or not responsive to conventional therapy has also been reported in patients receiving beta-blocker therapy [26–32].

An important point is that patients using beta-blockers have an increased risk of resistance to epinephrine during an anaphylaxis of any origin [31, 32]. As well as inhibiting the effects of epinephrine, beta-blockers may also increase the severity of anaphylaxis via effecting the allergic mediator release [31, 32]. The therapeutically administered dosage of epinephrine in these patients is recommended to be higher than the usual dose [31, 32]. Beta-blockers are advised to be used cautiously in patients with a history of anaphylactoid reaction of any origin [26, 32], or to be replaced with an alternative drug in patients especially undergoing venom immunotherapy [31]. Moreover, in patients with allergic disease like asthma, therapy options other than immunotherapy are suggested to be considered for treating the allergy if they are taking beta-blockers [31].

A nurse with a history of worsening hand eczema due to a solution containing labetalol and paraben developed contact anaphylactoid reaction without the presence of urticaria during open patch testing with the solution, which was attributed to labetalol as immediate- or delayed-response to paraben was negative in the standard patch testing [30].

Drug-Induced Lupus Erythematosus

Beta-blockers are not a frequent cause of lupus erythematosus, but single cases of SLE due to acebutolol [33], atenolol [34, 35], betaxolol [36], metoprolol [37], pindolol [38], propranolol [39], labetalol [40], and practolol [41] have been reported.

In most cases, skin eruption did not accompany SLE. The reaction may occur after months to years of therapy. A case of atenolol-induced SLE developing after 3 years of therapy was reported [34]. Positive antinuclear antibodies were reported to be seen in almost every patient, with frequent positivity of antihistone antibodies whereas anti-dsDNA was mostly negative [36]. Withdrawal of the drug was required for the resolution of symptoms, necessitating active treatment with corticosteroid and/or hydroxychloroquine in some cases.

A patient with subacute cutaneous lupus erythematosus due to acebutolol was reported showing positive antinuclear, antihistone, and Ro/SSA antibodies. The cutaneous lesions resolved 4 months after discontinuation of the drug and with concomitant hydroxychloroquine therapy [42].

A case of septal panniculitis with positive antinuclear antibodies and mild hypochromic normocytic anemia was reported during the use of atenolol without any other accompanying symptoms of lupus erythematosus. Atenolol was confirmed to be the cause of the reaction by the occurrence of panniculitis on reuse of the drug [43].

Peyronie's Disease

Beta-blockers such as practolol, propranolol, metoprolol, and labetalol have been reported to be associated with Peyronie's disease [37, 44, 45].

In a retrospective analysis of 146 patients with Peyronie's disease, 19 patients were using beta-blockers such as propranolol and practolol. Penile symptoms have been reported to develop 6 months after the initiation of therapy with beta-blockers [44]. Immunological factors for the practolol-induced cases and atherosclerosis/hypertension in propranolol-induced cases were suggested to play a role in the etiology [44].

Vasculitis

Beta-blockers like atenolol [46], acebutolol [47], sotalol [48], propranolol [49], and carvedilol [50] have been implicated to cause cutaneous vasculitis, mainly leukocytoclastic vasculitis. The eruption may be localized or generalized, and may appear in the form of palpable purpura, bullae, or ulcerations. Interestingly, the reaction has been reported to start within a day of initiating the therapy in a patient who has never used a beta-blocker agent before [50], and after 2 years of beta-blocker therapy in another case [49].

Peripheral Vascular Disease

Beta-blockers may induce *Raynaud's phenomenon* [51, 52]. Moreover, *cold extremities* are occasionally observed during therapy with beta-blockers such as propranolol, practolol, oxprenolol, metoprolol, atenolol, pindolol, and alprenolol [52, 53]. Development of *peripheral/digital gangrene* after cold extremities following the administration of beta-blockers such as metoprolol and propranolol+metoprolol was also reported [54, 55]. On the other hand, beta-blockers such as oxprenolol, atenolol, and propranolol have been reported to be responsible for the development of *skin necrosis* on the toes and/or soles without accompanying peripheral gangrene in patients with a lacking history of peripheral vascular disease. The reaction developed in the wintertime and resolved upon discontinuation of the offending beta-blocker [51]. It was indicated that patients complaining of cold extremities due to the use of beta-blockers in the wintertime should be carefully followed up for possible development of tissue damage [51].

Alopecia

Alopecia is a well-known side effect of beta-blockers. It was mainly reported with propranolol [56–58], metoprolol [59], and nadolol [60], but other beta-blockers may also cause hair loss [13].

Alopecia from beta-blockers is mostly described in the form of telogen effluvium that is reversible [56–59]. Moreover, diffuse alopecia accompanying a patchy infiltrative scalp dermatitis due to nadolol was also reported [60]. Topical corticosteroid therapy reduced the dermatitis, and regrowth of the hair was observed within 3 months of discontinuation of nadolol in this case.

Erythema Multiforme/Stevens–Johnson Syndrome/ Toxic Epidermal Necrolysis

These are among the rarely reported adverse cutaneous reactions to beta-blockers. Erythema multiforme in a patient receiving metoprolol therapy [61], Stevens–Johnson syndrome due to carvedilol [62], and propranolol [63], and a fatal toxic epidermal necrolysis case due to carvedilol [64] have been reported.

Fixed Drug Eruption

There are a few reports on fixed drug eruption due to beta-blockers like atenolol [65, 66], propranolol [67], and bisoprolol [68]. However, patch testing for confirming the reaction has rarely been performed. In one of the atenolol-induced cases, patch testing was positive in the previously affected site [66].

Nail Changes

Psoriatic nail changes may occur in patients receiving beta-blocker therapy, along with psoriasiform skin lesions [3]. On the other hand, isolated psoriatic nail changes without accompanying cutaneous lesions were also seen due to metoprolol therapy [69]. Rare cases of pincer nails were noted during beta-blocker therapy. Acebutolol [70] and metoprolol [71] were the reported causes of this reaction.

Pruritus

Pruritus can be seen during therapy with various beta-blockers [13, 14]. It usually accompanies different types of drug eruptions like lichenoid, urticarial or anaphylactoid reactions, erythema multiforme, or Stevens–Johnson syndrome [22–24, 28, 30, 61, 62].

Oral Mucosal Reactions

Xerostomia is an established class effect of beta-blockers [17]. Oral lichenoid lesions may be seen in patients using beta-blockers [24, 72]. A single case of aphthous ulcer was related to labetalol intake [73]. However, a case–control study revealed a significant association between beta-blocker therapy and the development of aphthous ulcers [74].

Other Reported Adverse Cutaneous Drug Reactions to Beta-Blockers

Pemphigoid has been associated with the use of atenolol [75], practolol, and nadolol [76]. *Photosensitivity* has been reported with tilisolol [77], but some other beta-blockers have also been implicated to be associated with photosensitivity [13]. *Acneiform eruption* was reported with propranolol and nadolol that were used in the therapy of migraine, the latter with possible cross-reaction to propranolol [78], but some other beta-blockers have also been implicated to be associated with acneiform lesions [13]. *Scalp tingling* was mainly observed during administration of labetalol [79–81]. *Generalized hyperpigmentation* was associated with oxprenolol in a single case [82]. Carvedilol was the cause of *occupational airborne contact dermatitis* together with simvastatin and zolpidem, all proven by patch testing, in a patient working in a pharmaceutical factory [83]. Atenolol-induced *pseudolymphoma* was reported in a case presenting with fever, lymphadenopathy, and generalized rash that would suggest drug rash with eosinophilia and systemic symptoms [84].

Beta-blockers are also found to be related with several other cutaneous adverse effects including *hyperhidrosis* and *purpura* [13].

References

1. Opie LH. Beta-blocking agents. In: Opie LH, Gersh BJ, editors. Drugs for the heart. 8th ed. Philadelphia: Elsevier Saunders; 2013.
2. Gold MH, Holy AK, Roenigk Jr HH. Beta-blocking drugs and psoriasis. A review of cutaneous side effects and retrospective analysis of their effects on psoriasis. J Am Acad Dermatol. 1988;19:837–41.
3. Abel EA, DiCicco LM, Orenberg EK, Fraki JE, Farber EM. Drugs in exacerbation of psoriasis. J Am Acad Dermatol. 1986;15:1007–22.
4. Jappe U, Uter W, de Padua CA, Herbst RA, Schnuch A. Allergic contact dermatitis due to beta-blockers in eye drops: a retrospective analysis of multicentre surveillance data 1993–2004. Acta Derm Venereol. 2006;86:509–14.
5. Basavaraj KH, Ashok NM, Rashmi R, Praveen TK. The role of drugs in the induction and/or exacerbation of psoriasis. Int J Dermatol. 2010;49:1351–61.
6. Dika E, Varotti C, Bardazzi F, Maibach HI. Drug-induced psoriasis: an evidence-based overview and the introduction of psoriatic drug eruption probability score. Cutan Ocul Toxicol. 2006;25:1–11.
7. White WB, Schulman P, McCabe EJ. Psoriasiform cutaneous eruptions induced by cetamolol hydrochloride. Arch Dermatol. 1986;122:857–8.
8. Hu CH, Miller AC, Peppercorn R, Farber EM. Generalized pustular psoriasis provoked by propranolol. Arch Dermatol. 1985;121:1326–7.
9. Palatsi R. A skin reaction to pindololum, a beta-blocking drug. Ann Clin Res. 1976;8: 239–40.
10. Jensen HA, Mikkelsen HI, Wadskov S, Sondergaard J. Cutaneous reactions to propranolol (Inderal). Acta Med Scand. 1976;199:363–7.
11. Wright P. Untoward effects associated with practolol administration: oculomucocutaneous syndrome. Br Med J. 1975;1:595–8.
12. Holt PJ, Waddington E. Oculocutaneous reaction to oxprenolol. Br Med J. 1975;2:539–40.
13. Litt JZ. Drug eruption reference manual. 19th ed. Boca Raton: CRC Press (Taylor and Francis Group); 2013.
14. Frishman WH, Brosnan BD, Grossman M, Dasgupta D, Sun AD. Adverse dermatologic effects of cardiovascular drug therapy: part I. Cardiol Rev. 2002;10:230–46.
15. Amos HE, Lake BG, Artis J. Possible role of antibody specific for a practolol metabolite in the pathogenesis of oculomucocutaneous syndrome. Br Med J. 1978;1:402–4.
16. Behan PO, Behan WM, Zacharias FJ, Nicholls JT. Immunological abnormalities in patients who had the oculomucocutaneous syndrome associated with practolol therapy. Lancet. 1976;2:984–7.
17. Torpet LA, Kragelund C, Reibel J, Nauntofte B. Oral adverse drug reactions to cardiovascular drugs. Crit Rev Oral Biol Med. 2004;15:28–46.
18. Gange RW, Jones EW. Bullous lichen planus caused by labetalol. Br Med J. 1978;1:816–7.
19. Massa MC, Jason SM, Gradini R, Welykyj S. Lichenoid drug eruption secondary to propranolol. Cutis. 1991;48:41–3.
20. O'Brien TJ, Lyall IG, Reid SS. Lichenoid eruption induced by sotalol. Australas J Dermatol. 1994;35:93–4.
21. Hawk JL. Lichenoid drug eruption induced by propranolol. Clin Exp Dermatol. 1980;5:93–6.
22. Nguyen DL, Wittich CM. Metoprolol-induced lichenoid dermatitis. J Gen Intern Med. 2011;26:1379–80.
23. Bodmer M, Egger SS, Hohenstein E, Beltraminelli H, Krähenbühl S. Lichenoid eruption associated with the use of nebivolol. Ann Pharmacother. 2006;40:1688–90.
24. Fessa C, Lim P, Kossard S, Richards S, Peñas PF. Lichen planus-like drug eruptions due to β-blockers: a case report and literature review. Am J Clin Dermatol. 2012;13:417–21.
25. Clayton R, Chaudhry S, Ali I, Cooper S, Hodgson T, Wojnarowska F. Mucosal (oral and vulval) lichen planus in women: are angiotensin-converting enzyme inhibitors protective,

and beta-blockers and non-steroidal anti-inflammatory drugs associated with the condition? Clin Exp Dermatol. 2010;35:384–7.
26. Krikorian RK, Quick A, Tal A. Angioedema following the intravenous administration of metoprolol. Chest. 1994;106:1922–3.
27. Seides SF, Ruskin JN, Damato AN. Propranolol-induced urticaria: successful therapy with tolamolol. Chest. 1975;67:496–7.
28. Ferree CE. Apparent anaphylaxis from labetalol. Ann Intern Med. 1986;104:729–30.
29. Hannaway PJ, Hopper GD. Severe anaphylaxis and drug-induced beta-blockade. N Engl J Med. 1983;308:1536.
30. Bause GS, Kugelman LC. Contact anaphylactoid response to labetalol. Contact Dermatitis. 1990;23:51.
31. Toogood JH. Beta-blocker therapy and the risk of anaphylaxis. CMAJ. 1987;136:929–33.
32. Goddet NS, Descatha A, Liberge O, Dolveck F, Boutet J, Baer M, et al. Paradoxical reaction to epinephrine induced by beta-blockers in an anaphylactic shock induced by penicillin. Eur J Emerg Med. 2006;13:358–60.
33. Record Jr NB. Acebutolol-induced pleuropulmonary lupus syndrome. Ann Intern Med. 1981;95:326–7.
34. McGuiness M, Frye RA, Deng JS. Atenolol induced systemic lupus erythematosus syndrome. J Am Acad Dermatol. 1997;37:298–9.
35. Gouet D, Marechaud R, Aucouturier P, Touchard G, Sudre Y, Preud'homme JL. Atenolol-induced lupus erythematosus. J Rheumatol. 1986;13:446–7.
36. Hardee JT, Roldan CA, Du Clos TW. Betaxolol and drug-induced lupus complicated by pericarditis and large pericardial effusion. West J Med. 1997;167:106–9.
37. Paladini G. Peyronie's disease and systemic lupus erythematosus syndrome associated with metoprolol administration: a case report. Int J Tissue React. 1981;3:95–8.
38. Bensaid J, Aldigier JC, Gualde N. Systemic lupus erythematosus syndrome induced by pindolol. Br Med J. 1979;1:1603–4.
39. Harrison T, Sisca TS, Wood WH. Case report. Propranolol-induced lupus syndrome? Postgrad Med. 1976;59:241–4.
40. Brown RC, Cooke J, Losowsky MS. SLE syndrome, probably induced by labetalol. Postgrad Med J. 1981;57:189–90.
41. Raftery EB, Denman AM. Systemic lupus erythematosus syndrome induced by practolol. Br Med J. 1973;2:452–5.
42. Fenniche S, Dhaoui A, Ammar FB, Benmously R, Marrak H, Mokhtar I. Acebutolol-induced subacute cutaneous lupus erythematosus. Skin Pharmacol Physiol. 2005;18:230–3.
43. Fragasso G, Ciboddo G, Pagnotta P, Chierchia SL. Septal panniculitis induced by atenolol–a case report. Angiology. 1998;49:499–502.
44. Pryor JP, Khan O. Beta blockers and Peyronie's disease. Lancet. 1979;1:331.
45. Kristensen BO. Labetalol-induced Peyronie's disease? A case report. Acta Med Scand. 1979;206:511–2.
46. Wolf R, Ophir J, Elman M, Krakowski A. Atenolol-induced cutaneous vasculitis. Cutis. 1989;43:231–3.
47. Ashford R, Staughton R, Brighton WD. Cutaneous vasculitis due to acebutolol. Lancet. 1977;2:462.
48. Rustmann WC, Carpenter MT, Harmon C, Botti CF. Leukocytoclastic vasculitis associated with sotalol therapy. J Am Acad Dermatol. 1998;38:111–2.
49. Iliopoulou A, Giannakopoulos G, Synetos A, Georgiou A, Chalkiadaki A. Leukocytoclastic vasculitis: is propranolol implicated? Pharmacotherapy. 2000;20:848–50.
50. Pavlović MD, Dragojević Simić V, Zolotarevski L, Zecević RD, Vesić S. Cutaneous vasculitis induced by carvedilol. J Eur Acad Dermatol Venereol. 2007;21:1004–5.
51. Gokal R, Dornan TL, Ledingham JG. Peripheral skin necrosis complicating beta-blockage. Br Med J. 1979;1:721–2.
52. Feleke E, Lyngstam O, Råstam L, Rydén L. Complaints of cold extremities among patients on antihypertensive treatment. Acta Med Scand. 1983;213:381–5.

53. Trash D, Grundman M, Cargill J, Christopher K. Letter: Cold extremities and beta-blockers. Br Med J. 1976;2:527–8.
54. Vale JA, Van de Pette SJ, Price TM. Peripheral gangrene complicating beta-blockade. Lancet. 1977;2:412.
55. Vale JA, Jefferys DB. Peripheral gangrene complicating beta-blockade. Lancet. 1978;1:1216.
56. Hilder RJ. Propranolol and alopecia. Cutis. 1979;24:63–4.
57. Martin CM, Southwick EG, Maibach HI. Propranolol induced alopecia. Am Heart J. 1973;86:236–7.
58. Scribner MD. Propranolol therapy. Arch Dermatol. 1977;113:1303.
59. Graeber CW, Lapkin RA. Metoprolol and alopecia. Cutis. 1981;28:633–4.
60. Shelley ED, Shelley WB. Alopecia and drug eruption of the scalp associated with a new beta-blocker, nadolol. Cutis. 1985;35:148–9.
61. Hong JA, Bisognano JD. Metoprolol succinate therapy associated with erythema multiforme. Cardiol J. 2009;16:82–3.
62. Kowalski BJ, Cody RJ. Stevens-Johnson syndrome associated with carvedilol therapy. Am J Cardiol. 1997;80:669–70.
63. Mukul, Verma G. Propranolol induced Steven-Johnson syndrome. J Assoc Physicians India. 1989;37:797–8.
64. Vlahovic-Palcevski V, Milic S, Hauser G, Protic A, Zupan Z, Reljic M, Stimac D. Toxic epidermal necrolysis associated with carvedilol treatment. Int J Clin Pharmacol Ther. 2010;48:549–51.
65. Palungwachira P, Palungwachira P. Fixed drug eruption due to atenolol: a case report. J Med Assoc Thai. 1999;82:1158–61.
66. Belhadjali H, Trimech O, Youssef M, Elhani I, Zili J. Fixed drug eruption induced by atenolol. Clin Cosmet Investig Dermatol. 2009;1:37–9.
67. Zaccaria E, Gualco F, Drago F, Rebora A. Fixed drug eruption due to propranolol. Acta Derm Venereol. 2006;86:371.
68. Giner Esparza MA, Miedes Pitarch E, Miquel Miquel FJ, Palop Larrea V. Fixed drug eruption and bisoprolol. Aten Primaria. 2009;41:351.
69. Gin A, Gin D, Sinclair R. Metoprolol-induced psoriatic nail disease. Australas J Dermatol. 2013;54:59–60.
70. Greiner D, Schofer H, Milbradt R. Reversible transverse overcurvature of the nails (pincer nails) after treatment with a beta-blocker. J Am Acad Dermatol. 1998;39:486–7.
71. Bostanci S, Ekmekci P, Akyol A, Peksari Y, Gurgey E. Pincer nail deformity: inherited and caused by a beta-blocker. Int J Dermatol. 2004;43:316–8.
72. Habbab KM, Moles DR, Porter SR. Potential oral manifestations of cardiovascular drugs. Oral Dis. 2010;16:769–73.
73. Pradalier A, Dry J, Baron JF. Aphthoid stomatitis induced by labetalol. Therapie. 1982;37:695–7.
74. Boulinguez S, Reix S, Bedane C, Debrock C, Bouyssou-Gauthier ML, Sparsa A, et al. Role of drug exposure in aphthous ulcers: a case-control study. Br J Dermatol. 2000;143:1261–5.
75. Kanjanabuch P, Arporniem S, Thamrat S, Thumasombut P. Mucous membrane pemphigoid in a patient with hypertension treated with atenolol: a case report. J Med Case Rep. 2012;6:373.
76. Stavropoulos PG, Soura E, Antoniou C. Drug-induced pemphigoid: a review of the literature. J Eur Acad Dermatol Venereol. 2014;28:1133–40. doi:10.1111/jdv.12366.
77. Miyauchi H, Horiki S, Horio T. Clinical and experimental photosensitivity reaction to tilisolol hydrochloride. Photodermatol Photoimmunol Photomed. 1994;10:255–8.
78. Bajwa ZH, Sami N, Flory C. Severe acne as a side effect of propranolol and nadolol in a migraineur. Headache. 1999;39:758–60.
79. Tcherdakoff P. Side-effects with long-term labetalol: an open study of 251 patients in a single centre. Pharmatherapeutica. 1983;3:342–8.
80. Hua AS, Thomas GW, Kincaid-Smith P. Scalp tingling in patients on labetalol. Lancet. 1977;2:295.

81. Bailey RR. Scalp tingling and difficulty in micturition in patients on labetalol. Lancet. 1977;2:720–1.
82. Harrower AD, Strong JA. Hyperpigmentation associated with oxprenolol administration. Br Med J. 1977;2:296.
83. Neumark M, Moshe S, Ingber A, Slodownik D. Occupational airborne contact dermatitis to simvastatin, carvedilol, and zolpidem. Contact Dermatitis. 2009;61:51–2.
84. Henderson CA, Shamy HK. Atenolol-induced pseudolymphoma. Clin Exp Dermatol. 1990;15:119–20.

Chapter 7
Class III Antiarrhythmic Drugs

Keywords Class III antiarrhythmic • Amiodarone • Photosensitivity • Hyperpigmentation • Lupus erythematosus • Angioedema/urticaria • Toxic epidermal necrolysis • Vasculitis • Iododerma

Class III antiarrhythmic drugs include amiodarone, bretylium, dofetilide, ibutilide, azimilide, and dronedarone. Among these, amiodarone is the most reported one to cause adverse cutaneous reactions. Amiodarone is a lipid soluble agent which accumulates in peripheral tissues including the adipose tissue, and the skin is one of the excretion ways of the drug. It has a very long half-life, up to 6 months [1], so it is stated that toxic side effects may also be seen after the withdrawal of the drug [2]. It is associated with many cutaneous side effects such as photosensitivity and pigmentation being the well-known ones.

Sotalol, which has also class III activity, is included in the chapter on beta-blockers. Adenosine and digitalis glycosides are other antiarrhythmic drugs that are discussed in Chap. 15.

The adverse cutaneous drug reactions described below are meant to be sorted by starting from the well-known reactions of class III antiarrhythmic drugs, particularly from amiodarone, to the lesser known ones. The major ones are summarized in Table 7.1.

Photosensitivity

Amiodarone is stated to be among the most common photosensitizing medications [3]. Photosensitivity reaction is suggested to be the most common cutaneous side effect of amiodarone [4].

It was described as a phototoxic reaction, induced mostly by UVA [5, 6]. However, reaction to both UVA and UVB wavelengths has also been reported [7]. The photosensitivity reaction was observed within 1 week to 4 months after starting therapy with amiodarone [5, 6, 8]. The reaction was reported to start with burning and stinging sensation as early as following 2–10 minutes of sun exposure [5]. Subsequent erythema developed on sun-exposed areas of the skin, and the reaction

E. Özkaya, K.D. Yazganoğlu, *Adverse Cutaneous Drug Reactions to Cardiovascular Drugs*, DOI 10.1007/978-1-4471-6536-1_7

Table 7.1 Major adverse cutaneous drug reactions with class III antiarrhythmic drugs

Adverse cutaneous drug reaction	Main inducers
Photosensitivity	Amiodarone, dronedarone
Hyperpigmentation	Amiodarone
Drug-induced lupus erythematosus (systemic lupus erythematosus)	Amiodarone
Angioedema/urticaria	Amiodarone
Toxic epidermal necrolysis	Amiodarone
Vasculitis	Amiodarone, dronedarone
Iododerma	Amiodarone

commonly faded within 1–2 days after avoiding sun exposure [5, 6, 8]. Amiodarone-induced photosensitivity usually resolves within months after discontinuation of the drug [3, 5]. However, persistent photosensitivity from amiodarone was reported in one case even 17 years after stopping the drug [8]. An interesting case of blistering dermatitis confined to the perioral area that occurred during summer months was attributed to amiodarone therapy. The patch test was weakly positive to balsam of Peru, but the reaction persisted in spite of omitting the allergen and resolved only after discontinuation of the drug [9].

Photosensitivity may also occur during dronedarone therapy [10]. Dronedarone seems to be less frequently involved in this type of reaction when compared to amiodarone [10].

Basal cell carcinomas were reported after amiodarone therapy arising in the skin sites related to amiodarone-induced photosensitivity including a sunburn reaction or in the skin sites related to amiodarone-induced pigmentation. However, they were also reported to occur on non-sun-exposed skin sites in patients generally having a history of normal sun exposure throughout their life, therefore a clear relationship between basal cell carcinomas and amiodarone therapy could not be established [11–13].

Hyperpigmentation

Slate-gray or blue-gray pigmentation on sun-exposed skin was observed with prolonged use of amiodarone therapy, approximately 1–2 years after starting therapy [6, 8, 14–16]. The reaction seems to be related especially with high doses of therapy [15]. Photosensitivity preceded the pigmentation in some cases [6, 8, 15]. Skin discoloration disappeared with reduction of the dose in some cases [15], but not in other ones [6, 16]. It was reported to resolve within 4 months to 3 years after discontinuation of the drug [8, 15, 17, 18].

Persistence of the photosensitivity and pigmentation was generally related to the tissue retention and slow elimination of the drug [7, 15, 19]. It was demonstrated that amiodarone and its metabolite desethylamiodarone were present in the skin of the patients receiving amiodarone [7]. They were detected in higher concentrations in sun-exposed pigmented areas than the nonpigmented skin [7]. Moreover, the skin biopsy of the patients revealed the presence of perivascular, yellow-brown, granular pigment in macrophages in the dermis compatible with lipofuscin deposition. Iodine-rich amiodarone and its metabolite have been suggested to be bound to lipofuscin within lysosomes of macrophages [7]. However, a recent report showed the absence of lipofuscin in the amiodarone-induced pigmented skin of a patient by electron microscopy, and indicated that the deposition of the drug in the skin was directly responsible for the pigmentation, and not the dermal lipofuscinosis [19].

Drug-Induced Lupus Erythematosus

Amiodarone has been reported to cause drug-induced systemic lupus erythematosus with or without accompanying skin involvement in several patients [20–23]. Malar rash was the prominent skin finding [20, 21, 23]. The reaction resolved after discontinuation of amiodarone even in the absence of additional specific therapy for lupus [20, 21, 23].

Angioedema/Urticaria

Facial angioedema appeared within a couple of weeks, and approximately 2 and 7 years after starting amiodarone therapy in three different cases [24, 25]. Oral rechallenge with amiodarone caused reappearance of the reaction [24, 25].

Angioedema was reported from amiodarone in a patient with previous history of an urticarial reaction to an iodinated radiocontrast agent [26]. Due to iodine content of amiodarone, it is contraindicated in patients with previous history of iodine allergy, but it is not clear if cross-sensitivity between iodine/iodinated agents and amiodarone really exists. According to a large retrospective study conducted in patients receiving amiodarone with previous allergy to iodine or iodinated contrast agents, the incidence of hypersensitivity reaction with amiodarone was documented as only 0.4 % [27].

Toxic Epidermal Necrolysis

Three cases of toxic epidermal necrolysis have been reported possibly due to amiodarone [28–30]. The reaction started within 3 days, 10 days, and 3 months after starting therapy with amiodarone, respectively, in each case. In the latter case, with the long latency period, the patient was on multidrug therapy and the authors were not totally sure that amiodarone was the definite inducer [28]. Another case lacked mucosal involvement [29]. The reaction was fatal in two cases [28, 30].

Pruritus

Pruritus is a nonspecific cutaneous adverse reaction of drugs. It was reported in patients receiving amiodarone or dronedarone therapy [31].

Other Reported Adverse Cutaneous Drug Reactions to Class III Antiarrhythmic Drugs

Leukocytoclastic vasculitis has been reported to occur due to amiodarone [32, 33] and dronedarone therapy [34].

Iododerma induced by amiodarone was reported [35, 36]. In one of the reported cases, multiple cutaneous irregular tumors with seropurulent discharge was diagnosed as iododerma associated with the use of amiodarone that had been given for 2 years. The reaction was attributed to iodine content of amiodarone [35]. The other patient developed iododerma after 14 months of therapy, and interestingly, experienced an exacerbation 3 months after withdrawal of amiodarone. Cyclosporine was used successfully in the treatment of iododerma in this patient [36].

Linear IgA dermatosis from amiodarone [37], *alopecia* due to amiodarone resolving after discontinuation of the drug and recurring after rechallenge [38], and *skin necrosis* secondary to amiodarone extravasation from a peripheral vein infusion were recorded [39]. *Psoriasis* [40] and *pseudoporphyria* [41] were other cutaneous side effects reported to be associated with amiodarone therapy. *Hyperhidrosis and dry skin*, probably as a result of amiodarone-induced hyperthyroidism/hypothyroidism have also been noted [4]. *Palmar erythema* with hepatic damage has been stated to occur with amiodarone [42].

Unspecified rash and *flushing* from bretylium [4]; *unspecified rash*, *angioedema*, *edema*, and *hyperhidrosis* from dofetilide [4, 31]; *bullous contact dermatitis* on the dorsum of the hands after contact exposure to ibutilide [43]; and *eczema* and *dermatitis* from dronedarone [31] were other reported side effects.

References

1. Opie LH. Beta-blocking agents. In: Opie LH, Gersh BJ, editors. Drugs for the heart. 8th ed. Philadelphia: Elsevier Saunders; 2013.
2. Klein AD, Pardo RJ, Gould E, Kerdel F. Blue-gray discoloration of the face. Amiodarone-induced cutaneous hyperpigmentation. Arch Dermatol. 1989;125(417):420–1.
3. Drucker AM, Rosen CF. Drug-induced photosensitivity: culprit drugs, management and prevention. Drug Saf. 2011;34:821–37.
4. Frishman WH, Brosnan BD, Grossman M, Dasgupta D, Sun DK. Adverse dermatologic effects of cardiovascular drug therapy: part II. Cardiol Rev. 2002;10:285–300.
5. Walter JF, Bradner H, Curtis GP. Amiodarone photosensitivity. Arch Dermatol. 1984;120: 1591–4.

6. Roupe G, Larko O, Olsson SB. Amiodarone photoreactions. Acta Derm Venereol. 1987;67:76–9.
7. Zachary CB, Slater DN, Holt DW, Storey GC, MacDonald DM. The pathogenesis of amiodarone-induced pigmentation and photosensitivity. Br J Dermatol. 1984;110:451–6.
8. Yones SS, O'Donoghue NB, Palmer RA, Menage Hdu P, Hawk JL. Persistent severe amiodarone-induced photosensitivity. Clin Exp Dermatol. 2005;30:500–2.
9. Shah N, Warnakulasuriya S. Amiodarone-induced peri-oral photosensitivity. J Oral Pathol Med. 2004;33:56–8.
10. Le Heuzey JY, De Ferrari GM, Radzik D, Santini M, Zhu J, Davy JM. A short-term, randomized, double-blind, parallel-group study to evaluate the efficacy and safety of dronedarone versus amiodarone in patients with persistent atrial fibrillation: the DIONYSOS study. J Cardiovasc Electrophysiol. 2010;21:597–605.
11. Monk BE. Basal cell carcinoma following amiodarone therapy. Br J Dermatol. 1995;133: 148–9.
12. Hall MA, Annas A, Nyman K, Talme T, Emtestam L. Basalioma after amiodarone therapy-not only in Britain. Br J Dermatol. 2004;151:932–3.
13. Maoz KB, Dvash S, Brenner S, Brenner S. Amiodarone-induced skin pigmentation and multiple basal-cell carcinomas. Int J Dermatol. 2009;48:1398–400.
14. Bahadir S, Apaydin R, Cobanoilu U, Kapicioilu Z, Ozoran Y, Gokce M, Alpay K. Amiodarone pigmentation, eye and thyroid alterations. J Eur Acad Dermatol Venereol. 2000;14: 194–5.
15. Kounis NG, Frangides C, Papadaki PJ, Zavras GM, Goudevenos J. Dose-dependent appearance and disappearance of amiodarone-induced skin pigmentation. Clin Cardiol. 1996;19: 592–4.
16. Ammann R, Braathen LR. Amiodarone pigmentation. Hautarzt. 1996;47:930–1.
17. Ioannides MA, Moutiris JA, Zambartas C. A case of pseudocyanotic coloring of skin after prolonged use of amiodarone. Int J Cardiol. 2003;90:345–6.
18. Blackshear JL, Randle HW. Reversibility of blue-gray cutaneous discoloration from amiodarone. Mayo Clin Proc. 1991;66:721–6.
19. Ammoury A, Michaud S, Paul C, Prost-Squarcioni C, Alvarez F, Lamant L, et al. Photodistribution of blue-gray hyperpigmentation after amiodarone treatment: molecular characterization of amiodarone in the skin. Arch Dermatol. 2008;144:92–6.
20. Susano R, Caminal L, Ramos D, Díaz B. Amiodarone induced lupus. Ann Rheum Dis. 1999;58:655–6.
21. Kundu AK. Amiodarone-induced systemic lupus erythematosus. J Assoc Physicians India. 2003;51:216–7.
22. Sheikhzadeh A, Schäfer U, Schnabel A. Drug-induced lupus erythematosus by amiodarone. Arch Intern Med. 2002;162:834–6.
23. Yachoui R, Saad W. Amiodarone-induced lupus-like syndrome. Am J Ther. 2013. [Epub ahead of print]. doi:10.1097/MJT.0b013e318296ee78.
24. Lahiri K, Malakar S, Sarma N. Amiodarone-induced angioedema: report of two cases. Indian J Dermatol Venereol Leprol. 2005;71:46–7.
25. Burches E, Garcia-Verdegay F, Ferrer M, Pelaez A. Amiodarone-induced angioedema. Allergy. 2000;55:1199–200.
26. Stafford L. Hypersensitivity reaction to amiodarone in a patient with a previous reaction to an iodinated radiocontrast agent. Ann Pharmacother. 2007;41:1310–4.
27. Lakshmanadoss U, Lindsley J, Glick D, Twilley CH, Lewin 3rd JJ, Marine JE. Incidence of amiodarone hypersensitivity in patients with previous allergy to iodine or iodinated contrast agents. Pharmacotherapy. 2012;32:618–22.
28. Yung A, Agnew K, Snow J, Oliver F. Two unusual cases of toxic epidermal necrolysis. Australas J Dermatol. 2002;43:35–8.
29. Chen A, Sauer W, Nguyen DT. A dire reaction: rash after amiodarone administration. Am J Med. 2013;126:301–3.
30. Bencini PL, Crosti C, Sala F, Bertani E, Nobili M. Toxic epidermal necrolysis and amiodarone treatment. Arch Dermatol. 1985;121:838.

31. Litt JZ. Drug eruption reference manual. 19th ed. Boca Raton: CRC Press (Taylor and Francis Group); 2013.
32. Staubli M, Zimmermann A, Bircher J. Amiodarone-induced vasculitis and polyserositis. Postgrad Med J. 1985;61:245–7.
33. Dootson G, Byatt C. Amiodarone-induced vasculitis and a review of the cutaneous side-effects of amiodarone. Clin Exp Dermatol. 1994;19:422–4.
34. Smith SM, Al-Bataineh M, Iorfido SB, Macfarlane J. A case report: Multaq-induced leukocytoclastic vasculitis. Am J Ther. 2014;21:e69–70. doi:10.1097/MJT.0b013e3182459c72.
35. Porters JE, Zantkuyl CF. Ioderma caused by amiodarone. Arch Dermatol. 1975;111:1656.
36. Ricci C, Krasovec M, Frenk E. Amiodarone induced iododerma treated by cyclosporine. Ann Dermatol Venereol. 1997;124:260–3.
37. Primka 3rd EJ, Liranzo MO, Bergfeld WF, Dijkstra JW. Amiodarone-induced linear IgA disease. J Am Acad Dermatol. 1994;31:809–11.
38. Ahmad S. Amiodarone and reversible alopecia. Arch Intern Med. 1995;155:1106.
39. Russell SJ, Saltissi S. Amiodarone induced skin necrosis. Heart. 2006;92:1395.
40. Basavaraj KH, Ashok NM, Rashmi R, Praveen TK. The role of drugs in the induction and/or exacerbation of psoriasis. Int J Dermatol. 2010;49:1351–61.
41. Parodi A, Guarrera M, Rebora A. Amiodarone-induced pseudoporphyria. Photodermatol. 1988;5:146–7.
42. Serrao R, Zirwas M, English JC. Palmar erythema. Am J Clin Dermatol. 2007;8:347–56.
43. Dodds ES, Oberg KC. Erythematous bullous lesions on the dorsa of the hands due to contact exposure to ibutilide fumarate for injection. Pharmacotherapy. 1998;18:880–2.

Chapter 8
Calcium Channel Blockers

Keywords Calcium channel blockers • Diltiazem • Verapamil • Nifedipine • Amlodipine • Flushing • Edema • Gingival hyperplasia • Gynecomastia • Photosensitivity • Hyperpigmentation • Acute generalized exanthematous pustulosis

Calcium channel blockers (CCBs) or calcium antagonists can be pharmacologically classified into different subgroups as benzothiazepines (diltiazem), phenylalkylamines (verapamil, gallopamil), dihydropyridines (nifedipine, nicardipine, nisoldipine, nimodipine, nitradipine, nilvadipine, nitrendipine, benidipine, felodipine, amlodipine, barnidipine, cilnidipine, efonidipine, manidipine, lacidipine, isradipine, lercanidipine, aranidipine, azelnidipine, pranidipine, clevidipine), and tetraols (mibefradil). Not classified within these subgroups, bepridil blocks sodium channels as well and monatepil has also alpha-1 adrenoreceptor blocking activity [1]. Diltiazem and verapamil are among the class IV antiarrhythmic drugs. Mibefradil was withdrawn from the market due to its potential side effects and drug interactions.

There are many cutaneous reactions associated with CCBs which are discussed below. The pharmacologic activity (vasodilatation, negative inotropic, and dromotropic action) of CCBs is responsible for their main adverse effects [1]. Adverse effects seem to be related with the degree of bioavailability of CCBs [1].

Adverse cutaneous drug reactions to diltiazem seem to constitute a significant proportion of its adverse effects [2]. According to an article analyzing adverse cutaneous drug reactions to diltiazem obtained from the reports (1966–1995) of Health Protection Branch (Canada), Adverse Drug Reaction Monitoring division, the number of diltiazem-induced adverse cutaneous drug reactions was reported to be higher than those induced by either nifedipine or verapamil, but the proportion of serious cutaneous adverse events (e.g., toxic epidermal necrolysis, Stevens–Johnson syndrome, drug hypersensitivity syndrome, erythroderma) did not differ between these drugs [2]. On the contrary, another study based on the reports of Food and Drug Administration (FDA)'s Division of Epidemiology and Drug Surveillance, and American Academy of Dermatology's Adverse Drug Reaction Reporting System demonstrated more serious reactions with diltiazem, but the authors suggested that this difference may be related with reporting bias [3].

E. Özkaya, K.D. Yazganoğlu, *Adverse Cutaneous Drug Reactions to Cardiovascular Drugs*, DOI 10.1007/978-1-4471-6536-1_8

Table 8.1 Major adverse cutaneous drug reactions with calcium channel blockers

Adverse cutaneous drug reaction	Main inducers
Peripheral edema	Dihydropyridines, diltiazem, verapamil
Flushing	Dihydropyridines, diltiazem, verapamil
Gingival hyperplasia	Nifedipine, diltiazem, verapamil, nicardipine, nimodipine, nitrendipine, felodipine, manidipine, amlodipine, isradipine
Gynecomastia	Verapamil, amlodipine, diltiazem, nifedipine
Maculopapular eruption	Diltiazem, nifedipine, verapamil, amlodipine, nimodipine
Photosensitivity	Diltiazem, nifedipine, nicardipine
Telangiectasia	Amlodipine, nifedipine, felodipine
Hyperpigmentation	Diltiazem
Acute generalized exanthematous pustulosis	Diltiazem
Drug-induced lupus erythematosus (mainly subacute cutaneous lupus erythematosus)	Diltiazem, verapamil, nifedipine, nitrendipine
Psoriasis/psoriasiform eruption	Nifedipine, felodipine, amlodipine, diltiazem
Erythromelalgia	Diltiazem, nifedipine, nicardipine, verapamil
Lichen planus/lichenoid eruption	Amlodipine, nifedipine, verapamil
Bullous eruption	
Pemphigus and bullous pemphigoid	Nifedipine
Linear IgA dermatosis	Amlodipine, verapamil
Erythema multiforme/Stevens–Johnson syndrome/toxic epidermal necrolysis	Diltiazem, amlodipine, nifedipine, verapamil
Erythroderma	Diltiazem, nifedipine, verapamil
DRESS	Diltiazem
Angioedema/urticaria	Diltiazem, nifedipine, verapamil, amlodipine, nicardipine
Purpura	Amlodipine, diltiazem, nifedipine
Eczematous eruption	Not specified

DRESS drug rash with eosinophilia and systemic symptoms

Cross-reactivity among CCBs has not yet been established clearly. While reactions suggesting cross-sensitivity between different subgroups of CCBs can be observed [4–6], it may not always be seen among the same subgroup [7].

The adverse cutaneous drug reactions described below are meant to be sorted by starting from the well-known reactions of CCBs to the lesser known ones. The major ones are summarized in Table 8.1.

Peripheral Edema

Ankle or pedal edema is one of the most common adverse effects that has been reported with dihydropyridine-type CCBs and also with diltiazem, verapamil, and mibefradil [1, 8–12]. It was stated to be a dose-dependent adverse effect, related with precapillary vasodilatation effect of CCBs leading to increased intracapillary pressure that is promoted when the patient is standing upright [10]. The incidence of adverse reactions which are associated with the vasodilatory effects including flushing and edema was reported to be higher with vasoselective dihydropyridines (nicardipine, isradipine, and amlodipine) than with diltiazem [8]. Moreover, the incidence of vasodilatory edema was stated to differ among dihydropyridine-type CCBs. With the use of lercanidipine and lacidipine, it was stated to be lesser than with amlodipine, nifedipine, felodipine, and isradipine [10, 11].

Flushing

Like pedal edema, flushing is also a common adverse effect that has been reported with CCBs, mostly with dihydropyridines, and also with diltiazem and verapamil due to peripheral vasodilatation [1, 8].

Gingival Hyperplasia

This is a well-documented adverse reaction of CCBs, mainly reported with diltiazem, verapamil, nifedipine, nicardipine, nimodipine, nitrendipine, felodipine, manidipine, amlodipine, and isradipine [1, 5, 7, 13–20].

The prevalence of gingival overgrowth differed among studies [13, 14]. Individuals using nifedipine were suggested to have a higher risk for developing gingival hyperplasia when compared with individuals using amlodipine or diltiazem [13]. Males taking nifedipine were found to be more likely to develop gingival hyperplasia than females [13]. The pathogenesis of gingival hyperplasia was linked to several factors including genetic predisposition, pharmacokinetic properties of the drugs, and factors related with periodontal variables and gingival inflammation [13, 14, 21].

Gingival changes usually improve upon discontinuation of the inducer drug. In a case of verapamil-induced gingival hyperplasia, resolution was seen following discontinuation of the drug, but recurrence was reported when diltiazem, belonging to another subgroup of CCB, was given [5]. On the other hand, the reaction induced by nifedipine was reported to resolve after initiating another dihydropyridine, namely, isradipine [7].

Gynecomastia

CCBs like amlodipine, diltiazem, verapamil, and nifedipine may cause gynecomastia [1, 22–25]. Gynecomastia can be unilateral [22–24] and may start even after years of therapy [23], and local tenderness may accompany [22].

In a study, the prevalence of hyperprolactinemia was found to be 8.5 % in male patients using verapamil [25]. The persistence of hyperprolactinemia during verapamil use and the normalization of prolactin levels upon cessation of verapamil therapy highly suggested the role of verapamil in the development of this condition [25]. Furthermore, the same study also revealed lower testosterone levels in patients using verapamil [25].

Maculopapular Eruption

Diltiazem [2, 3, 26–28], nifedipine [2, 3, 29], verapamil [2, 3], amlodipine [26], and nimodipine [30] were reported among the inducers of maculopapular drug eruption, also known as exanthematous eruption [2]. In fact, this is one of the most frequently reported adverse cutaneous drug reaction triggered by diltiazem, nifedipine, and verapamil [2, 3].

A patient suffering from a maculopapular eruption after diltiazem experienced the same cutaneous reaction with amlodipine after 3 days of discontinuation of diltiazem, suggesting a cross-reactivity between two different subgroups of CCBs [26]. However, the time between discontinuation of diltiazem and onset of amlodipine was too short questioning whether the eruption was related with diltiazem or amlodipine. Patch tests have been performed for the diagnosis and investigation of cross-reactivity in CCB-induced maculopapular drug eruption. Patch testing with diltiazem was positive in four cases who experienced a maculopapular eruption with diltiazem [27]. These cases were also patch tested with verapamil, nicardipine, nitrendipine, nimodipine, and nifedipine, and only verapamil was positive in one patient, but rechallenge was not performed with verapamil in this case [27]. Another patient with nimodipine-induced maculopapular eruption, which progressed to generalized eczema with oral mucosal lesions, reacted positively to nimodipine in patch testing, but test results were negative for amlodipine and nifedipine [30]. It was suggested that different lateral chains in the structure of amlodipine and nifedipine, two other drugs of the dihydropyridine subgroup, might be responsible for the absence of cross-reaction with nimodipine [30].

Photoinduced Reactions

Photoinduced reactions like photosensitivity, telangiectasia, and hyperpigmentation may be observed during therapy with some CCBs.

Photosensitivity reactions have been described with nifedipine [31], diltiazem [31, 32], and nicardipine [33]. Erythematous or maculopapular eruption was reported to develop on photoexposed areas [31]. Cross-reaction was suspected between nifedipine and diltiazem regarding photosensitivity [31]. One study showed positive UVA photopatch and photoscratch test results with nicardipine [33].

Telangiectases appearing on photoexposed skin, mainly on the face, have been reported particularly with dihydropyridine-type CCBs, especially amlodipine [34–36], but also with nifedipine [37] and felodipine [38]. The onset of telangiectases was reported to occur as early as 1 month after starting the CCB [34, 35], and resolution has been observed as early as 2 months after discontinuation of the drug [36, 38]. The eruption was not generally associated with any symptoms regarding phototoxicity or photoallergy. Rechallenge performed in a case of amlodipine-induced telangiectasia led to the recurrence of telangiectasia [36]. Vasodilatory effect of CCBs in addition to the actinic damage in vessels of the photoexposed sites was considered to be related with the development of telangiectasia [1, 38].

Felodipine was also implicated as a cause of a purpura-like discoloration with overlying telangiectases at a mastectomy site previously treated with radiotherapy, that was speculated to be related with the capillary fragility caused by felodipine and radiotherapy [39].

Diltiazem, mainly its extended-release form, was reported to be associated with another photoinduced reaction presenting as hyperpigmentation on sun-exposed sites, which was mostly observed in elderly African-American patients, but may also occur in other ethnic groups [40–45]. The hyperpigmentation was described as slate-gray, blue-gray, or dark brown in color that involved the face, neck, "V" area of the chest, distal parts of the arms, and rarely hands in a reticulated pattern or in patches. Patients were taking diltiazem for 6 months to 12.5 years before the hyperpigmentation developed [40–45]. Discontinuation of the drug resulted in slow, gradual resolution of the hyperpigmentation. A skin biopsy may show lichenoid dermatitis with pigmentary incontinence in the histopathology [40, 43, 44]. The mechanism of this reaction is obscure; it is not clear whether a drug metabolite causes the reaction or not [40]. The photospectrometry analysis could demonstrate a photosensitizing effect of diltiazem within the UVB spectrum [43]. Topical tacrolimus was reported to be effective in the management of the hyperpigmentation in some cases [45].

A patient was described to develop oral mucosal and cutaneous hyperpigmentation which was most prominent on the photoexposed areas, 1 year after starting amlodipine [46].

Acute Generalized Exanthematous Pustulosis

Diltiazem-induced acute generalized exanthematous pustulosis is well described in the literature [2, 47–52]. The onset of lesions was reported to occur within a range of 1 day to 3 weeks following therapy. Patch testing was found useful for identifying the culprit drug in acute generalized exanthematous pustulosis from diltiazem [47, 48, 51].

Drug-Induced Lupus Erythematosus

Diltiazem, verapamil, nifedipine, and nitrendipine were reported to cause drug-induced subacute cutaneous lupus erythematosus (SCLE) [53–56].

Papulosquamous, psoriasiform, or annular skin lesions usually on sun-exposed areas were observed in patients with drug-induced SCLE [53]. It was reported to start within 6 months to 5 years of CCB therapy [53–55]. Antinuclear antibody was present in most of the reported cases, but positivity of anti-Ro/SSA and anti- La/SSB antibodies was variable. Some patients showed only anti-Ro/SSA or anti- La/SSB, without the presence of antinuclear antibodies. Positivity of antihistone antibodies was also demonstrated in some [53]. Complete resolution was observed within 2–12 weeks after discontinuation of the drug, even without additional treatment.

It was speculated that Ro and La antigens were displaced to the surface of the keratinocytes due to the effect of CCBs on cytosolic calcium concentration, which subsequently resulted in the formation of autoantibodies. The attachment of antibodies to Ro and La antigens led then to keratinocyte injury by complement-mediated lysis and antibody-dependent cellular cytotoxicity [54].

Psoriasis/Psoriasiform Eruption

CCBs were found to be associated with the development of new-onset psoriasis and exacerbation of preexisting psoriasis [57]. Nifedipine, felodipine, amlodipine, and diltiazem were among the CCBs that were implicated to cause this type of reaction [3, 57, 58]. A case–control study found a long latency period (median 28 months, range 4–143 months) between the onset of CCB use and development or exacerbation of psoriasis [57]. However, almost half of the patients were concomitantly taking beta-blockers which might also have a contributory effect [57]. It was suggested that the pathogenesis could be related with the effect of CCBs on keratinocyte differentiation that is associated with intracellular calcium levels [57].

Erythromelalgia

Erythromelalgia is characterized by severe painful burning sensation associated with redness and increased skin temperature more commonly affecting the feet, but rarely involving the hands as well [59]. Primary erythromelalgia is an autosomal dominant condition, whereas erythromelalgia might also occur secondarily, and can be associated with myeloproliferative disorders, infectious diseases, diabetic neuropathy, or drugs [59]. The diagnosis depends on clinical findings and history of the patient, as there are no definitive diagnostic tests. CCBs including diltiazem [3], nifedipine [3, 60], nicardipine [61], and verapamil [62, 63] were reported among drugs inducing erythromelalgia.

The symptoms were reported to start within a wide range of time after commencing treatment with CCBs. It was reported to start 1 day [60], a few weeks [61], a few months [62], and even 5 years after initiating therapy [63]. Gradual resolution of the reaction was usually observed within 1–2 weeks after stopping the drug [62, 63].

The vasodilatation effect of CCBs was suggested to be responsible for the development of erythromelalgia [1]. On the contrary, CCBs like nifedipine and diltiazem were also used for the treatment of erythromelalgia because of their known therapeutic effect on microvascular ischemia [1, 59].

Lichen Planus/Lichenoid Eruption

This kind of eruption has been reported to occur with amlodipine [64, 65], nifedipine [66], and verapamil [3].

Widespread cutaneous lichenoid eruption and Wickham's striae in the oral cavity were described in a patient, 2 weeks after starting treatment with amlodipine [64]. This patient had a history of non-insulin-dependent diabetes mellitus and was suggested as a case of Grinspan's syndrome representing the triad of oral lichen planus, hypertension, and diabetes mellitus. Lesions improved with oral acitretin 30 mg daily for 5 weeks and additional potent topical corticosteroids, leaving residual hyperpigmentation. In another case of amlodipine-induced lichenoid eruption, the presence of transepidermal elimination of collagen with perforation in the histopathology suggested a perforating lichenoid reaction [65].

A patient under nifedipine therapy developed an erysipelas-like erythematous pruritic plaque on both shins which histopathologically showed a lichen planus-like eruption [66].

Bullous Eruption

Pemphigus and Pemphigoid

Nifedipine was reported to be associated with pemphigus foliaceus [67], pemphigus vulgaris [68], and bullous pemphigoid [69, 70], the latter presenting as pemphigoid nodularis in one case [69].

The pemphigus foliaceus lesions started within 3 months after commencement of nifedipine in the reported case. Direct and indirect immunofluorescence examinations were negative, and it was suggested that nifedipine directly caused acantholysis without formation of autoantibodies. Withdrawal of the drug and therapy with oral corticosteroids resulted in resolution of the reaction within 1 week. Readministration of nifedipine 10 days later confirmed that this drug was the causative agent of the reaction [67]. In another report, nifedipine was reported to be associated with the induction of pemphigus vulgaris in one case, and exacerbation of preexisting pemphigus in another one [68]. Both cases demonstrated tissue fixed and circulating antibodies in immunofluorescence examinations, supporting an immunological acantholysis.

In the case of bullous pemphigoid presenting as pemphigoid nodularis, the reaction occurred 3 months after starting treatment with nifedipine in a 70-year-old man [69]. Direct and indirect immunofluorescence findings were suggestive of pemphigoid; moreover, Western blot analysis revealed antibodies to the 230 kDa pemphigoid antigen. Pruritic papules and nodules on the back, trunk, limbs, face, and scalp, ulceration in the mouth, and dystrophy and pterygium unguis of the toes and fingers were the cutaneous findings. The lesions improved upon withdrawal of nifedipine, together with a decrease in the antibody titration, but complete resolution was not observed, so the authors suggested that this case was an example of an idiopathic bullous pemphigoid that nifedipine might have initiated [69].

Linear IgA Dermatosis

Amlodipine and verapamil were reported to be causative agents in two different reports of drug-induced linear IgA dermatosis [71, 72].

Erythema Multiforme/Stevens–Johnson Syndrome/ Toxic Epidermal Necrolysis

Erythema multiforme has been reported with diltiazem [2, 3, 73], verapamil [3], nifedipine [2, 3], and amlodipine [74], usually occurring within 2 days to 2 weeks of initiation of therapy [3]. A patient tolerated nifedipine without any reaction before and after the occurrence of erythema multiforme in the amlodipine-induced case [74]. Serious cutaneous eruptions like Stevens–Johnson syndrome/toxic epidermal necrolysis have been reported with diltiazem [2, 3], nifedipine [2, 3], verapamil [2, 3, 58], and amlodipine [75].

Erythroderma/Exfoliative Dermatitis

Erythroderma has been reported with diltiazem [2, 3, 6, 76], nifedipine [3], and verapamil [2, 3]. The reaction was reported to occur between 3 and 10 days after initiation of diltiazem in three cases, resolving within 7–12 days upon discontinuation of the drug [6]. The patients were patch tested with diltiazem, verapamil, and nifedipine, all belonging to different subgroups of CCBs. Patch testing with diltiazem was positive in all three patients. One patient showed an additional patch test positivity to nifedipine and another one to verapamil, suggesting a cross-reactivity [6].

Drug Rash with Eosinophilia and Systemic Symptoms

Diltiazem was reported to be associated with cutaneous reactions suggestive of drug rash with eosinophilia and systemic symptoms [2, 77–79]. The reaction occurred within 2–10 days after starting diltiazem.

Angioedema/Urticaria

Angioedema/urticaria was reported with diltiazem [2, 3, 80, 81], nifedipine [2, 3, 81], verapamil [2, 3, 80, 81], amlodipine [82–84], and nicardipine [84].

Pruritus

Pruritus is a nonspecific cutaneous adverse reaction of drugs. It was reported in patients receiving CCB therapy alone or mainly in the setting of different types of cutaneous eruptions [2, 3, 26, 66, 80, 85, 86].

Oral Mucosal Reactions

Gingival hyperplasia is the main oral mucosal reaction induced by CCBs and is described above. Xerostomia is another reported side effect with CCBs [87, 88]. Oral ulceration was also suggested to be caused by CCBs in isolated cases [89]. The lesions were located on the tongue. One was suspected to be caused by diltiazem as withdrawal of the drug resulted in healing of the ulceration; another one was suspected to be caused by verapamil, showing improvement after dose reduction and later discontinuation of the drug, but recurring after administration of diltiazem [89]. These cases, especially the second case might also be consistent with oral mucosal fixed drug eruption.

Other Reported Adverse Cutaneous Drug Reactions to Calcium Channel Blockers

Cutaneous vasculitis was reported in patients using diltiazem, nifedipine, and verapamil [3, 4, 90]. *Petechia* or *purpura*, not associated with vasculitis, has also been reported with the use of some CCBs like amlodipine [91, 92], diltiazem [85, 92], and nifedipine [92]. The lesions were usually scattered. They might occur as a component of pigmented purpuric dermatosis in some cases [85, 92]. Other than spontaneous occurrence, purpura may also be provoked by Hess testing. It was suggested that the mechanism of purpura could be related with a pharmacologic effect, rather than an idiosyncratic effect, and it could result from capillary fragility and capillary leakage of erythrocytes [92].

Two case–control studies revealed that chronic *eczematous eruption* in the elderly was significantly associated with the use of CCBs [93, 94]. Eczema during the use of nifedipine [3], and generalized eczema evolving from maculopapular eruption due to nimodipine were also reported [30].

Granuloma annulare-like eruption was suggested to be induced by amlodipine [95], whereas *interstitial granulomatous drug reaction* was reported to occur during the use of some CCBs like diltiazem, verapamil, and amlodipine [96, 97].

Some of the CCBs were linked to the development of other reactions like *acne* from verapamil and diltiazem [3]; *alopecia* by diltiazem, nifedipine, and verapamil [2, 3]; *erythema nodosum* due to nifedipine [3]; *lymphomatoid drug eruption* (CD30+ T cell pseudolymphoma) by amlodipine [98, 99]; *skin thickening* and *sensory loss of the feet* due to diltiazem [100]; *palmar hyperkeratosis* with verapamil [101]; *hair discoloration* with nifedipine [3]; *hirsutism* with diltiazem, nifedipine, and verapamil [3]; *melanonychia* and *periungual pigmentation* with amlodipine [102]; *nail dystrophy* with nifedipine and verapamil [3]; and *hyperhidrosis* with diltiazem, nifedipine, and verapamil [3].

References

1. Ioulios P, Charalampos M, Efrossini T. The spectrum of cutaneous reactions associated with calcium antagonists: a review of the literature and the possible etiopathogenic mechanisms. Dermatol Online J. 2003;9:6.
2. Knowles S, Gupta AK, Shear NH. The spectrum of cutaneous reactions associated with diltiazem: three cases and a review of the literature. J Am Acad Dermatol. 1998;38:201–6.
3. Stern R, Khalsa JH. Cutaneous adverse reactions associated with calcium channel blockers. Arch Intern Med. 1989;149:829–32.
4. Kuo M, Winiarski N, Garella S. Nonthrombocytopenic purpura associated sequentially with nifedipine and diltiazem. Ann Pharmacother. 1992;26:1089–90.
5. Giustiniani S, Robustelli della Cuna F, Marieni M. Hyperplastic gingivitis during diltiazem therapy. Int J Cardiol. 1987;15:247–9.
6. Gonzalo Garijo MA, Perez Calderon R, de Argila Fernandez-Duran D, Rangel Mayoral JF. Cutaneous reactions due to diltiazem and cross reactivity with other calcium channel blockers. Allergol Immunopathol (Madr). 2005;33:238–40.
7. Westbrook P, Bednarczyk EM, Carlson M, Sheehan H, Bissada NF. Regression of nifedipine-induced gingival hyperplasia following switch to a same class calcium channel blocker, isradipine. J Periodontol. 1997;68:645–50.
8. Kubota K, Pearce GL, Inman WH. Vasodilation-related adverse events in diltiazem and dihydropyridine calcium antagonists studied by prescription-event monitoring. Eur J Clin Pharmacol. 1995;48:1–7.
9. Messerli FH. Vasodilatory edema: a common side effect of antihypertensive therapy. Curr Cardiol Rep. 2002;4:479–82.
10. Messerli FH, Grossman E. Pedal edema–not all dihydropyridine calcium antagonists are created equal. Am J Hypertens. 2002;15:1019–20.

11. Leonetti G, Magnani B, Pessina AC, Rappelli A, Trimarco B, Zanchetti A, COHORT Study Group. Tolerability of long-term treatment with lercanidipine versus amlodipine and lacidipine in elderly hypertensives. Am J Hypertens. 2002;15:932–40.
12. Kobrin I, Charlon V, Lindberg E, Pordy R. Safety of mibefradil, a new once-a-day, selective T-type calcium channel antagonist. Am J Cardiol. 1997;80:40C–6.
13. Ellis JS, Seymour RA, Steele JG, Robertson P, Butler TJ, Thomason JM. Prevalence of gingival overgrowth induced by calcium channel blockers: a community-based study. J Periodontol. 1999;70:63–7.
14. Miranda J, Brunet L, Roset P, Berini L, Farre M. Prevalence and risk of gingival overgrowth in patients treated with diltiazem or verapamil. J Clin Periodontol. 2005;32:294–8.
15. Pascual-Castroviejo I, Pascual Pascual SI. Nicardipine-induced gingival hyperplasia. Neurologia. 1997;12:37–9.
16. Brown RS, Sein P, Corio R, Bottomley WK. Nitrendipine-induced gingival hyperplasia. First case report. Oral Surg Oral Med Oral Pathol. 1990;70:593–6.
17. Young PC, Turiansky GW, Sau P, Liebman MD, Benson PM. Felodipine-induced gingival hyperplasia. Cutis. 1998;62:41–3.
18. Ikawa K, Ikawa M, Shimauchi H, Iwakura M, Sakamoto S. Treatment of gingival overgrowth induced by manidipine administration. J Periodontol. 2002;73:115–22.
19. Morisaki I, Dol S, Ueda K, Amano A, Hayashi M, Mihara J. Amlodipine-induced gingival overgrowth: periodontal responses to stopping and restarting the drug. Spec Care Dentist. 2001;21:60–2.
20. Karnik R, Bhat KM, Bhat GS. Prevalence of gingival overgrowth among elderly patients under amlodipine therapy at a large Indian teaching hospital. Gerodontology. 2012;29: 209–13.
21. Prisant LM, Herman W. Calcium channel blocker induced gingival overgrowth. J Clin Hypertens (Greenwich). 2002;4:310–1.
22. Cornes PG, Hole AC. Amlodipine gynaecomastia. Breast. 2001;10:544–5.
23. Komine N, Takeda Y, Nakamata T. Amlodipine-induced gynecomastia in two patients on long-term hemodialysis therapy. Clin Exp Nephrol. 2003;7:85–6.
24. Otto C, Richter WO. Unilateral gynecomastia induced by treatment with diltiazem. Arch Intern Med. 1994;154:351.
25. Romeo JH, Dombrowski R, Kwak YS, Fuehrer S, Aron DC. Hyperprolactinaemia and verapamil: prevalence and potential association with hypogonadism in men. Clin Endocrinol (Oxf). 1996;45:571–5.
26. Baker BA, Cacchione JG. Dermatologic cross-sensitivity between diltiazem and amlodipine. Ann Pharmacother. 1994;28:118–9.
27. Cholez C, Trechot P, Schmutz JL, Faure G, Bene MC, Barbaud A. Maculopapular rash induced by diltiazem: allergological investigations in four patients and cross reactions between calcium channel blockers. Allergy. 2003;58:1207–9.
28. Heymann WR. Diltiazem-induced drug eruption sparing seborrheic keratoses. Cutis. 2000;66:129–30.
29. Parish LC, Witkowski JA. Truncal morbilliform eruption due to nifedipine. Cutis. 1992;49:113–4.
30. Nucera E, Schavino D, Roncallo C, de Pasquale T, Buonomo A, Pollastrini E, Patriarca G. Delayed-type allergy to oral nimodipine. Contact Dermatitis. 2002;47:246–7.
31. Seggev JS, Lagstein Z. Photosensitivity skin reactions to calcium channel blockers. J Allergy Clin Immunol. 1996;97:852–5.
32. Young L, Shehade SA, Chalmers RJ. Cutaneous reactions to diltiazem. Clin Exp Dermatol. 1990;15:467.
33. Conilleau V, Dompmartin A, Michel M, Verneuil L, Leroy D. Photoscratch testing in systemic drug-induced photosensitivity. Photodermatol Photoimmunol Photomed. 2000;16: 62–6.
34. Grabczynska SA, Cowley N. Amlodipine induced-photosensitivity presenting as telangiectasia. Br J Dermatol. 2000;142:1255–6.

35. Bakkour W, Haylett AK, Gibbs NK, Chalmers RJ, Rhodes LE. Photodistributed telangiectasia induced by calcium channel blockers: case report and review of the literature. Photodermatol Photoimmunol Photomed. 2013;29:272–5.
36. Byun JW, Bang CI, Yang BH, Han SH, Song HJ, Lee HS, et al. Photodistributed telangiectasia induced by amlodipine. Ann Dermatol. 2011;23 Suppl 1:S30–2.
37. Collins P, Ferguson J. Photodistributed nifedipine-induced facial telangiectasia. Br J Dermatol. 1993;129:630–3.
38. Silvestre JF, Albares MP, Carnero L, Botella R. Photodistributed felodipine-induced facial telangiectasia. J Am Acad Dermatol. 2001;45:323–4.
39. Al-Niaimi F, Lyon C. Felodipine-induced eruptive telangiectasia following mastectomy and radiotherapy. Br J Dermatol. 2010;162:210–1.
40. Scherschun L, Lee MW, Lim HW. Diltiazem-associated photodistributed hyperpigmentation: a review of 4 cases. Arch Dermatol. 2001;137:179–82.
41. Kuykendall-Ivy T, Collier SL, Johnson SM. Diltiazem-induced hyperpigmentation. Cutis. 2004;73:239–40.
42. Boyer M, Katta R, Markus R. Diltiazem-induced photodistributed hyperpigmentation. Dermatol Online J. 2003;9:10.
43. Saladi RN, Cohen SR, Phelps RG, Persaud AN, Rudikoff D. Diltiazem induces severe photodistributed hyperpigmentation: case series, histoimmunopathology, management, and review of the literature. Arch Dermatol. 2006;142:206–10.
44. Jaka A, López-Pestaña A, Tuneu A, Lobo C, López-Núñez M, Ormaechea N. Letter: photodistributed reticulated hyperpigmentation related to diltiazem. Dermatol Online J. 2011; 17:14.
45. Kubo Y, Fukumoto D, Ishigami T, Hida Y, Arase S. Diltiazem-associated photodistributed hyperpigmentation: report of two Japanese cases and published work review. J Dermatol. 2010;37:807–11.
46. Erbagci Z. Amlodipine associated hyperpigmentation. Saudi Med J. 2004;25:103–5.
47. Serrão V, Caldas Lopes L, Campos Lopes JM, Lobo L, Ferreira A. Acute generalized exanthematous pustulosis associated with diltiazem. Acta Med Port. 2008;21:99–102.
48. Wakelin SH, James MP. Diltiazem-induced acute generalised exanthematous pustulosis. Clin Exp Dermatol. 1995;20:341–4.
49. Janier M, Gerault MH, Carlotti A, Vignon MD, Daniel F. Acute generalized exanthematous pustulosis due to diltiazem. Br J Dermatol. 1993;129:354–5.
50. Lambert DG, Dalac S, Beer F, Chavannet P, Portier H. Acute generalized exanthematous pustular dermatitis induced by diltiazem. Br J Dermatol. 1988;118:308–9.
51. Vicente-Calleja JM, Aguirre A, Landa N, Crespo V, Gonzalez-Perez R, Diaz-Perez JL. Acute generalized exanthematous pustulosis due to diltiazem: confirmation by patch testing. Br J Dermatol. 1997;137:837–9.
52. Fernández-Ruiz M, López-Medrano F, García-Ruiz F, Rodríguez-Peralto JL. Diltiazem-induced acute generalized exanthemic pustulosis: a case and review of the literature. Actas Dermosifiliogr. 2009;100:725–7.
53. Gubinelli E, Cocuroccia B, Girolomoni G. Subacute cutaneous lupus erythematosus induced by nifedipine. J Cutan Med Surg. 2003;7:243–6.
54. Crowson AN, Magro CM. Subacute cutaneous lupus erythematosus arising in the setting of calcium channel blocker therapy. Hum Pathol. 1997;28:67–73.
55. Crowson AN, Magro CM. Diltiazem and subacute cutaneous lupus erythematosus-like lesions. N Engl J Med. 1995;333:1429.
56. Callen JP. Drug-induced subacute cutaneous lupus erythematosus. Lupus. 2010;19:1107–11.
57. Cohen AD, Kagen M, Friger M, Halevy S. Calcium channel blockers intake and psoriasis: a case-control study. Acta Derm Venereol. 2001;81:347–9.
58. Kitamura K, Kanasashi M, Suga C, Saito S, Yoshida S, Ikezawa Z. Cutaneous reactions induced by calcium channel blocker: high frequency of psoriasiform eruptions. J Dermatol. 1993;20:279–86.
59. Latessa V. Erythromelalgia: a rare microvascular disease. J Vasc Nurs. 2010;28:67–71.

60. Sunahara JF, Gora-Harper ML, Nash KS. Possible erythromelalgia-like syndrome associated with nifedipine in a patient with Raynaud's phenomenon. Ann Pharmacother. 1996;30:484–6.
61. Levesque H, Moore N, Wolfe LM, Courtois H. Erythromelalgia induced by nicardipine (inverse Raynaud's phenomenon?). BMJ. 1989;298:1252–3.
62. Drenth JP, Michiels JJ, Van Joost T, Vuzevski VD. Verapamil-induced secondary erythermalgia. Br J Dermatol. 1992;127:292–4.
63. Nanayakkara PW, van der Veldt AA, Simsek S, Smulders YM, Rauwerda JA. Verapamil-induced erythermalgia. Neth J Med. 2007;65:349–51.
64. Swale VJ, McGregor JM. Amlodipine-associated lichen planus. Br J Dermatol. 2001;144:920–1.
65. Lakshmi C, Srinivas CR, Ramachandran B, Pillai SB, Nirmala V. Perforating lichenoid reaction to amlodipine. Indian J Dermatol. 2008;53:98–9.
66. Leibovici V, Zlotogorski A, Heyman A, Kanner A, Melmed RN. Polymorphous drug eruption due to nifedipine. Cutis. 1988;41:367.
67. Kim SC, Won JH, Ahn SK. Pemphigus foliaceus induced by nifedipine. Acta Derm Venereol. 1993;73:210–1.
68. Brenner S, Golan H, Bialy-Golan A, Ruocco V. Lesion topography in two cases of nifedipine-related pemphigus. J Eur Acad Dermatol Venereol. 1999;13:123–6.
69. Ameen M, Harman KE, Black MM. Pemphigoid nodularis associated with nifedipine. Br J Dermatol. 2000;142:575–7.
70. Shachar E, Bialy-Golan A, Srebrnik A, Brenner S. "Two-step" drug-induced bullous pemphigoid. Int J Dermatol. 1998;37:938–9.
71. Schroeder D, Saada D, Rafaa M, Ingen-Housz-Oro S, Valeyrie-Allanore L, Sigal ML. Verapamil-induced linear IgA disease mimicking toxic epidermal necrolysis. Ann Dermatol Venereol. 2011;138:302–6.
72. Low L, Zaheri S, Wakelin S. Amlodipine-induced linear IgA disease. Clin Exp Dermatol. 2012;37:649–51.
73. Sanders CJ, Neumann HA. Erythema multiforme, Stevens-Johnson syndrome, and diltiazem. Lancet. 1993;341:967.
74. Bewley AP, Feher MD, Staughton RC. Erythema multiforme following substitution of amlopidine for nifedipine. BMJ. 1993;307:241.
75. Baetz BE, Patton ML, Guilday RE, Reigart CL, Ackerman BH. Amlodipine-induced toxic epidermal necrolysis. J Burn Care Res. 2011;32:e158–60.
76. Odeh M. Exfoliative dermatitis associated with diltiazem. J Toxicol Clin Toxicol. 1997;35:101–4.
77. Romano A, Pietrantonio F, Garcovich A, Rumi C, Bellocci F, Caradonna P, Barone C. Delayed hypersensitivity to diltiazem in two patients. Ann Allergy. 1992;69:31–2.
78. Scolnick B, Brinberg D. Diltiazem and generalized lymphadenopathy. Ann Intern Med. 1985;102:558.
79. Lavrijsen AP, Van Dijke C, Vermeer BJ. Diltiazem-associated exfoliative dermatitis in a patient with psoriasis. Acta Derm Venereol. 1986;66:536–8.
80. Sadick NS, Katz AS, Schreiber TL. Angioedema from calcium channel blockers. J Am Acad Dermatol. 1989;21:132–3.
81. Hedner T, Samuelsson O, Lindholm L, Andren L, Wiholm BE. Precipitation of angioedema by antihypertensive drugs. J Hypertens Suppl. 1991;9:360–1.
82. Southward J, Irvine E, Rabinovich M. Probable amlodipine-induced angioedema. Ann Pharmacother. 2009;43:772–6.
83. Hom KA, Hirsch R, Elluru RG. Antihypertensive drug-induced angioedema causing upper airway obstruction in children. Int J Pediatr Otorhinolaryngol. 2012;76:14–9.
84. Pierce WA, Hederman AD, Gordon CJ, Ostrenga AR, Herrington B. Angioedema associated with dihydropyridine calcium-channel blockers in a child with Burkitt lymphoma. Am J Health Syst Pharm. 2011;68:402–6.
85. Inui S, Itami S, Yoshikawa K. A case of lichenoid purpura possibly caused by diltiazem hydrochloride. J Dermatol. 2001;28:100–2.

86. Orme S, da Costa D. Generalised pruritus associated with amlodipine. BMJ. 1997;315:463.
87. Litt JZ. Drug eruption reference manual. 19th ed. Boca Raton: CRC Press (Taylor and Francis Group); 2013.
88. Torpet LA, Kragelund C, Reibel J, Nauntofte B. Oral adverse drug reactions to cardiovascular drugs. Crit Rev Oral Biol Med. 2004;15:28–46.
89. Cohen DM, Bhattacharyya I, Lydiatt WM. Recalcitrant oral ulcers caused by calcium channel blockers: diagnosis and treatment considerations. J Am Dent Assoc. 1999;130:1611–8.
90. Sheehan-Dare RA, Goodfield MJ. Widespread cutaneous vasculitis associated with diltiazem. Postgrad Med J. 1988;64:467–8.
91. Murthy MB, Murthy B. Amlodipine-induced petechial rash. J Postgrad Med. 2011;57:341–2.
92. Cox NH, Walsh ML, Robson RH. Purpura and bleeding due to calcium-channel blockers: an underestimated problem? Case reports and a pilot study. Clin Exp Dermatol. 2009;34:487–91.
93. Joly P, Benoit-Corven C, Baricault S, Lambert A, Hellot MF, Josset V, et al. Chronic eczematous eruptions of the elderly are associated with chronic exposure to calcium channel blockers: results from a case-control study. J Invest Dermatol. 2007;127:2766–71.
94. Summers EM, Bingham CS, Dahle KW, Sweeney C, Ying J, Sontheimer RD. Chronic eczematous eruptions in the aging: further support for an association with exposure to calcium channel blockers. JAMA Dermatol. 2013;149:814–8.
95. Lim AC, Hart K, Murrell D. A granuloma annulare-like eruption associated with the use of amlodipine. Australas J Dermatol. 2002;43:24–7.
96. Magro CM, Crowson AN, Schapiro BL. The interstitial granulomatous drug reaction: a distinctive clinical and pathological entity. J Cutan Pathol. 1998;25:72–8.
97. Magro CM, Cruz-Inigo AE, Votava H, Jacobs M, Wolfe D, Crowson AN. Drug-associated reversible granulomatous T cell dyscrasia: a distinct subset of the interstitial granulomatous drug reaction. J Cutan Pathol. 2010;37 Suppl 1:96–111.
98. Fukamachi S, Sugita K, Sawada Y, Bito T, Nakamura M, Tokura Y. Drug-induced CD30+ T cell pseudolymphoma. Eur J Dermatol. 2009;19:292–4.
99. Kabashima R, Orimo H, Hino R, Nakashima D, Kabashima K, Tokura Y. CD30-positive T-cell pseudolymphoma induced by amlodipine. J Eur Acad Dermatol Venereol. 2008;22:1522–4.
100. Ilia R, Goldfarb B, Gueron M. Skin thickening and sensory loss of the feet during diltiazem therapy. Int J Cardiol. 1992;35:115.
101. Major P. Verapamil as a cause of palmar hyperkeratosis. Tidsskr Nor Laegeforen. 1983;103:2061.
102. Sladden MJ, Mortimer NJ, Osborne JE. Longitudinal melanonychia and pseudo-Hutchinson sign associated with amlodipine. Br J Dermatol. 2005;153:219–20.

Chapter 9
Diuretics

Keywords Diuretic • Acetazolamide • Furosemide • Thiazide • Photosensitivity • Lupus • Lichenoid • Bullous pemphigoid • Pseudoporphyria • Acute generalized exanthematous pustulosis • Erythema multiforme/Stevens–Johnson syndrome • Vasculitis • Maculopapular

Diuretics can be classified into different subgroups such as carbonic anhydrase inhibitors (acetazolamide, dichlorphenamide), loop-active agents (furosemide, torsemide, bumetanide, ethacrynic acid), thiazide-type diuretics (chlorothiazide, hydrochlorothiazide, bendroflumethiazide, hydroflumethiazide, trichlormethiazide, benzthiazide, cyclopenthiazide), thiazide-like diuretics (chlorthalidone, indapamide, metolazone, xipamide), potassium-sparing agents such as mineralocorticoid antagonists (spironolactone, eplerenone), and sodium channel inhibitors (amiloride, triamterene).

Diuretics which contain a sulfonamide moiety include thiazide-type diuretics, thiazide-like diuretics, furosemide, bumetanide, torsemide, and acetazolamide [1].

Regarding adverse cutaneous drug reactions, cross-reactivity between sulfonamide antibiotics and sulfonamide diuretics has always been debated. It is generally believed that the arylamine (NH2) group at the para-position on the benzene ring, the so-called para-amino group, is responsible for the common delayed type hypersensitivity reactions and the possible cross-reactions of sulfonamide antibiotics [2]. A cross-reaction between sulfonamide antibiotics and sulfonamide diuretics seems therefore to be very unlikely, because sulfonamide diuretics contain a sulfonamide moiety but not an arylamine group [3]. On the other hand, the mechanism behind T cell recognition of sulfonamide drugs is not yet clearly understood [1]. Presuming that T cell recognition might be related to the sulfonamide moiety or some other functional groups, a cross-reaction between sulfonamide antibiotics and other sulfonamides lacking an arylamine group would be theoretically possible [4]. Indeed, a patient with indapamide-induced fixed drug eruption was reported to react with sulfamethoxazole and sulfadiazine, all confirmed by positive oral challenge test [5]. Interestingly, a patient with type I hypersensitivity reaction from sulfamethoxazole-trimethoprim presenting with angioedema/urticaria has been reported to show cross-reactivity to hydrochlorothiazide [6]. This would also not be expected to

E. Özkaya, K.D. Yazganoğlu, *Adverse Cutaneous Drug Reactions to Cardiovascular Drugs*, DOI 10.1007/978-1-4471-6536-1_9

occur, again because of the lack of the sulfonylarylamine structure and functional groups in hydrochlorothiazide that are believed to be required for type I immunologic reactions as well [1].

Moreover, hydrochlorothiazide was reported to show cross-reactivity to paraphenylenediamine in a patient [7]. Paraphenylenediamine also contains a para-amino group and is an important contact allergen that is present mainly in hair dyes and black henna products [8]. Hair dyes are the major source for occupational sensitization with p-phenylenediamine among hairdressers, whereas black henna temporary tattoos are the main source for nonoccupational sensitization. Although not proven, there might be a theoretical risk for patients who are sensitized with p-phenylenediamine, to develop a drug eruption with sulfonamides including thiazide diuretics, due to possible formation of some unknown intermediate substances during their metabolic process [8].

Diuretics were often used as combination drugs, so in some cases the main inducer of the adverse reactions was not clear. In fact, the possibility of a compound drug allergy cannot be excluded, if the drugs were not used or tested separately.

Adverse cutaneous drug reactions to acetazolamide have been mainly reported due to its systemic use in ophthalmology [9].

Other than its systemic use, spironolactone was incriminated to cause allergic contact dermatitis due to its topical use for other indications such as acne vulgaris and androgenetic alopecia [10, 11].

The adverse cutaneous drug reactions described below are meant to be sorted by starting from the well-known reactions of diuretics to the lesser known ones. The major ones are summarized in Table 9.1.

Photosensitivity

Photosensitivity is a well-established cutaneous side effect of thiazide diuretics, especially with hydrochlorothiazide (Figs. 1.45, 1.46, 1.48, 1.49 and 1.50). Other diuretics like torsemide or combination diuretics consisting of hydrochlorothiazide plus triamterene, or hydrochlorothiazide plus amiloride were also responsible for cutaneous photosensitivity [12–21].

The photosensitivity reaction usually presents as erythematous lesions with or without edema or papules on sun-exposed areas [13], and may show eczematous features in the histopathology [16]. However, the clinical appearance may also be lichenoid [14, 15, 21] or petechial [12]. Even an erythrodermic case has been reported [16]. Although the lesions were usually limited to the sun-exposed areas, they also involved the covered skin in some patients [13]. Pigmentation, particularly diffuse pigmentation on sun-exposed areas, was also reported that usually subsided after discontinuation of the drug [13].

The first reported case of diuretic-induced photosensitive drug eruption was due to chlorothiazide, presenting as non-pruritic petechial eruption on sun-exposed skin

Table 9.1 Major adverse cutaneous drug reactions with diuretics

Adverse cutaneous drug reaction	Main inducers
Photosensitivity	Thiazides (hydrochlorothiazide, others), xipamide
Drug-induced lupus erythematosus	
SCLE (mainly)	Hydrochlorothiazide, chlorothiazide, hydrochlorothiazide + triamterene
SLE	Hydrochlorothiazide
Bullous eruptions	
Bullous pemphigoid	Furosemide, spironolactone, bumetanide
Linear IgA dermatosis	Furosemide
Pemphigus vulgaris	Acetazolamide
Pemphigus foliaceus	Indapamide
Pseudoporphyria	Furosemide, bumetanide, chlorthalidone, hydrochlorothiazide + triamterene
Acute generalized exanthematous pustulosis	Hydrochlorothiazide, furosemide, acetazolamide
Erythema multiforme	Furosemide, indapamide + sertraline, spironolactone
Stevens–Johnson syndrome/toxic epidermal necrolysis	Hydrochlorothiazide, acetazolamide, indapamide, furosemide
Vasculitis	Thiazides, chlorthalidone, metolazone, furosemide, hydrochlorothiazide + amiloride
Lichen planus/lichenoid eruptions	Hydrochlorothiazide, furosemide, spironolactone
Angioedema/urticaria	Hydrochlorothiazide, chlorthalidone, indapamide, furosemide, acetazolamide, amiloride
Maculopapular eruption	Indapamide, acetazolamide, spironolactone
Interstitial granulomatous drug reaction	Furosemide
Sweet syndrome	Furosemide
Hypertrichosis	Acetazolamide

SCLE subacute cutaneous lupus erythematosus, *SLE* systemic lupus erythematosus

which developed 2 weeks after the drug intake, and resolved within 4 weeks following discontinuation of the drug [12].

The reaction was thought to be phototoxic [17], and it was postulated not to persist after drug withdrawal if a specific photodermatosis was not present or another photoactive drug was not used [13]. However, a photoallergic response may not be excluded, as photopatch testing was reported to be positive in some cases [18]. Interestingly, chronic photosensitivity was reported in patients due to thiazide intake even after the withdrawal of the drug [16]. The phototoxic potential of thiazide diuretics have been studied in 22 individuals by phototesting before and 2 weeks after therapy with hydrochlorothiazide or bendroflumethiazide [17]. The minimal erythemal doses for UVA by monochromator phototesting were found to be reduced in 13 subjects after receiving the diuretic. However, clinical photosensitivity was not observed in any of those cases [17].

Both the UVA and UVB wavebands were found to be responsible for thiazide-induced photosensitivity by phototesting [13, 16]. Lesions improved with only photoprotection without withdrawal of the drug in some cases [13]. However, discontinuation of the drug was required in most of the cases in order to achieve a complete resolution of the reaction [13]. On the other hand, as stated above, some cases continued to experience photosensitivity even after the withdrawal of the drug [16]. Development of actinic reticuloid was reported in one of these patients [16]. In the management of chronic photosensitivity persisting after withdrawal of the drug, PUVA (psoralen plus UVA radiation) therapy was tried. It was started along with an initial short course of high-dose corticosteroids in order to prevent an exacerbation of photosensitivity, and was generally successful to control the condition, except in a case who discontinued the PUVA treatment after a while [16].

Photo-onycholysis was reported to develop after 10 years of use of indapamide in a patient without accompanying photosensitivity at other skin sites. The reaction resolved within 4 months after discontinuation of the drug [22].

A patient was reported with photosensitivity who also developed photoleukoderma on sun-exposed sites, after the use of a combination drug consisting of losartan and hydrochlorothiazide. Photopatch test was positive with the drug [23]. The skin returned entirely to its normal color within 5 months after discontinuation of the drug and with topical use of tacrolimus and corticosteroids.

Photosensitivity was also reported with a combination drug of triamterene and xipamide showing positive photochallenge test [24]. The patient reacted with chlortalidone as well, suggesting that xipamide was the inducer, as xipamide and chlortalidone have a structural similarity [24, 25]. Another patient with xipamide-induced photoallergic drug eruption has also been reported [26].

Drug-Induced Lupus Erythematosus

Hydrochlorothiazide was reported to be the most often associated drug with subacute cutaneous lupus erythematosus (SCLE) [27]. Chlorothiazide and a combination of hydrochlorothiazide and triamterene were also implicated as causative drugs [27, 28].

In addition to the classic presentation of SCLE as annular scaly plaques mainly on the upper trunk, patients featuring cutaneous eruption like photodistributed erythema were also reported [29]. The reaction was reported to start within a few months or even up to a few years after the initiation of the drug [29, 30]. Positive antibodies to SSA/Ro antigen and antinuclear antibody positivity were demonstrated [29, 30]. Anti-SSA antibodies were found to remain positive in some patients after discontinuing hydrochlorothiazide. The reaction resolved within 2–8 weeks after the cessation of the drug [29, 30].

Apart from SCLE, systemic lupus erythematosus (SLE)-like dermatitis was also reported. A patient with persistent erythema on the face and arms with histopathological findings similar to lupus erythematosus was reported with persistent antinuclear antibody positivity even after 2 years of discontinuing hydrochlorothiazide. This case did not meet the criteria for the diagnosis of SLE, but later developed lupus pneumonitis [31]. Spironolactone was implicated to be the inducer of a cutaneous eruption that was clinically and histopathologically similar to SLE, but serologic findings for SLE were lacking [32].

Bullous Eruption

Bullous Pemphigoid

Among diuretics, furosemide and spironolactone are well-known drugs to be associated with the development of bullous pemphigoid [33–37]. Moreover, bullous pemphigoid due to bumetanide was also reported [38].

A multicenter prospective case–control study searching for a relation between chronically used medications and drug-induced bullous pemphigoid revealed that, among diuretics, only aldosterone antagonists increased the risk of bullous pemphigoid [39]. Another multicenter prospective case–control study evaluating potential risk factors for the development of bullous pemphigoid also found an association between chronic usage of spironolactone and the occurrence of bullous pemphigoid [40]. On the contrary, a recent study found an increased use of loop diuretics in bullous pemphigoid patients rather than spironolactone [41].

Linear IgA Dermatosis

Furosemide-induced linear IgA dermatosis seems to be extremely rare in the literature [42]. The eruption started as palmoplantar erythema and bullae 3 days after taking furosemide, and later progressed to involve the entire trunk, extremities, hard palate, and buccal mucosa. The diagnosis of linear IgA dermatosis was confirmed with histopathological and direct immunofluorescence findings. The lesions resolved after discontinuation of furosemide and a short-term therapy with dapsone [42].

Pemphigus

Acetazolamide was suspected as a cause of the relapse of pemphigus in few cases [43, 44]. In one report, it was reported that the patient had been using the drug for a month prior to the relapse of pemphigus vulgaris. The chemical amide group of acetazolamide was thought to play a causative role [43].

Pemphigus foliaceus was reported to be induced by indapamide [45, 46].

Pseudoporphyria

Drug-induced pseudoporphyria is characterized with skin fragility and blistering mainly on sun-exposed areas, resembling porphyria cutanea tarda [47]. Lesions heal with hyperpigmentation, scarring, and formation of milia. In contrast to porphyria cutanea tarda, porphyrin levels are normal in drug-induced cases [48].

It was reported during treatment with bumetanide [49], chlorthalidone [50], furosemide [51], and a combination drug of hydrochlorothiazide and triamterene [52].

Acute Generalized Exanthematous Pustulosis

Acute generalized exanthematous pustulosis (AGEP) was reported to occur with diuretics in several cases. Hydrochlorothiazide [53], furosemide [54], and acetazolamide [9] were reported to induce the eruption.

The reaction started within a few hours after the first dose of the drug in the furosemide-induced case, and resolved within 1 week after discontinuation of the drug [54]. The patient had a history of a previous skin eruption due to furosemide. A positive lymphocyte transformation test suggested an immunologic mechanism.

Hydrochlorothiazide-induced AGEP started after 6 days of treatment and cleared completely 6 days after stopping the drug in the reported case [53]. Fever and elevated liver function tests accompanied the reaction without eosinophilia. No confirmatory skin test was performed.

Acetazolamide, mainly used as systemic treatment in ophthalmology, was implicated as a causative agent in patients with AGEP. In a report including four patients, the reaction started within 1 day or two after the onset of medication [9]. Patch tests with acetazolamide revealed positive results in two of the three tested patients. The patient with negative patch test developed eczematous reaction on prick and intradermal test areas with acetazolamide after 2 and 4 days. The authors suggested that delayed readings of skin tests for immediate hypersensitivity, such as prick and intradermal tests, might be sensitive in the diagnosis of delayed hypersensitivity to acetazolamide [9].

Erythema Multiforme/Stevens–Johnson Syndrome/ Toxic Epidermal Necrolysis

Erythema multiforme or severe drug eruptions like Stevens–Johnson syndrome/ toxic epidermal necrolysis were reported to occur with some of the diuretics.

Furosemide [55, 56], indapamide plus sertraline [57], and spironolactone [58] were implicated to be the inducer drugs in cutaneous reactions reported as erythema multiforme. However, the clinical diagnosis of erythema multiforme was not confirmed histopathologically in some patients; moreover, the clinical or histopathological findings were not typical for erythema multiforme in some.

Stevens–Johnson syndrome has been reported to develop with the use of hydrochlorothiazide [59], acetazolamide [60, 61], indapamide [62, 63], and furosemide [64]; toxic epidermal necrolysis with indapamide [65, 66]; and severe bullous eruption mimicking toxic epidermal necrolysis with furosemide [67]. The reported Stevens–Johnson syndrome induced by acetazolamide was mainly related with its oral use in glaucoma treatment and was particularly observed in Asian patients. Moreover, as Stevens–Johnson syndrome was also reported with the use of another carbonic anhydrase inhibitor, methazolamide in Asian patients, and as the human leukocyte antigen (HLA) typing results of some of the Stevens–Johnson syndrome cases induced by either drug were positive for HLA-B59, a genetic susceptibility was suggested in these patients [61].

According to a case–control study, thiazide diuretics were not found to be associated with increased risk for Stevens–Johnson syndrome or toxic epidermal necrolysis [68]. Interestingly, a patient with a history of hypersensitivity to sulfonamide antibiotics was reported to tolerate hydrochlorothiazide for 16 months without any problems, but developed toxic epidermal necrolysis after indapamide intake [66].

Vasculitis

Cutaneous vasculitis, mainly leukocytoclastic vasculitis, was reported to occur with thiazides, hydrochlorothiazide + amiloride, chlorthalidone, furosemide, and metolazone [69–72].

In a case series of 25 patients presented as necrotizing cutaneous vasculitis, 24 were over 50 years old, 11 were using thiazides (most using chlorothiazide, others hydrochlorothiazide or trichlormethiazide), and 3 were on chlorthalidone therapy, but most of them were also taking other drugs. Positive rechallenge test with hydrochlorothiazide and later with chlorthalidone was yielded in one of the patients using hydrochlorothiazide [69].

In a patient with leukocytoclastic vasculitis who was taking several drugs including a combination drug of hydrochlorothiazide and amiloride, the eruption resolved upon discontinuation of the combination drug without any additional specific therapy for vasculitis [70].

Lichenoid Eruption

In addition to photodistributed lichenoid eruptions described above, non-photodistributed lichenoid skin reactions can also be seen with diuretics like hydrochlorothiazide, spironolactone, and furosemide [73–76]. Accompanying mucosal lesions were reported rarely [75]. Hypertrophic lichenoid pattern was reported in one case [76]. Patch test revealed positive results to the suspected offending drug in some cases, namely, in one case to spironolactone [73], and in another one to a combination drug containing hydrochlorothiazide and irbesartan [74]. Interestingly, patch test was not positive to single substances in the latter case, suggesting a compound allergy. One patient with lichenoid eruption probably induced by hydrochlorothiazide was administered furosemide that caused reappearance of the lesions which resolved upon discontinuation of furosemide, suggesting cross-sensitivity between the two drugs [75].

Angioedema/Urticaria

Angioedema/urticaria was reported with some of the diuretics [19] including indapamide [77], hydrochlorothiazide [6], acetazolamide [78], chlorthalidone [79], amiloride [20], and furosemide [80].

Maculopapular Eruption

Indapamide was implicated to be associated with maculopapular reactions in some patients. The reaction started from several days up to 15 days of administration. Fever accompanied in some cases; however, it was not reported in detail whether maculopapular eruption and fever were parts of a "drug rash with eosinophilia and systemic symptoms" in these cases [77].

Oral acetazolamide, mainly used in ophthalmology, was also implicated as a cause in maculopapular eruptions. In a report including seven patients with maculopapular eruption, the onset of the eruption was usually within 1 day after starting acetazolamide, except in one case whose eruption started after 5 days of drug intake [9]. Concomitant mucosal lesions were reported in one case. Patch test to acetazolamide was positive in five of the six tested patients. The patient with a negative patch test, namely the same patient who had experienced acetazolamide-induced AGEP in another setting of drug use as described above, developed eczematous reaction on prick and intradermal test areas with acetazolamide after 2 and 4 days. The authors suggested that delayed readings of skin tests for immediate hypersensitivity such as prick and intradermal tests might be sensitive in the diagnosis of delayed hypersensitivity to acetazolamide [9].

A case of maculopapular eruption due to systemic administration of spironolactone was reported. Further confirmatory tests including patch test and rechallenge with the drug yielded positive results [81].

Pruritus

Pruritus is a nonspecific cutaneous adverse reaction of drugs. It was also reported in patients receiving diuretics [19]. It usually accompanies different types of cutaneous drug eruptions [14, 16, 34, 73–76].

Other Reported Adverse Cutaneous Drug Reactions to Diuretics

Sweet syndrome was reported to be associated with furosemide [82, 83]. In the reported two cases, the reaction started within 3 days and 6 weeks of furosemide therapy, respectively, and resolved after the cessation of the drug [82, 83].

Interstitial granulomatous drug reaction was described during the use of furosemide that resolved after the withdrawal of the drug [84, 85].

Psoriasiform eruption with chlorthalidone [86] and *pustular psoriasis* precipitated with acetazolamide [87] were also reported.

Pityriasis rosea-like eruption was reported in patients using hydrochlorothiazide in combination with other drugs, mainly angiotensin-converting enzyme inhibitors [88].

A case of *papuloerythroderma of Ofuji* was reported with the use of furosemide. Furosemide was confirmed to be the culprit drug by a positive rechallenge test [89].

Fixed drug eruption was reported to be induced by indapamide [5].

Eczematous eruption was seen during the use of angiotensin-converting enzyme inhibitors or angiotensin II receptor blockers combined to hydrochlorothiazide [90].

Symmetrical drug-related intertriginous and flexural exanthema was reported to be induced by telmisartan–hydrochlorothiazide [91].

Spironolactone was reported to be associated with reactions like *xerosis*, *chloasma-like pigmentation*, and *gynecomastia/breast enlargement* [92, 93].

Generalized erythematous rash was reported with indapamide that might be suggestive of *erythroderma* [77].

Thrombocytopenic or nonthrombocytopenic *purpura* may be observed during the use of some diuretic drugs, mainly thiazides and furosemide [19].

Apart from their systemic use as cardiovascular medications, topical use of spironolactone and acetazolamide was implicated as a cause of *allergic contact dermatitis* in some cases [10, 11, 94].

Cold extremities are among the reported side effects of diuretics [95].

A case of *lymphomatoid drug eruption* was associated with the use of a combination drug containing hydrochlorothiazide and amiloride [96]. In a prospective study, hydrochlorothiazide was suggested as an antigenic trigger for mycosis fungoides in a small subset of patients [97].

Acetazolamide was reported among the frequent inducers of *hypertrichosis* [98].

Xerostomia is also a reported side effect with diuretics [99].

References

1. Boehringer SK. Sulfa drugs and sulfa-allergic patient. Pharm Lett/Prescr Lett. 2005;21: 211113.
2. Lee AG, Johnson KK, Green DL, Rife JP, Limon L. Sulfonamide cross-reactivity: fact or fiction? Ann Pharmacother. 2005;39:290–301.
3. Garg A, Smith W. Sulfur allergies can be misleading. J Pharm Pract Res. 2013;43:332.
4. Brackett CC, Singh H, Block JH. Likelihood and mechanisms of cross-allergenicity between sulfonamide antibiotics and other drugs containing a sulfonamide functional group. Pharmacotherapy. 2004;24:856–70.
5. De Barrio M, Tornero P, Zubeldia JM, Sierra Z, Matheu V, Herrero T. Fixed drug eruption induced by indapamide. Cross-reactivity with sulfonamides. J Investig Allergol Clin Immunol. 1998;8:253–5.
6. Ruscin JM, Page 2nd RL, Scott J. Hydrochlorothiazide-induced angioedema in a patient allergic to sulfonamide antibiotics: evidence from a case report and a review of the literature. Am J Geriatr Pharmacother. 2006;4:325–9.

7. Jacob SE, Zapolanski T, Chayavichitsilp P. Sensitivity to para-phenylenediamine and intolerance to hydrochlorothiazide. Dermatitis. 2008;19:E44–5.
8. Ozkaya E, Yazganoğlu KD. Henna stone: a lesser-known solid material from which to obtain black henna paste. Contact Dermatitis. 2013;69:386.
9. Jachiet M, Bellon N, Assier H, Amsler E, Gaouar H, Pecquet C, et al. Cutaneous adverse drug reaction to oral acetazolamide and skin tests. Dermatology. 2013;226:347–52. doi:10.1159/000350939.
10. Corazza M, Strumia R, Lombardi AR, Virgili A. Allergic contact dermatitis from spironolactone. Contact Dermatitis. 1996;35:365–6.
11. Aguirre A, Manzano D, Zabala R, Eizaguirre X, Diaz-Perez JL. Allergic contact dermatitis from spironolactone. Contact Dermatitis. 1994;30:312.
12. Norins A. Chlorothiazide drug eruption involving photosensitization. AMA Arch Derm. 1959;79:592.
13. Addo HA, Ferguson J, Frain-Bell W. Thiazide-induced photosensitivity: a study of 33 subjects. Br J Dermatol. 1987;116:749–60.
14. Johnston GA. Thiazide-induced lichenoid photosensitivity. Clin Exp Dermatol. 2002;27:670–2.
15. Byrd DR, Ahmed I. Photosensitive lichenoid reaction to torsemide–a loop diuretic. Mayo Clin Proc. 1997;72:930–1.
16. Robinson HN, Morison WL, Hood AF. Thiazide diuretic therapy and chronic photosensitivity. Arch Dermatol. 1985;121:522–4.
17. Diffey BL, Langtry J. Phototoxic potential of thiazide diuretics in normal subjects. Arch Dermatol. 1989;125:1355–8.
18. Wagner SN, Welke F, Goos M. Occupational UVA-induced allergic photodermatitis in a welder due to hydrochlorothiazide and ramipril. Contact Dermatitis. 2000;43:245–6.
19. Frishman WH, Brosnan BD, Grossman M, Dasgupta D, Sun DK. Adverse dermatologic effects of cardiovascular drug therapy: part II. Cardiol Rev. 2002;10:285–300.
20. Litt JZ. Drug eruption reference manual. 19th ed. Boca Raton: CRC Press (Taylor and Francis Group); 2013.
21. Almeyda J, Levantine A. Drug reactions. XVI. Lichenoid drug eruptions. Br J Dermatol. 1971;85:604–7.
22. Rutherford T, Sinclair R. Photo-onycholysis due to indapamide. Australas J Dermatol. 2007;48:35–6.
23. Masuoka E, Bito T, Shimizu H, Nishigori C. Dysfunction of melanocytes in photoleukomelanoderma following photosensitivity caused by hydrochlorothiazide. Photodermatol Photoimmunol Photomed. 2011;27:328–30.
24. Lehmann P, Hölzle E, Plewig G. Photoallergy to Neotri and cross reaction to tenoretic–detection by systemic photoprovocation. Hautarzt. 1988;39:38–41.
25. Prichard BN, Brogden RN. Xipamide. A review of its pharmacodynamic and pharmacokinetic properties and therapeutic efficacy. Drugs. 1985;30:313–32.
26. Schauder S. Photosensitivity following enoxacin and xipamide: combined phototoxic and photo-allergic reaction to enoxacin, photo-allergic reaction to xipamide with subsequent transient light reaction. Z Hautkr. 1990;65:253–62.
27. Callen JP. Drug-induced subacute cutaneous lupus erythematosus. Lupus. 2010;19:1107–11.
28. Darken M, McBurney EI. Subacute cutaneous lupus erythematosus-like drug eruption due to combination diuretic hydrochlorothiazide and triamterene. J Am Acad Dermatol. 1988;18: 38–42.
29. Srivastava M, Rencic A, Diglio G, Santana H, Bonitz P, Watson R, et al. Drug-induced, Ro/SSA-positive cutaneous lupus erythematosus. Arch Dermatol. 2003;139:45–9.
30. Reed BR, Huff JC, Jones SK, Orton PW, Lee LA, Norris DA. Subacute cutaneous lupus erythematosus associated with hydrochlorothiazide therapy. Ann Intern Med. 1985;103:49–51.
31. Goodrich AL, Kohn SR. Hydrochlorothiazide-induced lupus erythematosus: a new variant? J Am Acad Dermatol. 1993;28:1001–2.

32. Uddin MS, Lynfield YL, Grosberg SJ, Stiefler R. Cutaneous reaction to spironolactone resembling lupus erythematosus. Cutis. 1979;24:198–200.
33. Stavropoulos PG, Soura E, Antoniou C. Drug-induced pemphigoid: a review of the literature. J Eur Acad Dermatol Venereol. 2014;28:1133–40. doi:10.1111/jdv.12366.
34. Fellner MJ, Katz JM. Occurrence of bullous pemphigoid after furosemide therapy. Arch Dermatol. 1976;112:75–7.
35. Modeste AB, Cordel N, Courville P, Gilbert D, Lauret P, Joly P. Bullous pemphigoid induced by spironolactone. Ann Dermatol Venereol. 2002;129:56–8.
36. Grange F, Scrivener Y, Koessler A, Straub P, Guillaume JC. Spironolactone-induced pemphigoid. Ann Dermatol Venereol. 1997;124:700–2.
37. Baz K, Ikizoglu G, Kaya TI, Koca A. Furosemide-induced bullous pemphigoid. J Eur Acad Dermatol Venereol. 2002;16:81–2.
38. Boulinguez S, Bernard P, Bedane C, le Brun V, Bonnetblanc JM. Bullous pemphigoid induced by bumetanide. Br J Dermatol. 1998;138:548–9.
39. Bastuji-Garin S, Joly P, Picard-Dahan C, Bernard P, Vaillant L, Pauwels C, et al. Drugs associated with bullous pemphigoid. A case-control study. Arch Dermatol. 1996;132:272–6.
40. Bastuji-Garin S, Joly P, Lemordant P, Sparsa A, Bedane C, Delaporte E, et al. Risk factors for bullous pemphigoid in the elderly: a prospective case-control study. J Invest Dermatol. 2011;131:637–43.
41. Lloyd-Lavery A, Chi CC, Wojnarowska F, Taghipour K. The associations between bullous pemphigoid and drug use: a UK case-control study. JAMA Dermatol. 2013;149:58–62.
42. Cerottini JP, Ricci C, Guggisberg D, Panizzon RG. Drug-induced linear IgA bullous dermatosis probably induced by furosemide. J Am Acad Dermatol. 1999;41:103–5.
43. Lo Schiavo A, Sangiuliano S, Puca RV, Brunetti G, Ruocco E. Pemphigus relapse and acetazolamide, a drug with an active amide group: a casual or causal relationship? J Eur Acad Dermatol Venereol. 2009;23:716–7.
44. Schmutz JL, Barbaud A, Trechot P. Pemphigus relapse and acetazolamide. Ann Dermatol Venereol. 2010;137:500.
45. Bayramgürler D, Erçin C, Apaydin R, Unal G. Indapamide-induced pemphigus foliaceus. J Dermatolog Treat. 2001;12:175–7.
46. Schmutz JL, Barbaud A, Trechot P. Indapamide-induced pemphigus foliaceus a sulfurous affair? Ann Dermatol Venereol. 2002;129:1085.
47. Al-Niaimi F. Drug eruptions in dermatology. Expert Rev Dermatol. 2011;6:273–86.
48. Ramsay CA. Drug induced pseudoporphyria. J Rheumatol. 1991;18:799–800.
49. Leitao EA, Person JR. Bumetanide-induced pseudoporphyria. J Am Acad Dermatol. 1990;23:129–30.
50. Baker EJ, Reed KD, Dixon SL. Chlorthalidone-induced pseudoporphyria: clinical and microscopic findings of a case. J Am Acad Dermatol. 1989;21:1026–9.
51. Breier F, Feldmann R, Pelzl M, Gschnait F. Pseudoporphyria cutanea tarda induced by furosemide in a patient undergoing peritoneal dialysis. Dermatology. 1998;197:271–3.
52. Motley RJ. Pseudoporphyria due to dyazide in a patient with vitiligo. BMJ. 1990;300:1468.
53. Petavy-Catala C, Martin L, Fontes V, Lorette G, Vaillant L. Hydrochlorothiazide-induced acute generalized exanthematous pustulosis. Acta Derm Venereol. 2001;81:209.
54. Noce R, Paredes BE, Pichler WJ, Krahenbuhl S. Acute generalized exanthematic pustulosis (AGEP) in a patient treated with furosemide. Am J Med Sci. 2000;320:331–3.
55. Gibson TP, Blue P. Erythema multiforme and furosemide therapy. JAMA. 1970;212:1709.
56. Zugerman C, La Voo EJ. Erythema multiforme caused by oral furosemide. Arch Dermatol. 1980;116:518–9.
57. Gales BJ, Gales MA. Erythema multiforme and angioedema with indapamide and sertraline. Am J Hosp Pharm. 1994;51:118–9.
58. Greenberger PA, Lazar HP. Readministration of spironolactone in the spironolactone-intolerant patient. N Engl Reg Allergy Proc. 1986;7:343–5.
59. Ting HC, Adam BA. Stevens-Johnson syndrome. A review of 34 cases. Int J Dermatol. 1985;24:587–91.

60. Ogasawara K, Tomitsuka N, Kobayashi M, Komoribayashi N, Fukuda T, Saitoh H, et al. Stevens-Johnson syndrome associated with intravenous acetazolamide administration for evaluation of cerebrovascular reactivity. Case report. Neurol Med Chir (Tokyo). 2006;46:161–3.
61. Her Y, Kil MS, Park JH, Kim CW, Kim SS. Stevens-Johnson syndrome induced by acetazolamide. J Dermatol. 2011;38:272–5.
62. Spinler SA, Globus NJ, Raymond JZ, Lancefield ML. Indapamide-associated Stevens-Johnson syndrome. Cutis. 1992;50:200–2.
63. Sanz-Muñoz C, Martínez-Morán C, Torrero-Antón MV, Miranda-Romero A. Indapamide-associated Stevens-Johnson syndrome. Actas Dermosifiliogr. 2008;99:321–2.
64. Wright AA, Vesta KS, Stark JE, Smith WJ. Stevens-Johnson syndrome associated with furosemide: a case report. J Pharm Pract. 2010;23:367–70.
65. Black RJ, Murphy P, Robinson TJ, Scott KW. Toxic epidermal necrolysis associated with indapamide. BMJ. 1990;301:1280–1.
66. Partanen J, Pohjola-Sintonen S, Makijarvi M, Harma M. Toxic epidermal necrolysis due to indapamide. Arch Dermatol. 1993;129:793.
67. Mebazaa A, Zaïem A, Béji S, El Héni I, El Euch D, Mokni M, et al. Bullous eruption in a patient treated with low dose of furosemide for lupic glomerulonephritis. Therapie. 2011;66:183–4.
68. Roujeau JC, Kelly JP, Naldi L, Rzany B, Stern RS, Anderson T, et al. Medication use and the risk of Stevens-Johnson syndrome or toxic epidermal necrolysis. N Engl J Med. 1995;333:1600–7.
69. Björnberg A, Gisslen H. Thiazides: a cause of necrotising vasculitis? Lancet. 1965;2:982–3.
70. Grunwald MH, Halevy S, Livni E. Allergic vasculitis induced by hydrochlorothiazide: confirmation by mast cell degranulation test. Isr J Med Sci. 1989;25:572–4.
71. Hendricks WM, Ader RS. Furosemide-induced cutaneous necrotizing vasculitis. Arch Dermatol. 1977;113:375.
72. Cox NH, Hodkin P. Vasculitis due to metolazone. Postgrad Med J. 1991;67:860.
73. Schon MP, Tebbe B, Trautmann C, Orfanos CE. Lichenoid drug eruption induced by spironolactone. Acta Derm Venereol. 1994;74:476.
74. Pfab F, Athanasiadis GI, Kollmar A, Ring J, Ollert M. Lichenoid drug eruption due to an antihypertonic drug containing irbesartan and hydrochlorothiazide. Allergy. 2006;61:786–7.
75. Aouam K, Ali HB, Youssef M, Chaabane A, Hamdi MH, Boughattas NA, Zili JE. Lichenoid eruption associated with hydrochlorothiazide and possible cross reactivity to furosemide. Therapie. 2009;64:344–7.
76. Arias-Santiago S, Aneiros-Fernandez J, Aceituno-Madera P, Burkhardt-Perez P, Naranjo Sintes R. Hypertrophic lichenoid eruption due to furosemide. Acta Derm Venereol. 2010;90:78–9.
77. Stricker BH, Biriell C. Skin reactions and fever with indapamide. Br Med J (Clin Res Ed). 1987;295:1313–4.
78. Lee AG, Anderson R, Kardon RH, Wall M. Presumed "sulfa allergy" in patients with intracranial hypertension treated with acetazolamide or furosemide: cross-reactivity, myth or reality? Am J Ophthalmol. 2004;138:114–8.
79. Piller LB, Ford CE, Davis BR, Nwachuku C, Black HR, Oparil S, et al. Incidence and predictors of angioedema in elderly hypertensive patients at high risk for cardiovascular disease: a report from the Antihypertensive and Lipid-Lowering Treatment to Prevent Heart Attack Trial (ALLHAT). J Clin Hypertens (Greenwich). 2006;8:649–56.
80. Domínguez-Ortega J, Martínez-Alonso JC, Domínguez-Ortega C, Fuentes MJ, Frades A, Fernández-Colino T. Anaphylaxis to oral furosemide. Allergol Immunopathol (Madr). 2003;31:345–7.
81. Alonso JC, Ortega FJ, Gonzalo MJ, Palla PS. Cutaneous reaction to oral spironolactone with positive patch test. Contact Dermatitis. 2002;47:178–9.
82. Govindarajan G, Bashir Q, Kuppuswamy S, Brooks C. Sweet syndrome associated with furosemide. South Med J. 2005;98:570–2.
83. Cobb MW. Furosemide-induced eruption simulating Sweet's syndrome. J Am Acad Dermatol. 1989;21:339–43.

84. Perrin C, Lacour JP, Castanet J, Michiels JF. Interstitial granulomatous drug reaction with a histological pattern of interstitial granulomatous dermatitis. Am J Dermatopathol. 2001;23:295–8.
85. Magro CM, Crowson AN, Schapiro BL. The interstitial granulomatous drug reaction: a distinctive clinical and pathological entity. J Cutan Pathol. 1998;25:72–8.
86. Wolf R, Dorfman B, Krakowski A. Psoriasiform eruption induced by captopril and chlorthalidone. Cutis. 1987;40:162–4.
87. Kuroda K, Kojima T, Tanabe E, Fujita M, Shinkai H. Pustular psoriasis precipitated by acetazolamide. J Dermatol. 1995;22:784–7.
88. Atzori L, Pinna AL, Ferreli C, Aste N. Pityriasis rosea-like adverse reaction: review of the literature and experience of an Italian drug-surveillance center. Dermatol Online J. 2006;12:1.
89. Sugita K, Kabashima K, Nakashima D, Tokura Y. Papuloerythroderma of Ofuji induced by furosemide. J Am Acad Dermatol. 2008;58(2 Suppl):S54–5.
90. Vena GA, Cassano N, Coco V, De Simone C. Eczematous reactions due to angiotensin-converting enzyme inhibitors or angiotensin II receptor blockers. Immunopharmacol Immunotoxicol. 2013;35:447–50.
91. Ferreira O, Mota A, Morais P, Cunha AP, Azevedo F. Symmetrical drug-related intertriginous and flexural exanthema (SDRIFE) induced by telmisartan-hydrochlorothiazide. Cutan Ocul Toxicol. 2010;29:293–5.
92. Hughes BR, Cunliffe WJ. Tolerance of spironolactone. Br J Dermatol. 1988;118:687–91.
93. Shaw JC. Low-dose adjunctive spironolactone in the treatment of acne in women: a retrospective analysis of 85 consecutively treated patients. J Am Acad Dermatol. 2000;43:498–502.
94. Daveluy A, Vial T, Marty L, Miremont-Salamé G, Moore N, Haramburu F. Contact dermatitis caused by acetazolamide under occlusion. Presse Med. 2007;36(12Pt 1):1756–8.
95. Feleke E, Lyngstam O, Råstam L, Rydén L. Complaints of cold extremities among patients on antihypertensive treatment. Acta Med Scand. 1983;213:381–5.
96. Kardaun SH, Scheffer E, Vermeer BJ. Drug-induced pseudolymphomatous skin reactions. Br J Dermatol. 1988;118:545–52.
97. Jahan-Tigh RR, Huen AO, Lee GL, Pozadzides JV, Liu P, Duvic M. Hydrochlorothiazide and cutaneous T cell lymphoma: prospective analysis and case series. Cancer. 2013;119:825–31. doi:10.1002/cncr.27740.
98. Valeyrie-Allanore L, Sassolas B, Roujeau JC. Drug-induced skin, nail and hair disorders. Drug Saf. 2007;30:1011–30.
99. Torpet LA, Kragelund C, Reibel J, Nauntofte B. Oral adverse drug reactions to cardiovascular drugs. Crit Rev Oral Biol Med. 2004;15:28–46.

Chapter 10
Vasodilatory Drugs

Keywords Vasodilatory • Hydralazine • Minoxidil • Nitrate • Nitroglycerin patch • Nicorandil • Flushing • Edema • Hypertrichosis • Lupus erythematosus • Vasculitis • Erythroderma • Contact dermatitis • Mucocutaneous ulcer

Vasodilatory drugs include bosentan, diazoxide, epoprostenol, fenoldopam, hydralazine, minoxidil, nitrates such as isosorbide dinitrate, isosorbide mononitrate, nitroglycerin (glyceryl trinitrate), pentaerythritol tetranitrate, nitroprusside, nesiritide, nicorandil, and phosphodiesterase inhibitors such as cilostazol, amrinone, milrinone, enoximone, and sildenafil citrate. Sildenafil is mainly used for the treatment of erectile dysfunction.

Flushing [1–5] and *edema* [3, 5, 6] may be seen with various vasodilators and seem to be the most common reactions that may be observed with these agents due to their vasodilatory effects.

Other adverse cutaneous drug reactions described below are meant to be sorted by starting from the well-known reactions of vasodilatory drugs to the lesser known ones. The major ones are summarized in Table 10.1.

Hypertrichosis

One of the most common reactions occurring with diazoxide [7–9] and minoxidil therapy [6, 10, 11] is hypertrichosis.

The incidence of hypertrichosis with diazoxide seems to be higher in children due to long-term treatment of hypoglycemia [7]. Hypertrichosis was reported to be noticed after several months of therapy with diazoxide [7, 9]. It was reported to involve almost all vellus hairs, including the face, trunk, and limbs. There was a correlation between the increase in hair growth and dosage, but not exclusively, as hypertrichosis appeared even at low doses [9]. The drug was reported to initiate the anagen phase of the hair growth and to change the hairs to be larger and longer than vellus hairs [9].

E. Özkaya, K.D. Yazganoğlu, *Adverse Cutaneous Drug Reactions to Cardiovascular Drugs*, DOI 10.1007/978-1-4471-6536-1_10

Table 10.1 Major adverse cutaneous drug reactions with vasodilatory drugs

Adverse cutaneous drug reaction	Main inducers
Flushing	Most of the vasodilators
Edema	Most of the vasodilators
Hypertrichosis	Diazoxide, minoxidil
Drug-induced lupus erythematosus (mainly systemic lupus erythematosus)	Hydralazine
Vasculitis	Hydralazine (usually ANCA positive), epoprostenol, bosentan
Contact dermatitis	Transdermal nitroglycerin
Erythema multiforme/Stevens–Johnson syndrome/toxic epidermal necrolysis	Transdermal nitroglycerin, minoxidil, sildenafil
Mucocutaneous ulceration	Nicorandil
Erythroderma	Epoprostenol, pentaerythritol tetranitrate–glyceryl trinitrate
Generalized erythema	Epoprostenol, bosentan
Maculopapular eruption	Isosorbide dinitrate, bosentan
DRESS	Bosentan
Lichen planus/lichenoid eruption	Sildenafil
Fixed drug eruption	Hydralazine, sildenafil

DRESS drug rash with eosinophilia and systemic symptoms, *ANCA* antineutrophil cytoplasmic autoantibody

Minoxidil-induced hypertrichosis due to its systemic use was reported to begin after 1 month of therapy, with slow regression upon discontinuation of the drug [6]. This side effect on systemic use led to the topical use of minoxidil in the treatment of androgenetic alopecia [10]. Minoxidil-induced hypertrichosis usually starts from the face and may then involve the trunk and extremities. The mechanism of hypertrichosis due to minoxidil is not clear, but it was suggested to be probably related with increased cutaneous blood flow, in addition to its effect on hair cycling, ie., by causing premature termination of telogen and prolongation of anagen, along with an increase in hair follicle size, or its ability to open the potassium channels in the hair follicles, the latter lacking a clear demonstration [11].

Drug-Induced Lupus Erythematosus

Drug-induced systemic lupus erythematosus (SLE) is a well-known adverse reaction of hydralazine. Hydralazine is stated to be among the highest-risk drugs implicated to cause SLE with an incidence of 5–8 % [12], occurring within the first year of therapy while using the same doses. This effect was particularly seen in slow acetylators of the drug [1] and also in HLA-DR4-positive individuals [12].

The incidence of SLE was reported to be higher in women [1, 13], and it was dose dependent [13]. The symptoms tended to develop as early as after 1 month of therapy [13]. The incidence of positivity of antinuclear antibody (ANA) test was reported to be higher than the incidence of hydralazine-induced SLE after 3 years of therapy [1]; in other words, a considerable number of patients had only ANA positivity without any clinical findings. Rapid acetylators of hydralazine were reported to develop ANA slower than slow acetylators, but the proportion of positivity was reported to be similar after 3 years of treatment [1].

The reported mucocutaneous features of hydralazine-induced SLE included facial rash [1, 13], vasculitis [1, 13–15], Sweet syndrome [16], ulcerated lesions of the larynx due to necrotizing vasculitis [17], pyoderma-gangrenosum-like ulcers [18], orogenital ulcers [19], cutaneous ulcerations without evidence of vasculitis, and purpura especially on sun-exposed areas [19].

Minoxidil may also cause SLE-like syndrome, in rare instances [20].

Vasculitis

Cutaneous vasculitis including necrotizing and leukocytoclastic vasculitis was reported to be induced by hydralazine with or without associated hydralazine-induced SLE [1, 13–15, 19, 21, 22]. Cutaneous lesions included maculopapular eruption, purpuric lesions, and/or ulcerations in different cases.

Hydralazine was found to be associated particularly with antineutrophil cytoplasmic autoantibody (ANCA) vasculitis [21, 22]. It might also be associated with other autoantibodies like ANA, antihistone, anti-double stranded DNA (anti-dsDNA), or antiphospholipid antibodies [21]. In one case with hydralazine-induced cutaneous vasculitis, the patient developed purplish rash on the lower extremities, livedo reticularis, acrocyanosis, and digital ischemia that evolved into digital gangrene and required partial amputation [21]. Leukocytoclastic vasculitis was found histopathologically in biopsy specimens of the amputated tissue. ANA, anti-dsDNA, ANCA, and anticardiolipin antibody were positive in this patient as well as factor V Leiden mutation [21]. In another report, a suspected case of hydralazine-induced cutaneous vasculitis (without histopathological confirmation) presented with livedo reticularis, erythematous and urticarial lesions, facial telangiectasia, and acrocyanosis. ANA was negative in this case, but the authors suspected of SLE [13].

Bosentan was also suggested as a cause of necrotizing leukocytoclastic vasculitis in a patient [23]. Leukocytoclastic vasculitis was reported during the administration of intravenous epoprostenol in several patients [2].

Contact Dermatitis

Contact dermatitis that might be irritant or allergic in nature was reported due to the local use of transdermal nitroglycerin patch. It may occur due to the transdermal patch material or nitroglycerin itself [24, 25].

Contact dermatitis manifesting as an erythema multiforme-like eruption starting on the application site of a nitroglycerin patch was reported to progress into generalized erythema multiforme in one case [26]. Severe maculopapular eruption developed in a patient after intravenous administration of isosorbide dinitrate who had allergic contact dermatitis from topical application of the cross-reacting nitroglycerin used as transdermal patch [25].

Topical application of minoxidil may cause irritant contact dermatitis, allergic contact dermatitis, or an exacerbation of seborrheic dermatitis [27]. Allergic contact dermatitis from topical minoxidil solution is mostly due to propylene glycol, which is present as an emulsifier in the preparation, and rarely to minoxidil itself [27–29].

Erythema Multiforme/Stevens–Johnson Syndrome/Toxic Epidermal Necrolysis

Generalized erythema multiforme developed in a patient with contact dermatitis from a nitroglycerin patch, starting as an erythema multiforme-like eruption on the application site of the patch [26].

Stevens–Johnson syndrome [30], severe erythematous and bullous eruption [31], and toxic epidermal necrolysis [32] were reported due to minoxidil therapy in isolated cases.

A case of toxic epidermal necrolysis associated with high-dose sildenafil intake was reported [33].

Erythroderma

Erythroderma, which is characterized by widespread confluent erythema that is often associated with desquamation, involving more than 80 % of the body surface, was reported with epoprostenol, and was accompanied by fever [34].

A patient was described with erythroderma developing after 8 years use of pentaerythritol tetranitrate (Peritrate) and glyceryl trinitrate; readministration of both drugs caused recurrence of the eruption confirming the drugs as the culprits of the reaction [35].

Apart from erythroderma, there are several reports of generalized erythematous reactions without associated desquamation, due to epoprostenol and bosentan [2, 36, 37]. Cases with generalized erythema, histopathologically revealing spongiotic dermatitis, were reported, which were suggested to be induced by epoprostenol [2]. Bosentan was reported as an inducer of painful generalized persistent patchy erythema with edema in a patient [36].

Drug-Induced Ulceration

Drug-induced mucocutaneous ulceration is a well-described effect of nicorandil, a nicotinamide ester, that was reported in many instances but still seems to be underreported [38]. Ulcerations may involve oral, perianal, perivulvar, and penile sites as well as fragile cutaneous sites like surgical wounds and peristomal areas or rarely intact skin [39–42]. The ulcerations were described as painful, well-circumscribed, aphthous or "punched out," shallow or deep lesions. The latency time between the onset of the drug therapy and the development of ulceration could exceed a year and be sometimes as long as several years. Healing of the ulcers usually required several weeks or months following discontinuation of the drug. The relationship with dosage and duration of therapy was not clear; long-term treatments or increase in drug dosage seemed to be contributory in some cases. Several different mechanisms were proposed for the occurrence of the nicorandil-associated ulcers including vascular steal phenomenon, direct toxicity of the drug, and abnormal distribution of nicotinic acid due to its accumulation outside the endogenous pool of nicotinamide adenine dinucleotide phosphate [40, 43–45].

Maculopapular Eruption

Maculopapular eruption was reported with isosorbide dinitrate [25] and bosentan [46] in isolated cases. Severe maculopapular eruption developed in a patient after intravenous administration of isosorbide dinitrate who had allergic contact dermatitis to topical application of cross-reacting nitroglycerin as transdermal patch [25]. In the bosentan-induced case, patch test and delayed reading of intradermal skin test with bosentan were negative, but lymphocyte transformation test was positive [46]. Moreover, rechallenge with bosentan was performed that caused drug rash with eosinophilia and systemic symptoms (DRESS) [46].

Drug Rash with Eosinophilia and Systemic Symptoms

Bosentan was suspected as the inducer drug in two cases [46, 47]. A patient initially presenting with maculopapular eruption, who showed negative results in patch test and delayed reading of intradermal skin tests to bosentan, but had positive lymphocyte transformation test, was rechallenged with bosentan that caused DRESS [46]. The other patient had a history of previous allergy to co-trimoxazole and several other drugs, and the authors suspected that the sulfonamide moiety of bosentan could have a contributing effect on the cutaneous reaction [47].

Generalized erythema with fever and eosinophilia was reported in another patient suggesting DRESS [37]. The drug reaction was confirmed with positive rechallenge test to bosentan [37].

Pruritus

Pruritus is a nonspecific cutaneous adverse reaction of drugs. It was reported to occur in some patients receiving vasodilator therapy, usually accompanying different types of drug eruptions [2, 15, 26, 34, 48].

Other Reported Adverse Cutaneous Drug Reactions to Vasodilators

Lichenoid drug eruptions were reported in men with intermittent intake of sildenafil for sexual enhancement. The drug reaction was confirmed by the rechallenge test with sildenafil in the reported cases [48, 49].

Fixed drug eruption was reported to be caused by hydralazine that was confirmed with oral provocation test [50], and by sildenafil, that recurred on reintake of the drug [51].

Hyperhidrosis seems to be a common adverse effect seen especially with epoprostenol but also with other vasodilators including isosorbide dinitrate, isosorbide mononitrate, nitroglycerin, nitroprusside, nesiritide, and sildenafil [5]. *Nail discoloration* may develop during the use of amrinone [52]. *Xerosis* was linked to cilostazol, minoxidil, and amrinone [5, 52, 53]; *angioedema/urticaria* to several vasodilators like cilostazol, hydralazine, nitroglycerin, minoxidil, bosentan, epoprostenol, and sildenafil [5, 53]; *anaphylactoid reactions* to milrinone, minoxidil, and nitroglycerin [5]; *bleeding/purpura/ecchymoses* to cilostazol [5]; *purpura* to nitroglycerin [5]; *xerostomia* to isosorbide dinitrate, nitroglycerin, and sildenafil [5]; and *rosacea* exacerbation to nitroglycerin [5].

References

1. Mansilla-Tinoco R, Harland SJ, Ryan PJ, Bernstein RM, Dollery CT, Hughes GR, et al. Hydralazine, antinuclear antibodies, and the lupus syndrome. Br Med J (Clin Res Ed). 1982;284:936–9.
2. Myers SA, Ahearn GS, Angelica Selim M, Tapson VF. Cutaneous findings in patients with pulmonary arterial hypertension receiving long-term epoprostenol therapy. J Am Acad Dermatol. 2004;51:98–102.
3. Hsu HH, Chen JS, Chen RJ, Ko WJ, Kuo SW, Wu ET, et al. Long-term outcome and effects of oral bosentan therapy in Taiwanese patients with advanced idiopathic pulmonary arterial hypertension. Respir Med. 2007;101:1556–62.

4. Wijitsettakul U, Pempongkosol S. The efficacy and safety of on-demand Elonza; a generic product of sildenafil in Thai men with erectile dysfunction. J Med Assoc Thai. 2013;96: 683–8.
5. Litt JZ. Drug eruption reference manual. 19th ed. Boca Raton: CRC Press (Taylor and Francis Group); 2013.
6. Nawar T, Nolin L, Plante GE, Caron C, Montambault P. Long-term treatment of severe hypertension with minoxidil. Can Med Assoc J. 1977;117:1178–82.
7. Salido R, Gómez-García FJ, Garnacho-Saucedo G, Galán-Gutiérrez M. Acquired generalized hypertrichosis due to diazoxide. Actas Dermosifiliogr. 2013;104:166–7.
8. Menter MA. Hypertrichosis lanuginosa and a lichenoid eruption due to diazoxide therapy. Proc R Soc Med. 1973;66:326–7.
9. Koblenzer PJ, Baker L. Hypertrichosis lanuginosa associated with diazoxide therapy in prepubertal children: a clinicopathologic study. Ann N Y Acad Sci. 1968;150:373–82.
10. Dawber RP, Rundegren J. Hypertrichosis in females applying minoxidil topical solution and in normal controls. J Eur Acad Dermatol Venereol. 2003;17:271–5.
11. Messenger AG, Rundegren J. Minoxidil: mechanisms of action on hair growth. Br J Dermatol. 2004;150:186–94.
12. Vedove CD, Del Giglio M, Schena D, Girolomoni G. Drug-induced lupus erythematosus. Arch Dermatol Res. 2009;301:99–105.
13. Cameron HA, Ramsay LE. The lupus syndrome induced by hydralazine: a common complication with low dose treatment. Br Med J (Clin Res Ed). 1984;289:410–2.
14. Bernstein RM, Egerton-Vernon J, Webster J. Hydralazine-induced cutaneous vasculitis. Br Med J. 1980;280:156–7.
15. Finlay AY, Statham B, Knight AG. Hydralazine-induced necrotising vasculitis. Br Med J (Clin Res Ed). 1981;282:1703–4.
16. Cartee TV, Chen SC. Sweet syndrome associated with hydralazine-induced lupus erythematosus. Cutis. 2012;89:121–4.
17. Weiser GA, Forouhar FA, White WB. Hydralazine hoarseness. A new appearance of drug-induced systemic lupus erythematosus. Arch Intern Med. 1984;144:2271–2.
18. Peterson LL. Hydralazine-induced systemic lupus erythematosus presenting as pyoderma gangrenosum-like ulcers. J Am Acad Dermatol. 1984;10:379–84.
19. Neville E, Graham PY, Brewis RA. Orogenital ulcers, SLE and hydralazine. Postgrad Med J. 1981;57:378–9.
20. Hoffman B, Tunkel AR, Shuman M, Popkin M, Seth R. Minoxidil-induced systemic lupus erythematosus. Arch Intern Med. 1987;147:599–600.
21. Yokogawa N, Vivino FB. Hydralazine-induced autoimmune disease: comparison to idiopathic lupus and ANCA-positive vasculitis. Mod Rheumatol. 2009;19:338–47.
22. Pendergraft WF, Niles JL. Trojan horses: drug culprits associated with antineutrophil cytoplasmic autoantibody (ANCA) vasculitis. Curr Opin Rheumatol. 2014;26:42–9.
23. Gasser S, Kuhn M, Speich R. Severe necrotising leucocytoclastic vasculitis in a patient taking bosentan. BMJ. 2004;329:430.
24. Kounis NG, Zavras GM, Papadaki PJ, Soufras GD, Poulos EA, Goudevenos J, et al. Allergic reactions to local glyceryl trinitrate administration. Br J Clin Pract. 1996;50:437–9.
25. Aquilina S, Felice H, Boffa MJ. Allergic reactions to glyceryl trinitrate and isosorbide dinitrate demonstrating cross-sensitivity. Clin Exp Dermatol. 2002;27:700–2.
26. Silvestre JF, Betlloch I, Guijarro J, Albares MP, Vergara G. Erythema-multiforme-like eruption on the application site of a nitroglycerin patch, followed by widespread erythema multiforme. Contact Dermatitis. 2001;45:299–300.
27. Friedman ES, Friedman PM, Cohen DE, Washenik K. Allergic contact dermatitis to topical minoxidil solution: etiology and treatment. J Am Acad Dermatol. 2002;46:309–12.
28. Rodríguez-Martín M, Sáez-Rodríguez M, Carnerero-Rodríguez A, Cabrera de Paz R, Sidro-Sarto M, Pérez-Robayna N, et al. Pustular allergic contact dermatitis from topical minoxidil 5%. J Eur Acad Dermatol Venereol. 2007;21:701–2.
29. Corazza M, Borghi A, Ricci M, Sarno O, Virgili A. Patch testing in allergic contact dermatitis from minoxidil. Dermatitis. 2010;21:217–8.

30. DiSantis DJ, Flanagan J. Minoxidil-induced Stevens-Johnson syndrome. Arch Intern Med. 1981;141:1515.
31. Ackerman BH, Townsend ME, Golden W, Bryan AB. Pruritic rash with actinic keratosis and impending exfoliation in a patient with hypertension managed with minoxidil. Drug Intell Clin Pharm. 1988;22:702–3.
32. Karaoui LR, Chahine-Chakhtoura C. Fatal toxic epidermal necrolysis associated with minoxidil. Pharmacotherapy. 2009;29:460–7.
33. Al-Shouli S, Abouchala N, Bogusz MJ, Al Tufail M, Thestrup-Pedersen K. Toxic epidermal necrolysis associated with high intake of sildenafil and its response to infliximab. Acta Derm Venereol. 2005;85:534–5.
34. Ahearn GS, Selim MA, Tapson VF. Severe erythroderma as a complication of continuous epoprostenol therapy. Chest. 2002;122:378–80.
35. Ryan FP. Erythroderma due to peritrate and glyceryl trinitrate. Br J Dermatol. 1972;87: 498–500.
36. Gallardo F, Gil A, Comín J, Molina L, Iglesias M, Pujol RM. Persistent painful indurated erythema secondary to bosentan. Acta Derm Venereol. 2006;86:186–7.
37. Nagai Y, Yamanaka M, Nishimura S, Nakano A, Hasegawa A, Ishikawa O. Drug eruption due to bosentan in a patient with systemic sclerosis. Mod Rheumatol. 2006;16:188–90.
38. Smith VM, Lyon CC. Results of an electronic survey of British Association of Dermatologists members: nicorandil ulceration. Br J Dermatol. 2013;168:1136–7.
39. Yap T, Philippou P, Perry M, Lam W, Corbishley C, Watkin N. Nicorandil-induced penile ulcerations: a case series. BJU Int. 2011;107:268–71.
40. Claeys A, Weber-Muller F, Trechot P, Cuny JF, Georges MY, Barbaud A, Schmutz JL. Cutaneous, perivulvar and perianal ulcerations induced by nicorandil. Br J Dermatol. 2006;155:494–6.
41. Ogden S, Mukasa Y, Lyon CC, Coulson IH. Nicorandil-induced peristomal ulcers: is nicorandil also associated with gastrointestinal fistula formation? Br J Dermatol. 2007;156:608–9.
42. Yamamoto K, Matsusue Y, Horita S, Minamiguchi M, Komatsu Y, Kirita T. Nicorandil-induced oral ulceration: report of 3 cases and review of the Japanese literature. Oral Surg Oral Med Oral Pathol Oral Radiol Endod. 2011;112:754–9.
43. Watson A, Al-Ozairi O, Fraser A, Loudon M, O'Kelly T. Nicorandil associated anal ulceration. Lancet. 2002;360:546–7.
44. Trechot P, Barbaud A, Petitpain N, Claeys A, Schmutz JL. Nicorandil and ulcerations: a NAD/NADP and nicotinic acid-dependent side-effect? Br J Dermatol. 2008;158:1150–1.
45. Trechot P, Jouzeau JY, Brouillard C, Scala-Bertola J, Petitpain N, Cuny JF, et al. Role of nicotinic acid and nicotinamide in nicorandil-induced ulcerations: from hypothesis to demonstration. Int Wound J. 2013. doi:10.1111/iwj.12147.
46. Romano A, Giovannetti A, Caruso C, Rosato E, Pierdominici M, Salsano F. Delayed hypersensitivity to bosentan. Allergy. 2009;64:499–501.
47. Allanore Y, Moachon L, Maury E, Isvy A, Kahan A. Bosentan-induced drug reaction with eosinophilia and systemic symptoms (DRESS) syndrome. J Rheumatol. 2010;37:1077–8.
48. Goldman BD. Lichenoid drug reaction due to sildenafil. Cutis. 2000;65:282–3.
49. Antiga E, Melani L, Cardinali C, Giomi B, Caproni M, Francalanci S, Fabbri P. A case of lichenoid drug eruption associated with sildenafil citratus. J Dermatol. 2005;32:972–5.
50. Sehgal VN, Gangwani OP. Hydralazine-induced fixed drug eruption. Int J Dermatol. 1986;25:394.
51. Ghosh SK, Bandyopadhyay D. Nonpigmenting mucosal fixed drug eruption due to sildenafil citrate. J Sex Med. 2009;6:3500–1.
52. Wilsmhurst PT, Webb-Peploe MM. Side effects of amrinone therapy. Br Heart J. 1983;49: 447–51.
53. Frishman WH, Brosnan BD, Grossman M, Dasgupta D, Sun DK. Adverse dermatologic effects of cardiovascular drug therapy: part III. Cardiol Rev. 2002;10:337–48.

Chapter 11
Lipid-Lowering Drugs

Keywords Lipid lowering • Statins • Fibrate • Niacin • Nicotinic acid • Dermatomyositis • Lupus erythematosus • Eczema • Eosinophilic fasciitis • Acanthosis nigricans • Xerosis • Photosensitivity • Lichenoid • Angioedema/urticaria • Alopecia

Lipid-lowering drugs include 3-hydroxy-3-methylglutaryl coenzyme A (HMG-CoA) reductase inhibitors (statins such as simvastatin, atorvastatin, pravastatin, fluvastatin, lovastatin, cerivastatin, rosuvastatin, pitavastatin), fibric acids (fibrates such as fenofibrate, clofibrate, gemfibrozil, bezafibrate, and ciprofibrate), bile acid sequestrants (resins) (cholestyramine, colestipol, and colesevelam), and others (nicotinic acid [niacin], nicotinic acid analogs like xanthinol nicotinate and acipimox, and cholesterol absorption inhibitor such as ezetimibe). Lipid-lowering drugs inhibit different steps in the cholesterol synthesis.

Statins

Statins are used in the treatment of hyperlipidemias as they suppress cholesterol synthesis in the liver. First-generation statins are simvastatin, lovastatin, and pravastatin, and second-generation statins are atorvastatin and fluvastatin. The former ones have a similar chemical structure, while the latter ones do not [1]. On the other hand, simvastatin and lovastatin are prodrugs that are hydrolyzed into the active forms [2]. Cerivastatin is no longer used because of its side effects.

The adverse cutaneous drug reactions described below are meant to be sorted by starting from the well-known reactions of statins to the lesser known ones. The major ones are summarized in Table 11.1.

E. Özkaya, K.D. Yazganoğlu, *Adverse Cutaneous Drug Reactions to Cardiovascular Drugs*, DOI 10.1007/978-1-4471-6536-1_11

Table 11.1 Major adverse cutaneous drug reactions with statins

Adverse cutaneous drug reaction	Main inducers
Lichenoid eruption	Simvastatin, pravastatin, fluvastatin, lovastatin
Dermatomyositis	Simvastatin, atorvastatin, lovastatin, fluvastatin, pravastatin
Drug-induced lupus erythematosus	
Systemic lupus erythematosus	Simvastatin, atorvastatin, pravastatin, fluvastatin, lovastatin, cerivastatin, rosuvastatin
Subacute cutaneous lupus erythematosus	Simvastatin, pravastatin
Eczematous eruption	Simvastatin, pravastatin
Xerosis/ichthyosis	Atorvastatin, simvastatin, fluvastatin, pravastatin
Eosinophilic fasciitis	Simvastatin, atorvastatin
Photosensitivity	Atorvastatin, simvastatin, and pravastatin
Bullous eruption	
Lichen planus pemphigoides	Simvastatin
Linear IgA dermatosis	Atorvastatin
Angioedema/urticaria	Most of the statins
Interstitial granulomatous drug reaction	Atorvastatin, lovastatin, pravastatin+propranolol
Vasculitis	Simvastatin
Alopecia	Atorvastatin, lovastatin, fluvastatin, pravastatin, simvastatin

Lichenoid Eruption

Lichenoid eruptions with or without mucosal involvement have been observed with pravastatin [3, 4], simvastatin [5], fluvastatin, and lovastatin [6]. The cutaneous lesions were pigmented [4], or photodistributed on the arms and hands [3]. Mucosal lesions were localized to the oral mucosa presenting with white streaks [5, 6].

The reaction occurred within 3 weeks to 4 months after initiation of therapy and mostly resolved within 3 weeks to 9 months after discontinuation of the culprit drug [3–6]. Rechallenge was tried with the same drug (pravastatin) in one case which caused reappearance of the lesions [3]. Interestingly, in a patient with fluvastatin-induced lichenoid eruption, administration of lovastatin caused reappearance of the rash [6], pointing out to a possible cross-reactivity.

Dermatomyositis

Myopathy and rhabdomyolysis are well-known side effects of statin therapy. On the other hand, statins may induce dermatomyositis and also lupus suggesting a statin-induced autoimmunity [1]. Simvastatin [7–9], atorvastatin [10], lovastatin [11], fluvastatin [12], and pravastatin [13] have been reported to be associated with dermatomyositis. Typical cutaneous findings of dermatomyositis including heliotrope rash and Gottron papules are usually present [8–11], but not in every case [7]. The reaction can start after several months to several years of statin therapy. Antinuclear antibody may be found positive in some cases [1, 9, 10], and high plasma levels of antinuclear antibody were reported to be seen for a long time after the withdrawal of the drug [10].

Due to the development of lupus or dermatomyositis in some patients treated with statins, it was suggested that screening for plasma creatine kinase levels and antinuclear antibody could be helpful if skin rash and unexplained fatigue were present [10]. However, amyopathic form of dermatomyositis, namely, "dermatomyositis sine myositis" may occur as well [9]; thus, creatine kinase levels may be normal. The reaction may show a benign course, namely, showing resolution without necessitating immunosuppressive therapy [8, 10, 12], or it may persist even after withdrawal of the drug, and immunosuppressive therapies might be necessary [7].

Drug-Induced Lupus Erythematosus

There are many reports indicating the association of statin use and autoimmune diseases like systemic lupus erythematosus (SLE) and dermatomyositis. Among these, SLE has been more commonly reported. Almost every statin, like simvastatin, atorvastatin, pravastatin, fluvastatin, lovastatin, cerivastatin, and rosuvastatin have been indicated as triggers of SLE [1, 14, 15], but simvastatin-induced cases seem to be more commonly reported. Systemic as well as subacute cutaneous lupus erythematosus (SCLE) may occur with statins, but reported cases of SCLE were less than the systemic form [1, 14]. Simvastatin and pravastatin were among the inducer statins in the SCLE cases [16–19].

A long latency period between the initiation of therapy and the onset of the reaction may be observed in statin-induced SLE. The reaction has been reported to start after a week to even 6 years of therapy [1, 14]. Therefore, it may sometimes be difficult to consider the drug as the inducer of the reaction. It is indeed more difficult if the patient is on multidrug regimen.

Skin findings of the patients with statin-induced SLE were mostly absent or mild such as only facial rash, or only phosensitivity, or localized, slightly erythematous scaly lesions [1]. On the other hand, patients with SCLE had almost always skin features like photodistributed erythema or annular scaly erythematosus lesions [1, 17–19]. SLE and SCLE from statins presented with erythemato-papulous rash in a photodistributed fashion or a diffuse annular–polycyclic rash in a previous report. Alopecia was also reported. The authors stated that most of their patients showed features of SCLE [15].

Serologic findings included the presence of antinuclear antibodies both in SLE and SCLE cases. Anti-dsDNA antibodies were reported either as positive or negative, and antihistone antibodies were lacking in some cases of SLE [1, 14]. Anti-Ro/SSA was positive mainly in patients with SCLE [17–19].

The cessation of the drug generally led to slow resolution of the reaction and required immunosuppressive therapy in most of the SLE cases. A case with fatal outcome was also reported [1]. Serologic improvement was even slower than the clinical one. On the other hand, patients with SCLE were mainly followed up with sunscreens or treated with local medications [1, 17]. Rechallenge was positive in a simvastatin-induced case of SCLE [19].

The pathogenesis of statin-induced autoimmune reactions is not clear. Their effect on cellular apoptosis, on T lymphocytes (shifting of the balance from T helper 1 to T helper 2 that causes an increase in the reactivity of B cells and production of antibodies), and on secretion of IL-12 and IL-18 in monocytes has been postulated [1, 14, 20]. On the other hand, it was speculated that statins have only a progressive effect on a preexisting autoimmunity, thus causing a clinically apparent autoimmune disease rather than being the direct cause of the autoimmune reaction [14].

Eczematous Eruption

Generalized eczema has been reported from simvastatin and pravastatin [2, 21], and localized nummular eczema from pravastatin [21]. Scaling or xerosis accompanied in some cases [2]. The reaction started within a few weeks to 6 months after initiation of therapy and resolved within several weeks after cessation of the drug, either upon treatment with oral and/or topical corticosteroids or only with emollients.

Patch test was performed in the patient presenting with nummular eczema from pravastatin and revealed a positive result [21], indicating that the reaction was allergic. On the other hand, it was suggested that eczematous reactions and xerosis observed with statins were associated with direct inhibition of HMG-CoA reductase in the epidermis. This would cause an alteration of the stratum corneum lipid content and a defect in the skin barrier function, which would then lead to an increase in transepidermal water loss, dryness and eczematous lesions [2].

Simvastatin was reported as a cause of occupational contact dermatitis in several patients working in pharmaceutical companies. Occupational airborne contact dermatitis was reported in two patients presenting with facial and neck eczema [22]. Occupational exposure to simvastatin caused allergic contact dermatitis of the eyelids in another case [23]. These reactions were further confirmed by patch test [22, 23]. Simvastatin was the cause of occupational airborne contact dermatitis on the face together with carvedilol and zolpidem in another patient, all proven by patch testing [24]. Dose increase caused an exacerbation of the eczema in one patient using simvastatin suggesting that the reaction might be dose dependent [2].

Xerosis

Xerosis was implicated to occur with the use of statins, mostly atorvastatin, simvastatin, and fluvastatin [25]. It was suggested that eczematous reactions and xerosis observed with statins were the result of the alteration of the stratum corneum lipid content and defect in the skin barrier function, caused by the direct inhibition of HMG-CoA reductase in the epidermis. The subsequent increase in transepidermal water loss would lead to dryness and eczematous lesions [2]. Therefore, atopic individuals could be at more risk for experiencing these side effects [2]. A patient with acquired ichthyosis from pravastatin [26] and another one from lovastatin [27] has also been reported. On the contrary, a recent review argued that systemic statins did not seem to alter skin cholesterol significantly nor transepidermal water loss and permeability barrier of the skin [28].

Eosinophilic Fasciitis

Eosinophilic fasciitis usually presents with symmetrical swelling and induration of the skin and subcutaneous tissues starting from the proximal extremities, sometimes involving the neck or chest, and it is associated with peripheral eosinophilia [29]. Four cases of statin-induced eosinophilic fasciitis have been reported to our knowledge. Simvastatin was the inducer statin in three cases [29–31] and atorvastatin in one case [32].

The reaction started within usually 1–4 weeks after therapy with statin [29, 31, 32], but it was reported to develop even after 18 months [30]. The relationship between the reaction and the drug as a possible inducer is difficult to establish in patients with eosinophilic fasciitis, because the reaction does not immediately resolve after discontinuation of the drug and may even be progressive [32]. Indeed, systemic corticosteroid therapy was required in all of the reported patients [29–32], together with methotrexate in two cases [31, 32].

Photosensitivity

Photosensitivity reactions have been rarely reported with statins showing abnormal phototest findings. Atorvastatin [33], simvastatin, and pravastatin [34] were among the inducer drugs. Persistent photosensitivity leading to *chronic actinic dermatitis* due to simvastatin was also reported [35, 36]. The reaction was confirmed by positive photopatch testing and rechallenge with phototesting in one patient [36].

Bullous Eruptions

Lichen Planus Pemphigoides

Lichen planus pemphigoides was reported to develop in a patient 1 month after commencing simvastatin, and resolved completely within 3 months with discontinuation of the medication [37].

Linear IgA Dermatosis

Linear IgA dermatosis started after 2 weeks use of atorvastatin in a patient, disappeared on discontinuation of the drug, and reappeared after readministration, necessitating systemic corticosteroid and dapsone therapy [38].

Pruritus

Pruritus is a nonspecific cutaneous adverse reaction of drugs. It was reported in patients receiving statin therapy, mainly accompanying different types of drug eruptions [2, 3, 5, 6, 21, 37].

Other Reported Adverse Cutaneous Drug Reactions to Statins

Atorvastatin was suggested to induce *angioedema/urticaria* and *dermographism* in a patient [39]. In another patient, it was reported to cause chronic urticaria. The reaction resolved 10 days after discontinuation of atorvastatin, and scratch testing was positive with the drug [40]. Other statins including rosuvastatin, simvastatin, pravastatin, fluvastatin, and lovastatin were also implicated to cause angioedema/urticaria or anaphylactoid reactions [25].

Interstitial granulomatous drug reaction with atorvastatin, lovastatin, and in one case with a combination drug that contained pravastatin and propranolol was reported [41–43].

Cutaneous vasculitis was reported with the use of simvastatin. A combination drug, simvastatin–ezetimibe, was implicated as a cause of cutaneous vasculitis in a patient who showed positive results for antineutrophil cytoplasmic antibody, and antimyeloperoxidase, antinuclear, and anti-Ro/SSA antibodies. This might be considered as another example of statin-induced autoimmunity [44]. Withdrawal of the drug and treatment with colchicine led to resolution of the symptoms within 6 weeks. Antinuclear and anti-Ro/SSA antibodies were negative after several months, but antimyeloperoxidase antibodies were still positive after 11 months of discontinuation of the drug [44]. A patient with simvastatin-induced *urticarial vasculitis* tolerated atorvastatin without any skin eruption [45].

A *psoriasiform drug eruption* was associated with pravastatin in a patient with no history of preexisting psoriasis. It was reported to resolve after discontinuation of the drug but reappeared a few days later although the patient did not take the medicine again. The authors speculated that the psoriasiform drug eruption converted into psoriasis de novo [46].

A possible relationship was reported between pravastatin therapy and necrotic *skin ulcers* located on the ears and elbows [47]. *Radiation recall dermatitis* developing 1 year after radiotherapy was reported to occur within several days of simvastatin use [48]. A skin ulcer on the radiation area, corresponding to the pressure site of the brassière strings, was also reported in this case.

Erythema multiforme from rosuvastatin [49] and *toxic epidermal necrolysis* from atorvastatin were reported, the latter developing after 4 days of therapy [50].

One case of *acute generalized exanthematous pustulosis* has been reported in association with simvastatin [51]. The reaction started after 2 weeks of therapy and resolved within a few weeks after the cessation of the drug. The reaction was confirmed by a positive rechallenge test.

Patients were reported with *porphyria cutanea tarda* from simvastatin and pravastatin [52, 53].

Drug rash with eosinophilia and systemic symptoms has been reported with atorvastatin [54].

Spiny keratoderma presenting with multiple keratotic projections involving the palms and soles has been reported in patients using simvastatin, often in individuals working with their hand in manual labor [55].

Simvastatin was reported to cause *acral cutaneous vesiculobullous and pustular eruption* located on the distal arms, lower legs, and hands that was pruritic and purpuric as well, and revealed nonspecific and different histopathological changes on three different biopsies in 1 year such as spongiotic, lichenoid, and vasculitic [56].

Other reported reactions included *cheilitis* from simvastatin [57], and *alopecia* with atorvastatin [58], lovastatin, fluvastatin, pravastatin, and simvastatin [25]. *Edema* may also be seen with atorvastatin, rosuvastatin, simvastatin, and pravastatin [25].

Fibrates

Among fibrates, fenofibrate was reported to be associated most commonly with skin reactions which were indicated as the most frequent reason for the withdrawal of the drug [59].

Photosensitivity

Photosensitivity reactions, usually presenting with eczematous morphology, were reported mainly with fenofibrate, a benzophenone derivative [60–64]. Some have been reproduced by systemic photochallenge or photopatch testing either with UVA or UVB radiation or both [60, 61, 63, 64], and also by photoscratch testing [62]. It was suggested that the concentration of the drug for photopatch testing should be higher than 1 %, or even higher than 5 % [60]. On the other hand, systemic photochallenge was regarded as a more appropriate test to determine the fenofibrate-induced photosensitivity [61, 65]. The negative photopatch test results were also attributed to the possibility that the drug metabolite could have caused the reaction [61, 62].

A cross-photosensitization might occur between systemically administered fenofibrate and topically applied ketoprofen, which is another benzophenone-containing drug [64].

Bezafibrate has also been reported to induce photosensitivity in one patient [64].

Angioedema/Urticaria

Angioedema/urticaria may occur with bezafibrate, fenofibrate, clofibrate, and gemfibrozil [25, 59, 66], while anaphylactic/anaphylactoid reactions were reported from bezafibrate and gemfibrozil [25, 59, 67]. The late-onset reaction with bezafibrate both for angioedema [66] and anaphylaxis [67] was rather interesting and was partly attributed to the slow-release form of the drug [66, 67].

Other Reported Adverse Cutaneous Drug Reactions to Fibrates

Maculopapular eruption associated with high fever and facial edema from clofibrate was reported suggesting drug rash with eosinophilia and systemic symptoms that was confirmed with rechallenge [68].

Erythema multiforme was reported from clofibrate that was confirmed by rechallenge [69]. *Stevens–Johnson syndrome* was reported with clofibrate [70] and bezafibrate [71].

Clofibrate was implicated to be a cause of *SLE-like syndrome* in a patient manifesting with oral ulcers but no skin rash [72].

A patient developing *facial erythematous, edematous eruption* with burning sensation 1 month after using a combination drug containing clofibrate and androsterone was reported to have the same reaction after readministration of the drug 2 years later [73].

Pigmented purpuric dermatosis induced by bezafibrate [74] and *exacerbation of psoriasis* with gemfibrozil [75] were also reported.

Palmar erythema with hepatic damage has been stated to occur with gemfibrozil [76]. Other reported cutaneous reactions induced by fibrates included *alopecia*, *xerosis*, or *ichthyosis* and nonspecific reactions such as *pruritus* [25, 59].

Bile Acid Resins

Cholestyramine and colestipol have been linked to reactions like edema, exanthema, or urticaria [25, 59]. *Palmar erythema* with hepatic damage has been implicated with cholestyramine [76].

Other Lipid-Lowering Drugs

Niacin

Niacin (nicotinic acid) and its analog, acipimox, were reported to induce *flushing* [77, 78]. Flushing was implicated as the most common cutaneous reaction with niacin due to its vasodilatory effect mediated by prostaglandin D2, that might require the withdrawal of the drug. A recent study revealed a high incidence of a pruritic cutaneous eruption in patients treated with a combination drug, namely, extended-release niacin/laropiprant [77]. Laropiprant was used to reduce the flushing effect caused by niacin; 14 % of 201 patients were reported to experience mainly a *maculopapular* or *urticarial* cutaneous eruption that revealed spongiotic dermatitis by histopathological examination. In one of the patients, blistering reaction was observed. However, no confirmatory tests were performed to identify the culprit drug. This combination drug was also implicated as a cause of *bullous drug eruption* revealing subepidermal blisters in the histopathology. Negative direct immunofluorescence findings excluded the possibility of bullous pemphigoid [79]. Xanthinol nicotinate, a potent form of niacin that is used for vasodilatory effects in vascular disorders, was reported to cause a pruritic erythematous eruption that progressed to severe bullous reaction in another patient who also had negative direct immunofluorescence findings excluding the possibility of bullous pemphigoid [80].

Xerosis/ichthyosis is an established side effect of niacin via alteration in epidermal cholesterol metabolism [81].

Another well-known reaction of niacin is the development of *acanthosis nigricans* [82–84]. It generally develops after several months of niacin intake and resolves within weeks to months upon discontinuation of the drug [82–84]. Resolution was also observed in a case upon substitution of niacin to its analog, acipimox [84]. The development of acanthosis nigricans from niacin was implicated to be related with the effect of niacin on inducing insulin resistance and its effect on the alteration of epidermal lipids [82].

Fixed drug eruption [85], *dry hair, pruritus, urticaria, edema,* and *hyperhidrosis* are other adverse cutaneous effects of niacin use [25, 59, 82].

Ezetimibe

A combination drug, simvastatin–ezetimibe, was implicated as a cause of *cutaneous vasculitis* in a patient with positivity of antineutrophil cytoplasmic antibody and antimyeloperoxidase, antinuclear, and anti-Ro/SSA antibodies [44]. Ezetimibe was also linked to skin reactions like *angioedema/urticaria* [25].

References

1. Noël B. Lupus erythematosus and other autoimmune diseases related to statin therapy: a systematic review. J Eur Acad Dermatol Venereol. 2007;21:17–24.
2. Krasovec M, Elsner P, Burg G. Generalized eczematous skin rash possibly due to HMG-CoA reductase inhibitors. Dermatology. 1993;186:248–52.
3. Keough GC, Richardson TT, Grabski WJ. Pravastatin-induced lichenoid drug eruption. Cutis. 1998;61:98–100.
4. Pua VS, Scolyer RA, Barnetson RS. Pravastatin-induced lichenoid drug eruption. Australas J Dermatol. 2006;47:57–9.
5. Roger D, Rolle F, Labrousse F, Brosset A, Bonnetblanc JM. Simvastatin-induced lichenoid drug eruption. Clin Exp Dermatol. 1994;19:88–9.
6. Sebok B, Toth M, Anga B, Harangi F, Schneider I. Lichenoid drug eruption with HMG-CoA reductase inhibitors (fluvastatin and lovastatin). Acta Derm Venereol. 2004;84:229–30.
7. Vasconcelos OM, Campbell WW. Dermatomyositis-like syndrome and HMG-CoA reductase inhibitor (statin) intake. Muscle Nerve. 2004;30:803–7.
8. Inhoff O, Peitsch WK, Paredes BE, Goerdt S, Goebeler M. Simvastatin-induced amyopathic dermatomyositis. Br J Dermatol. 2009;161:206–8.
9. Zaraa IR, Labbène I, Mrabet D, Zribi H, Chelly I, Zitouna M, et al. Simvastatin-induced dermatomyositis in a 50-year-old man. BMJ Case Rep. 2011;2011. doi:10.1136/bcr.02.2011.3832.
10. Noel B, Cerottini JP, Panizzon RG. Atorvastatin-induced dermatomyositis. Am J Med. 2001;110:670–1.
11. Rodriguez-Garcia JL, Serrano Commino M. Lovastatin-associated dermatomyositis. Postgrad Med J. 1996;72:694.
12. Thual N, Penven K, Chevallier JM, Dompmartin A, Leroy D. Fluvastatin-induced dermatomyositis. Ann Dermatol Venereol. 2005;132(12 Pt 1):996–9.
13. Zuech P, Pauwels C, Duthoit C, Méry L, Somogyi A, Louboutin A, Veyssier-Belot C. Pravastatin-induced dermatomyositis. Rev Med Interne. 2005;26:897–902.
14. de Jong HJ, Tervaert JW, Saldi SR, Vandebriel RJ, Souverein PC, Meyboom RH, et al. Association between statin use and lupus-like syndrome using spontaneous reports. Semin Arthritis Rheum. 2011;41:373–81.
15. Moulis G, Béné J, Sommet A, Sailler L, Lapeyre-Mestre M, Montastruc JL. French Association of PharmacoVigilance Centres. Statin-induced lupus: a case/non-case study in a nationwide pharmacovigilance database. Lupus. 2012;21:885–9.
16. Noel B, Panizzon RG. Lupus-like syndrome associated with statin therapy. Dermatology. 2004;208:276–7.
17. Srivastava M, Rencic A, Diglio G, Santana H, Bonitz P, Watson R, et al. Drug-induced, Ro/SSA-positive cutaneous lupus erythematosus. Arch Dermatol. 2003;139:45–9.
18. Rüger RD, Simon JC, Treudler R. Subacute-cutaneous lupus erythematosus induced by Simvastatin. J Dtsch Dermatol Ges. 2011;9:54–5.
19. Suchak R, Benson K, Swale V. Statin-induced Ro/SSa-positive subacute cutaneous lupus erythematosus. Clin Exp Dermatol. 2007;32:589–91.

20. Park SJ, Shin JI. Role of interleukin-12 and - 18 in lupus-like syndrome patients with statin use: comment on: Association between statin use and lupus-like syndrome using spontaneous reports. Semin Arthritis Rheum. 2012;41:e2–3.
21. de Boer EM, Bruynzeel DP. Allergy to pravastatin. Contact Dermatitis. 1994;30:238.
22. Peramiquel L, Serra E, Dalmau J, Vila AT, Mascaró JM, Alomar A. Occupational contact dermatitis from simvastatin. Contact Dermatitis. 2005;52:286–7.
23. Field S, Bourke B, Hazelwood E, Bourke JF. Simvastatin – occupational contact dermatitis. Contact Dermatitis. 2007;57:282–3.
24. Neumark M, Moshe S, Ingber A, Slodownik D. Occupational airborne contact dermatitis to simvastatin, carvedilol, and zolpidem. Contact Dermatitis. 2009;61:51–2.
25. Litt JZ. Drug eruption reference manual. 19th ed. Boca Raton: CRC Press (Taylor and Francis Group); 2013.
26. Sparsa A, Boulinguez S, Le Brun V, Roux C, Bonnetblanc JM, Bedane C. Acquired ichthyosis with pravastatin. J Eur Acad Dermatol Venereol. 2007;21:549–50.
27. Baykal C, Korkmaz Y, Kavak A. Lovastatin-induced, acquired ichthyosis. Eur J Dermatol. 1996;6:581–3.
28. Jowkar F, Namazi MR. Statins in dermatology. Int J Dermatol. 2010;49:1235–43.
29. Dugonik A, Belič M, Miljković J. Eosinophilic fasciitis. Acta Dermatovenerol Alp Panonica Adriat. 2003;12:72–5.
30. Choquet-Kastylevsky G, Kanitakis J, Dumas V, Descotes J, Faure M, Claudy A. Eosinophilic fasciitis and simvastatin. Arch Intern Med. 2001;161:1456–7.
31. Serrano-Grau P, Mascaró-Galy JM, Iranzo P. Eosinophilic fasciitis after taking simvastatin. Actas Dermosifiliogr. 2008;99:420–1.
32. DeGiovanni C, Chard M, Woollons A. Eosinophilic fasciitis secondary to treatment with atorvastatin. Clin Exp Dermatol. 2006;31:131–2.
33. Marguery MC, Chouini-Lalanne N, Drugeon C, Gadroy A, Bayle P, Journe F, et al. UV-B phototoxic effects induced by atorvastatin. Arch Dermatol. 2006;142:1082–4.
34. Rodríguez-Pazos L, Sánchez-Aguilar D, Rodríguez-Granados MT, Pereiro-Ferreirós MM, Toribio J. Erythema multiforme photoinduced by statins. Photodermatol Photoimmunol Photomed. 2010;26:216–8.
35. Holme SA, Pearse AD, Anstey AV. Chronic actinic dermatitis secondary to simvastatin. Photodermatol Photoimmunol Photomed. 2002;18:313–4.
36. Granados MT, de la Torre C, Cruces MJ, Piñeiro G. Chronic actinic dermatitis due to simvastatin. Contact Dermatitis. 1998;38:294–5.
37. Stoebner PE, Michot C, Ligeron C, Durand L, Meynadier J, Meunier L. Simvastatin-induced lichen planus pemphigoides. Ann Dermatol Venereol. 2003;130(2 Pt 1):187–90.
38. Konig C, Eickert A, Scharfetter-Kochanek K, Krieg T, Hunzelmann N. Linear IgA bullous dermatosis induced by atorvastatin. J Am Acad Dermatol. 2001;44:689–92.
39. Adcock BB, Hornsby LB, Jenkins K. Dermographism: an adverse effect of atorvastatin. J Am Board Fam Pract. 2001;14:148–51.
40. Anliker MD, Wüthrich B. Chronic urticaria to atorvastatin. Allergy. 2002;57:366.
41. Hernández N, Peñate Y, Borrego L. Generalized erythematous-violaceous plaques in a patient with a history of dyslipidemia. Interstitial granulomatous drug reaction (IGDR). Int J Dermatol. 2013;52:393–4.
42. Magro CM, Crowson AN, Schapiro BL. The interstitial granulomatous drug reaction: a distinctive clinical and pathological entity. J Cutan Pathol. 1998;25:72–8.
43. Magro CM, Cruz-Inigo AE, Votava H, Jacobs M, Wolfe D, Crowson AN. Drug-associated reversible granulomatous T cell dyscrasia: a distinct subset of the interstitial granulomatous drug reaction. J Cutan Pathol. 2010;37 Suppl 1:96–111.
44. Sen D, Rosenstein ED, Kramer N. ANCA-positive vasculitis associated with simvastatin/ezetimibe: expanding the spectrum of statin-induced autoimmunity? Int J Rheum Dis. 2010; 13:e29–31.
45. Bellini V, Assalve D, Lisi P. Urticarial vasculitis from simvastatin: what is the alternative drug? Dermatitis. 2010;21:223–4.

46. Yamamoto M, Ikeda M, Kodama H, Sano S. Transition of psoriasiform drug eruption to psoriasis de novo evidenced by histopathology. J Dermatol. 2008;35:732–6.
47. Fernández-Torres R, del Pozo J, Almagro M, Yebra-Pimentel MT, Fernández-Jorge B, Mazaira M, Fonseca E. Skin ulcers and myopathy associated with pravastatin therapy. Clin Exp Dermatol. 2009;34:e237–8.
48. Abadir R, Liebmann J. Radiation reaction recall following simvastatin therapy: a new observation. Clin Oncol (R Coll Radiol). 1995;7:325–6.
49. Rivera Irigoín R, Nicolau Ramis J, Terrasa Sagrista F, Masmiquel Comas L. Rosuvastatin-induced erythema multiforme. Med Clin (Barc). 2013;140:523–4.
50. Pfeiffer CM, Kazenoff S, Rothberg HD. Toxic epidermal necrolysis from atorvastatin. JAMA. 1998;279:1613–4.
51. Oskay T, Kutluay L. Acute generalized exanthematous pustulosis induced by simvastatin. Clin Exp Dermatol. 2003;28:558–9.
52. Perrot JL, Guy C, Bour Guichenez G, Amigues O, Servoz J, Cambazard F. Porphyria cutanea tarda induced by HMG CoA reductase inhibitors: simvastatin, pravastatin. Ann Dermatol Venereol. 1994;121:817–9.
53. Schindl A, Trautinger F, Pernerstorfer-Schön H, Konnaris C, Hönigsmann H. Porphyria cutanea tarda induced by the use of pravastatin. Arch Dermatol. 1998;134:1305–6.
54. Gressier L, Pruvost-Balland C, Dubertret L, Viguier M. Atorvastatin-induced drug reaction with eosinophilia and systemic symptoms (DRESS). Ann Dermatol Venereol. 2009;136:50–3.
55. Horton SL, Hashimoto K, Toi Y, Miner JE, Mehregan D, Fligiel A, et al. Spiny keratoderma: a common under-reported dermatosis. J Dermatol. 1998;25:353–61.
56. Adams AE, Bobrove AM, Gilliam AC. Statins and "chameleon-like" cutaneous eruptions: simvastatin-induced acral cutaneous vesiculobullous and pustular eruption in a 70-year-old man. J Cutan Med Surg. 2010;14:207–11.
57. Mehregan DR, Mehregan DA, Pakideh S. Cheilitis due to treatment with simvastatin. Cutis. 1998;62:197–8.
58. Segal AS. Alopecia associated with atorvastatin. Am J Med. 2002;113:171.
59. Frishman WH, Brosnan BD, Grossman M, Dasgupta D, Sun DK. Adverse dermatologic effects of cardiovascular drug therapy: part III. Cardiol Rev. 2002;10:337–48.
60. Machet L, Vaillant L, Jan V, Lorette G. Fenofibrate-induced photosensitivity: value of photopatch testing. J Am Acad Dermatol. 1997;37:808–9.
61. Leenutaphong V, Manuskiatti W. Fenofibrate-induced photosensitivity. J Am Acad Dermatol. 1996;35:775–7.
62. Conilleau V, Dompmartin A, Michel M, Verneuil L, Leroy D. Photoscratch testing in systemic drug-induced photosensitivity. Photodermatol Photoimmunol Photomed. 2000;16:62–6.
63. Hong JB, Wang SH, Chu CY. Fenofibrate-induced photosensitivity-a case report and literature review. Dermatol Sin. 2009;27:37–43.
64. Serrano G, Fortea JM, Latasa JM, Millan F, Janes C, Bosca F, Miranda MA. Photosensitivity induced by fibric acid derivatives and its relation to photocontact dermatitis to ketoprofen. J Am Acad Dermatol. 1992;27:204–8.
65. Leenutaphong V. Reply: Fenofibrate-induced photosensitivity: value of photopatch testing. J Am Acad Dermatol. 1997;37:809.
66. Frendo M, Theuma R, Fava S. Delayed bezafibrate-induced angio-oedema in a 68-year-old man. Br J Clin Pharmacol. 2007;64:560–1.
67. de Barrio M, Matheu V, Baeza ML, Tornero P, Rubio M, Zubeldia JM. Bezafibrate-induced anaphylactic shock: unusual clinical presentation. J Investig Allergol Clin Immunol. 2001;11:53–5.
68. Arif MA, Vahrman J. Letter: skin eruption due to clofibrate. Lancet. 1975;2:1202.
69. Murata Y, Tani M, Amano M. Erythema multiforme due to clofibrate. J Am Acad Dermatol. 1988;18:381–2.
70. Wong SS. Stevens-Johnson syndrome induced by clofibrate. Acta Derm Venereol. 1994;74:475.
71. Sawamura D, Umeki K. Stevens-Johnson syndrome associated with bezafibrate. Acta Derm Venereol. 2000;80:457.
72. Howard EJ, Brown SM. Letter: clofibrate-induced antinuclear factor and lupus-like syndrome. JAMA. 1973;226:1358–9.

73. Orgain ES, Bogdonoff MD, Cain C. Clofibrate and androsterone effect on serum lipids. Arch Intern Med. 1967;119:80–5.
74. Yung A, Goulden V. Pigmented purpuric dermatosis (capillaritis) induced by bezafibrate. J Am Acad Dermatol. 2005;53:168–9.
75. Fisher DA, Elias PM, LeBoit PL. Exacerbation of psoriasis by the hypolipidemic agent, gemfibrozil. Arch Dermatol. 1988;124:854–5.
76. Serrao R, Zirwas M, English JC. Palmar erythema. Am J Clin Dermatol. 2007;8:347–56.
77. Yang YL, Hu M, Chang M, Tomlinson B. A high incidence of exanthematous eruption associated with niacin/laropiprant combination in Hong Kong Chinese patients. J Clin Pharm Ther. 2013;38:528–32.
78. Pontiroli AE, Fattor B, Pozza G, Pianezzola E, Strolin Benedetti M, Musatti L. Acipimox-induced facial skin flush: frequency, thermographic evaluation and relationship to plasma acipimox level. Eur J Clin Pharmacol. 1992;43:145–8.
79. Ho SA, Aw DC. Bullous drug eruption secondary to nicotinic acid/laropiprant. Ann Acad Med Singapore. 2012;41:134–5.
80. Mehta V, Vasanth V, Balachandran C. Xanthinol nicotinate induced bullous drug eruption. J Pak Assoc Dermatol. 2009;19:124–5.
81. Williams ML, Feingold KR, Grubauer G, Elias PM. Ichthyosis induced by cholesterol-lowering drugs. Implications for epidermal cholesterol homeostasis. Arch Dermatol. 1987;123:1535–8.
82. Stals H, Vercammen C, Peeters C, Morren MA. Acanthosis nigricans caused by nicotinic acid: case report and review of the literature. Dermatology. 1994;189:203–6.
83. Tromovitch TA, Jacobs PH, Kern S. Acanthosis nigricans-like lesions from nicotinic acid. Arch Dermatol. 1964;89:222–3.
84. Coates P, Shuttleworth D, Rees A. Resolution of nicotinic acid-induced acanthosis nigricans by substitution of an analogue (acipimox) in a patient with type V hyperlipidaemia. Br J Dermatol. 1992;126:412–4.
85. Nelson LM. Fixed drug eruptions; a report of two cases, one caused by niacin, the other by cocaine. Calif Med. 1955;82:127–8.

Chapter 12
Platelet Inhibitors

Keywords Platelet inhibitors • Aspirin • Acetylsalicylic acid • Ticlopidine • Clopidogrel • Prasugrel • Angioedema/urticaria • Maculopapular • Thrombotic thrombocytopenic purpura • Lichenoid • Lupus erythematosus • Drug rash with eosinophilia and systemic symptoms • Erythema multiforme/Stevens–Johnson syndrome/toxic epidermal necrolysis • Fixed drug eruption

The cutaneous adverse effects of aspirin (acetylsalicylic acid), dipyridamole, ticagrelor, cangrelor; thienopyridine derivatives such as ticlopidine, clopidogrel, and prasugrel; and platelet glycoprotein IIb/IIIa receptor antagonists such as abciximab, tirofiban, and eptifibatide are reviewed in this chapter. Aspirin is more commonly associated with cutaneous reactions due to its use as a nonsteroidal antiinflammatory drug.

The adverse cutaneous drug reactions described below are meant to be sorted by starting from the well-known reactions of platelet inhibitors to the lesser known ones. The major ones are summarized in Table 12.1.

Angioedema/Urticaria

Urticaria with or without angioedema were reported with aspirin [1, 2], ticlopidine [3], clopidogrel [4–6], and prasugrel [7]. Aspirin [2, 8], abciximab [9], and dipyridamole [10] have also been reported to cause anaphylactoid reactions. Different from anaphylaxis that is an IgE-mediated immune reaction, anaphylactoid reactions are non-IgE-mediated pseudoallergic reactions.

Urticaria and angioedema are among the most common adverse cutaneous reactions of aspirin. The prevalence of aspirin-induced urticaria was stated to vary from 0.07 to 0.2 % in the general population [1]. On the other hand, aspirin has been reported to aggravate urticaria in 20–30 % of patients with chronic urticaria in a dose-related manner [1, 2]. The onset of urticaria varied from 15 minutes to 24 hours following aspirin intake, and the resolution of the reaction was stated to occur mostly in a few days but could also take up to 2 weeks [2].

The mechanism of aspirin-related urticaria is mostly attributed to its cyclooxygenase-1 (COX-1) inhibition effect. The resulting inhibition of prostaglandin D2 and E2 might then facilitate cutaneous mast cell degranulation and histamine

E. Özkaya, K.D. Yazganoğlu, *Adverse Cutaneous Drug Reactions to Cardiovascular Drugs*, DOI 10.1007/978-1-4471-6536-1_12

Table 12.1 Major adverse cutaneous drug reactions with platelet inhibitors

Adverse cutaneous drug reaction	Main inducers
Angioedema/urticaria	Aspirin, ticlopidine, clopidogrel, prasugrel
Anaphylactoid reaction	Aspirin, abciximab, dipyridamole
Maculopapular eruption	Ticlopidine, clopidogrel, prasugrel
Bleeding/purpura	Aspirin, ticlopidine, clopidogrel, prasugrel, abciximab, tirofiban, eptifibatide
Thrombotic thrombocytopenic purpura	Ticlopidine, clopidogrel, prasugrel
Lichenoid eruption	Aspirin, ticlopidine, clopidogrel
Drug-induced lupus erythematosus	Ticlopidine
DRESS	Ticlopidine, clopidogrel, aspirin
Erythema multiforme/Stevens–Johnson syndrome/toxic epidermal necrolysis	Aspirin, ticlopidine
Fixed drug eruption	Ticlopidine, clopidogrel, aspirin
Vasculitis	Ticlopidine, clopidogrel
Acute generalized exanthematous pustulosis	Aspirin, ticlopidine, clopidogrel
Serum sickness-like reaction	Ticlopidine, clopidogrel

DRESS drug rash with eosinophilia and systemic symptoms

release [1]. Another suggested mechanism was the diversion of arachidonic acid metabolism from prostaglandins to leukotrienes that was supported by an improvement of aspirin-related urticaria with leukotriene receptor antagonists [1].

As aspirin causes a non-immunologic activation and degranulation of mast cells, skin prick tests with aspirin are usually negative, and there are no detectable aspirin-specific IgEs in the sera of patients with aspirin-related urticaria. An exceptional case has been reported with aspirin-induced angioedema who showed specific IgE antibodies to an acetylsalicylic acid–human serum albumin conjugate [11].

Urticaria was among the most common adverse cutaneous reactions from ticlopidine, too [3]. Notably, in some cases with urticaria suggested to be induced by ticlopidine, the reaction was reported to resolve with antihistamines despite continuation of the drug [3]. Urticaria was reported to start between 4 and 21 days after initiation of ticlopidine [3].

In clopidogrel-associated angioedema/urticaria, the reaction was stated to start within 1 day of therapy, and systemic corticosteroids without discontinuation of the drug were effective in the management of these patients [6].

Maculopapular Eruption

Maculopapular eruption was reported to occur with ticlopidine [3, 12], clopidogrel [6, 12], and prasugrel [13–15].

Urticarial and maculopapular eruption were reported among the most common adverse cutaneous reactions to ticlopidine [3]. Notably, in some cases with maculopapular eruption suggested to be induced by ticlopidine, the reaction was reported to resolve with antihistamine or corticosteroid therapy despite continuation of the drug [3].

Generalized maculopapular eruptions, stated as exanthematous rash, were seen during clopidogrel use, usually within 1 week after starting therapy. In fact, they were reported to be the most common adverse cutaneous reaction during clopidogrel therapy. Treatment with systemic corticosteroids without discontinuation of the drug was found to be effective in the management of these patients [6]. A patient with maculopapular eruption from prasugrel was also treated with systemic corticosteroids without necessitating drug withdrawal [13].

Cross-reactivity between thienopyridine derivatives, ticlopidine and clopidogrel, were suggested to be possible and reported to be seen especially in mild reactions like rash, but not in life-threatening allergic reactions. The data were based on clinical history of the patients using both drugs [16]. Another study about cutaneous adverse reactions in patients using clopidogrel demonstrated cross-reactivity for ticlopidine, prasugrel, or more rarely for both drugs according to patch test or intradermal skin test results. However, oral provocation tests with ticlopidine or prasugrel were not performed [6]. Desensitization protocols for clopidogrel were suggested [17].

Bleeding/Purpura

Bleeding complications such as hemorrhage, bruising or hematoma are common especially with aspirin, clopidogrel and prasugrel [15, 18]. Clopidogrel was mainly associated with hemorrhage, whereas a stronger association was suggested for gastrointestinal bleeding with aspirin [18].

Thrombocytopenia can be seen during therapy with ticlopidine [19, 20], clopidogrel [21, 22], abciximab [23], tirofiban [23], and eptifibatide [24].

Hematologic adverse effects of ticlopidine are common and may be fatal. Thrombotic thrombocytopenic purpura, a life-threatening disease, can occur with ticlopidine [19, 20]. It was reported to occur usually within 3 months of therapy; therefore, close monitoring was advised in this period [19].

Thrombotic thrombocytopenic purpura was also reported with other thienopyridine derivatives such as clopidogrel and prasugrel [22, 25]. Different from the ticlopidine-induced cases, the reaction was stated to occur generally within 2 weeks of initiation of therapy with clopidogrel [22].

Patients using aspirin are at risk of developing bruising [26], and generalized purpura was reported to occur during the use of a combination drug containing acetylsalicylic acid and acetaminophen with concomitant intake of alcohol. It was suggested to develop as a result of platelet dysfunction caused by aspirin, that was enhanced by alcohol [27]. Ecchymoses can also occur during clopidogrel treatment as a result of thrombocytopenia without association of thrombotic thrombocytopenic purpura [21].

Lichenoid Eruption

Lichenoid eruption can occur with clopidogrel [28], ticlopidine [29], and acetylsalicylic acid [30].

Photosensitive lichenoid eruption localized on the face, neck, and extensor forearms starting within a month of clopidogrel therapy, and resolving within 4 weeks after discontinuation of the drug was reported [28]. Lesions reappeared on two different administrations [28]. Preexisting oral reticular lichen planus progressing to erosive lesions within 1 week after initiation of clopidogrel was reported. The erosive lesions were stated to disappear with discontinuation of the drug and additional systemic corticosteroid therapy, whereas reticular lesions showed persistence [31].

A case of lichen planus-like drug eruption developing approximately after 2 months of therapy with ticlopidine was reported. Patch test with ticlopidine was negative in this case, but oral rechallenge test was positive confirming ticlopidine as the causative drug [29].

Generalized lichenoid eruption without mucosal involvement was reported to occur after one month of therapy with acetylsalicylic acid. The reaction resolved within 3 weeks after discontinuation of the therapy but reappeared after readministration of the drug, suggesting that acetylsalicylic acid was the culprit agent [30].

Drug-Induced Lupus Erythematosus

Ticlopidine was reported to cause drug-induced systemic lupus erythematosus (SLE) in several cases [32–34]. An isolated case of subacute cutaneous lupus erythematosus associated with ticlopidine was also reported [35]. All patients were relatively elderly individuals.

Drug-induced SLE was usually reported to start as early as 2 weeks after the initiation of ticlopidine, but a long latency period up to 1–4 years was also reported in some cases [32–34]. Antinuclear antibodies and antihistone antibodies were detected in all patients. Clinical improvement was only seen after discontinuation of the drug with additional systemic therapy with corticosteroids, methotrexate or hydroxychloroquine in some cases. However, resolution was slow in some patients [32–34]. On the other hand, serologic improvement was not seen in every case in a follow-up period of 9–10 months [34]. Dermatologic findings of SLE were very rarely present in the reported cases; a pruritic urticarial rash on photoexposed areas like the face, chest, shoulders, and arms was described in one of them [32].

Drug Rash with Eosinophilia and Systemic Symptoms

Drug rash with eosinophilia and systemic symptoms (DRESS) was reported with clopidogrel [36, 37], ticlopidine [38], and aspirin [39]. The reaction started after 10 to approximately 15 days of drug administration in clopidogrel- and ticlopidine-induced cases. Hematologic abnormalities like pancytopenia or neutropenia usually accompanied. The reaction was called as a "systemic inflammatory response syndrome" in one case with clopidogrel-induced reaction who had normal hematologic parameters [40].

Aspirin was confirmed to be the culprit drug in a patient with DRESS by means of patch testing and lymphocyte stimulation test [39]. Patch test was positive with aspirin at concentrations of 10 and 20 % in petrolatum.

Erythema Multiforme/Stevens–Johnson Syndrome/ Toxic Epidermal Necrolysis

Erythema multiforme-like eruption was suggested to be induced by ticlopidine [3], Stevens–Johnson syndrome by aspirin [41], and toxic epidermal necrolysis by ticlopidine [42]. A case–control study conducted in four countries in Europe from 1989 to 1995 revealed that the risk of development of Stevens–Johnson syndrome or toxic epidermal necrolysis was not substantially increased by the use of acetylsalicylic acid and other salicylates [43].

Fixed Drug Eruption

Fixed drug eruption was reported with ticlopidine [3, 44], clopidogrel [6, 45], and aspirin [46]. Lesional patch test and oral challenge test were performed in one of the ticlopidine-induced cases, and revealed positive results for both, confirming ticlopidine as the inducer drug [44]. In one of the cases with clopidogrel-induced fixed drug eruption, oral challenge test was performed revealing positive reaction, thus confirming clopidogrel as the inducer drug [45]. Oral provocation was also positive in the case of aspirin-induced fixed drug eruption [46].

Vasculitis

Leukocytoclastic vasculitis has been reported with ticlopidine [47] and clopidogrel [48, 49] in isolated cases. Interestingly, in clopidogrel-associated cases, vasculitis occurred as a relatively early reaction starting after 4 days of therapy in one patient [48], and as a late reaction developing after 1 year of therapy with clopidogrel in another one [49].

Acute Generalized Exanthematous Pustulosis

Acute generalized exanthematous pustulosis was reported with the use of acetylsalicylic acid [50], clopidogrel [51], and ticlopidine [52]. Patch test with ticlopidine revealed positive result in the latter case.

Serum Sickness-Like Reaction

Maculopapular or urticarial rash in addition to arthralgias/arthritis with or without fever was reported due to clopidogrel [53] and ticlopidine [54]. The authors called this reaction as a "serum sickness-like reaction" in the clopidogrel-associated case [53]. They further suggested that the ticlopidine-associated case [54] was an example of this reaction as well, although it was regarded as drug-induced hypersensitivity vasculitis in the original report.

Pruritus

Pruritus is a nonspecific cutaneous adverse reaction of drugs. It was reported in patients receiving platelet inhibitor therapy, mainly accompanying different types of drug eruptions [3, 5, 6, 10, 30, 44, 55, 56].

Other Reported Adverse Cutaneous Drug Reactions to Platelet Inhibitors

Eczematous drug eruption caused by dipyridamole was reported. The reaction was seen during the use of a combination drug of dipyridamole and acetylsalicylic acid. Patch test revealed positive result with the combination drug, whereas oral rechallenge with acetylsalicylic acid was negative, excluding acetylsalicylic acid as the cause [56].

An attack of suberythrodermic *pustular psoriasis* was reported in a patient with a previous history of psoriasis that developed during the use of clopidogrel and captopril. The reaction reappeared after readministration of clopidogrel, suggesting that clopidogrel was the causative drug [57]. Clopidogrel was linked to exacerbation of palmoplantar pustular psoriasis in one case [58]. The risk of psoriasis or psoriatic arthritis was not clearly associated with aspirin intake according to the results of a cohort study [59].

Ticlopidine was suggested to be responsible for a reaction manifesting initially as a pruritic mild rash but, after discontinuation of the drug, progressing to *erythroderma* with fever within 4 days [60]. *Erythromelalgia-like eruption* was reported with ticlopidine [3].

A case of *papuloerythroderma of Ofuji* was reported to be caused by aspirin according to positive rechallenge test and positive lymphocyte stimulation test results. Patch test was negative in this patient [55]. *Bullous pemphigoid* was reported to be induced by aspirin in a patient [61]. *Mucosal burn* was reported to develop from chewable aspirin [62].

Localized cutaneous reactions such as erythematous and desquamative rash on the face, focal erythema of the neck, symmetrical bilateral erythematous rash in the axilla, symmetrical bilateral desquamation of the palms, and symmetrical bilateral hyperkeratotic psoriasiform lesions on the soles have been reported during the use of clopidogrel [6].

References

1. Gollapudi RR, Teirstein PS, Stevenson DD, Simon RA. Aspirin sensitivity: implications for patients with coronary artery disease. JAMA. 2004;292:3017–23.
2. Grattan CE. Aspirin sensitivity and urticaria. Clin Exp Dermatol. 2003;28:123–7.
3. Yosipovitch G, Rechavia E, Feinmesser M, David M. Adverse cutaneous reactions to ticlopidine in patients with coronary stents. J Am Acad Dermatol. 1999;41:473–6.
4. Khambekar SK, Kovac J, Gershlick AH. Clopidogrel induced urticarial rash in a patient with left main stem percutaneous coronary intervention: management issues. Heart. 2004;90:e14.
5. Gowda RM, Misra D, Khan IA. Hypersensitivity skin rash: an adverse drug reaction to clopidogrel loading dose. Int J Cardiol. 2004;95:333.
6. Cheema AN, Mohammad A, Hong T, Jakubovic HR, Parmar GS, Sharieff W, et al. Characterization of clopidogrel hypersensitivity reactions and management with oral steroids without clopidogrel discontinuation. J Am Coll Cardiol. 2011;58:1445–54.
7. Báez-Montiel BB, Gutiérrez-Islas E, Herrera-Ontañón JR, Turabián JL. To enlighten and to dazzle: a case of an inadequate prescription of prasugrel with an adverse reaction of urticaria. Aten Primaria. 2013;45:64–5.
8. Berkes EA. Anaphylactic and anaphylactoid reactions to aspirin and other NSAIDs. Clin Rev Allergy Immunol. 2003;24:137–48.
9. Pharand C, Palisaitis DA, Hamel D. Potential anaphylactic shock with abciximab readministration. Pharmacotherapy. 2002;22:380–3.
10. Angelides S, Van der Wall H, Freedman SB. Acute reaction to dipyridamole during myocardial scintigraphy. N Engl J Med. 1999;340:394.
11. Blanca M, Perez E, Garcia JJ, Miranda A, Terrados S, Vega JM, Suau R. Angioedema and IgE antibodies to aspirin: a case report. Ann Allergy. 1989;62:295–8.
12. Makkar K, Wilensky RL, Julien MB, Herrmann HC, Spinler SA. Rash with both clopidogrel and ticlopidine in two patients following percutaneous coronary intervention with drug-eluting stents. Ann Pharmacother. 2006;40:1204–7.
13. Yang DC, Feldman DN, Kim LK, Minutello RM, Bergman G, Wong SC, Swaminathan RV. A strategy of 'treating through' a prasugrel-induced rash. Int J Cardiol. 2013;168:4381–2.
14. Raccah BH, Shalit M, Danenberg HD. Allergic reaction to prasugrel and cross-reactivity with clopidogrel. Int J Cardiol. 2012;157:e48–9.
15. Nanau RM, Delzor F, Neuman MG. Efficacy and safety of Prasugrel in acute coronary syndrome patients. Clin Biochem. 2014;47:516–28. doi:10.1016/j.clinbiochem.2014.03.005.
16. Lokhandwala JO, Best PJ, Butterfield JH, Skelding KA, Scott T, Blankenship JC, et al. Frequency of allergic or hematologic adverse reactions to ticlopidine among patients with allergic or hematologic adverse reactions to clopidogrel. Circ Cardiovasc Interv. 2009;2:348–51.

17. Owen P, Garner J, Hergott L, Page 2nd RL. Clopidogrel desensitization: case report and review of published protocols. Pharmacotherapy. 2008;28:259–70.
18. Tamura T, Sakaeda T, Kadoyama K, Okuno Y. Aspirin- and clopidogrel-associated bleeding complications: data mining of the public version of the FDA adverse event reporting system, AERS. Int J Med Sci. 2012;9:441–6. doi:10.7150/ijms.4549.
19. Bennett CL, Davidson CJ, Raisch DW, Weinberg PD, Bennett RH, Feldman MD. Thrombotic thrombocytopenic purpura associated with ticlopidine in the setting of coronary artery stents and stroke prevention. Arch Intern Med. 1999;159:2524–8.
20. Paradiso-Hardy FL, Angelo CM, Lanctot KL, Cohen EA. Hematologic dyscrasia associated with ticlopidine therapy: evidence for causality. CMAJ. 2000;163:1463–4.
21. Briguori C, Manganelli F, Picardi M, Villari B, Ricciardelli B. Thrombocytopenia and purpura-like lesions associated with clopidogrel. Ital Heart J. 2001;2:935–7.
22. Bennett CL, Connors JM, Carwile JM, Moake JL, Bell WR, Tarantolo SR, et al. Thrombotic thrombocytopenic purpura associated with clopidogrel. N Engl J Med. 2000;342:1773–7.
23. Merlini PA, Rossi M, Menozzi A, Buratti S, Brennan DM, Moliterno DJ, et al. Thrombocytopenia caused by abciximab or tirofiban and its association with clinical outcome in patients undergoing coronary stenting. Circulation. 2004;109:2203–6.
24. Graidis C, Golias C, Dimitriadis D, Dimitriadis G, Bitsis T, Dimitrelos I, et al. Eptifibatide-induced acute profound thrombocytopenia: a case report. BMC Res Notes. 2014;7:107.
25. Jacob S, Dunn BL, Qureshi ZP, Bandarenko N, Kwaan HC, Pandey DK, et al. Ticlopidine-, clopidogrel-, and prasugrel-associated thrombotic thrombocytopenic purpura: a 20-year review from the Southern Network on Adverse Reactions (SONAR). Semin Thromb Hemost. 2012;38:845–53.
26. Frishman WH, Brosnan BD, Grossman M, Dasgupta D, Sun DK. Adverse dermatologic effects of cardiovascular drug therapy: part III. Cardiol Rev. 2002;10:337–48.
27. Tsuda T, Okamoto Y, Sakaguchi R, Katayama N, Hara I, Hayashi H, Ota K. Purpura due to aspirin-induced platelet dysfunction aggravated by drinking alcohol. J Int Med Res. 2001;29:374–80.
28. Dogra S, Kanwar AJ. Clopidogrel bisulphate-induced photosensitive lichenoid eruption: first report. Br J Dermatol. 2003;148:609–10.
29. Kurokawa I, Umehara M, Nishijima S. Lichen planus-type drug eruption resulting from ticlopidine. Int J Dermatol. 2005;44:436–7.
30. Ruiz Villaverde R, Blasco Melguizo J, Mendoza Guil F, Martin Sanchez MC, Naranjo Sintes R. Generalized lichen planus-like eruption due to acetylsalicylic acid. J Eur Acad Dermatol Venereol. 2003;17:470–2.
31. Guijarro Guijarro B, Lopez Sanchez AF. Lichenoid reaction caused by clopidogrel, a new antiplatelet drug. Med Oral. 2003;8:33–7.
32. Braun-Moscovici Y, Schapira D, Balbir-Gurman A, Sevilia R, Nahir AM. Ticlopidine-induced lupus. J Clin Rheumatol. 2001;7:102–5.
33. Yokoyama T, Usui T, Kiyama K, Nakashima R, Yukawa N, Kawabata D, et al. Two cases of late-onset drug-induced lupus erythematosus caused by ticlopidine in elderly men. Mod Rheumatol. 2010;20:405–9.
34. Spiera RF, Berman RS, Werner AJ, Spiera H. Ticlopidine-induced lupus: a report of 4 cases. Arch Intern Med. 2002;162:2240–3.
35. Reich A, Bialynicki-Birula R, Szepietowski JC. Drug-induced subacute cutaneous lupus erythematosus resulting from ticlopidine. Int J Dermatol. 2006;45:1112–4.
36. Doogue MP, Begg EJ, Bridgman P. Clopidogrel hypersensitivity syndrome with rash, fever, and neutropenia. Mayo Clin Proc. 2005;80:1368–70.
37. Comert A, Akgun S, Civelek A, Kavala M, Sarigul S, Yildirim T, Arsan S. Clopidogrel-induced hypersensitivity syndrome associated with febrile pancytopenia. Int J Dermatol. 2005;44:882–4.
38. Ceylan C, Kirimli O, Akarsu M, Undar B, Güneri S. Early ticlopidine-induced hepatic dysfunction, dermatitis and irreversible aplastic anemia after coronary artery stenting. Am J Hematol. 1998;59:260.

39. Kawakami T, Fujita A, Takeuchi S, Muto S, Soma Y. Drug-induced hypersensitivity syndrome: drug reaction with eosinophilia and systemic symptoms (DRESS) syndrome induced by aspirin treatment of Kawasaki disease. J Am Acad Dermatol. 2009;60:146–9.
40. Wolf I, Mouallem M, Rath S, Farfel Z. Clopidogrel-induced systemic inflammatory response syndrome. Mayo Clin Proc. 2003;78:618–20.
41. Ting HC, Adam BA. Stevens-Johnson syndrome. A review of 34 cases. Int J Dermatol. 1985;24:587–91.
42. Strippoli D, Russo G, Simonetti V, Motolese A. Lyell syndrome due to ticlopidine. G Ital Dermatol Venereol. 2011;146:497–500.
43. Kaufman DW, Kelly JP. Acetylsalicylic acid and other salicylates in relation to Stevens-Johnson syndrome and toxic epidermal necrolysis. Br J Clin Pharmacol. 2001;51:174–6.
44. Garcia CM, Carmena R, Garcia R, Berges P, Camacho E, Cotter MP, de la Hoz B. Fixed drug eruption from ticlopidine, with positive lesional patch test. Contact Dermatitis. 2001; 44:40–1.
45. Ghosh SK, Bandyopadhyay D. Clopidogrel-induced fixed drug eruption. J Eur Acad Dermatol Venereol. 2009;23:1202–3.
46. Chan HL. Fixed drug eruptions. A study of 20 occurrences in Singapore. Int J Dermatol. 1984;23:607–9.
47. Pintor E, Sanmartin M, Azcona L, Hernandez R, Fernandez-Cruz A, Macaya C. Leukocytoclastic vasculitis associated with ticlopidine. Rev Esp Cardiol. 2001;54:114–6.
48. Erpolat S, Nazli Y, Colak N, Yenidunya S. Leucocytoclastic vasculitis associated with clopidogrel. Cutan Ocul Toxicol. 2012;31:171–3.
49. Shetty RK, Madken M, Naha K, Vivek G. Leucocytoclastic vasculitis as a late complication of clopidogrel therapy. BMJ Case Rep. 2013;17:2013.
50. Ballmer-Weber BK, Widmer M, Burg G. Acetylsalicylic acid-induced generalized pustulosis. Schweiz Med Wochenschr. 1993;123:542–6.
51. Ellerbroek JC, Cleveland MG. Clopidogrel-associated acute generalized exanthematous pustulosis. Cutis. 2011;87:181–5.
52. Cannavo SP, Borgia F, Guarneri F, Vaccaro M. Acute generalized exanthematous pustulosis following use of ticlopidine. Br J Dermatol. 2000;142:577–8.
53. Phillips EJ, Knowles SR, Shear NH. Serum sickness-like reaction associated with clopidogrel. Br J Clin Pharmacol. 2003;56:583.
54. Dakik HA, Salti I, Haidar R, Uthman IW. Drug points: ticlopidine associated with acute arthritis. BMJ. 2002;324:27.
55. Sugita K, Koga C, Yoshiki R, Izu K, Tokura Y. Papuloerythroderma caused by aspirin. Arch Dermatol. 2006;142:792–3.
56. Salava A, Alanko K, Hyry H. Dipyridamole-induced eczematous drug eruption with positive patch test reaction. Contact Dermatitis. 2012;67:103–4.
57. Meissner M, Beier C, Wolter M, Kaufmann R, Gille J. Suberythrodermic pustular psoriasis induced by clopidogrel. Br J Dermatol. 2006;155:630–1.
58. Mahajan VK, Khatri G, Prabha N, Abhinav C, Sharma V. Clopidogrel: a possible exacerbating factor for psoriasis. Indian J Pharmacol. 2014;46:123–4.
59. Wu S, Han J, Qureshi AA. Use of aspirin, nonsteroidal anti-inflammatory drugs, and aceta-minophen (paracetamol), and risk of psoriasis and psoriatic arthritis: A Cohort Study. Acta Derm Venereol. 2014. doi:10.2340/00015555-1855.
60. Hsi DH, Mock DJ, Rocco Jr TA. Toxic erythroderma due to ticlopidine. N Engl J Med. 1999;340:1212.
61. Durdu M, Baba M, Seçkin D. A case of bullous pemphigoid induced by aspirin. J Am Acad Dermatol. 2011;65:443–4.
62. Maron F. Mucosal burn resulting from chewable aspirin: report of case. J Am Dent Assoc. 1989;119:279–80.

Chapter 13
Thrombolytics

Keywords Thrombolytic • Fibrinolytic • Plasminogen • Anistreplase • Streptokinase • Purpura • Angioedema/urticaria • Vasculitis • Serum sickness-like reaction • Cholesterol embolism

Thrombolytic (fibrinolytic) agents include alteplase (tissue plasminogen activator), anistreplase (anisoylated plasminogen streptokinase activator complex), reteplase, streptokinase, tenecteplase, and urokinase.

The adverse cutaneous drug reactions described below are meant to be sorted by starting from the well-known reactions of thrombolytics to the lesser known ones. The major ones are summarized in Table 13.1.

Purpura

Thrombolytic agents are plasminogen activators that play a role in conversion of plasminogen to the active proteolytic enzyme plasmin which lyses the fibrin of a blood clot. The clot may be physiologic or a pathologic thrombus. Systemic activation of the fibrinolytic mechanism and degradation of physiologic clot at sites of vascular injury that has healed incompletely are associated with increased risk of hemorrhage as an adverse effect of these drugs [1].

Occurrence of ecchymoses or purpura is not unusual with these drugs [2, 3]. Localized purpuric lesions developing after administration of intravenous streptokinase, and resolving spontaneously within a few days, were reported [4].

Table 13.1 Major adverse cutaneous drug reactions with thrombolytics

Adverse cutaneous drug reaction	Main inducers
Purpura/ecchymosis	Class effect
Angioedema/urticaria	Streptokinase, alteplase, reteplase, and urokinase
Vasculitis	Streptokinase, anistreplase
Serum sickness-like reaction	Streptokinase
Cholesterol embolism	Streptokinase, alteplase
Maculopapular eruption	Anistreplase

E. Özkaya, K.D. Yazganoğlu, *Adverse Cutaneous Drug Reactions to Cardiovascular Drugs*, DOI 10.1007/978-1-4471-6536-1_13

Subcutaneous hematomas may occur after mild trauma in patients using these agents [5]. Massive subfascial hematoma presenting as cutaneous ecchymosis associated with a sudden fall in hemoglobin after the administration of alteplase for acute myocardial infarction was reported in a case [6].

Angioedema/Urticaria

Angioedema or urticaria or life-threatening anaphylactic/anaphylactoid reactions were reported with thrombolytic agents like streptokinase, alteplase, reteplase, and urokinase [7–12]. Even endogenous proteins such as alteplase and urokinase, which are considered as low antigenic fibrinolytics, were reported to be associated with anaphylactic/anaphylactoid reactions [8–11]. In fact, alteplase seemed to be the most common cause of allergic reactions among thrombolytics [12].

Vasculitis

Cutaneous vasculitis was reported in several cases due to streptokinase and anistreplase presented mainly as leukocytoclastic vasculitis [13–16]. Vasculitic lesions were reported to develop in six of 253 patients treated with anistreplase [14]. It started between 7 and 15 days after administration of the drug. Accompanying arthropathy, urinary abnormalities, and gastrointestinal involvement were seen in some of the patients [14]. Interestingly, cutaneous vasculitis was reported to develop immediately on the day of streptokinase administration in a patient [16]. As streptokinase is produced from streptococci, it was suggested that a presensitization to streptococcal antigens with antibody formation could be present in this patient leading to a cross-reaction with streptokinase and causing a rapid immune response [16].

Serum Sickness-Like Reaction

Drug-induced cutaneous vasculitis may also be part of a so-called serum sickness-like reaction (SSLR), especially if it is associated with arthralgia/arthritis and often fever. However, vasculitis and fever are not consistent findings in the reported cases of SSLR. Dermatologic lesions may be variable such as palpable purpura with/without hemorrhagic vesicles, urticarial lesions, or erythema multiforme-like lesions in SSLR [17]. Moreover, gastrointestinal disturbances, lymphadenopathy, low complement levels, circulating immune complexes, and proteinuria associated with renal involvement that would be expected in true serum sickness are usually absent or rarely reported in drug-induced SSLR [17, 18]. In cases with detected circulating immune complexes to drugs, the condition is better termed as drug-induced serum sickness reaction.

Drug-induced SSLR or serum sickness reaction presenting as urticarial or purpuric lesions in addition to arthralgias/arthritis with/without fever has been reported to occur mainly with streptokinase therapy [19–23]. The eruption was reported to occur within 7–9 days following streptokinase administration [20–23]. Histopathology of purpuric lesions was performed in some cases, showing vasculitic changes [22, 23]. Urinary abnormalities like hematuria and proteinuria and even renal failure were reported to develop in some [21, 22]. As an interesting finding, circulating immune complexes, detected as a cryoglobulin, were demonstrated in the serum of a patient, comprising antistreptokinase, streptokinase, and C3. The reaction was therefore considered as an immune complex-mediated type III hypersensitivity reaction with elevation of circulating immune complexes or antibodies to streptokinase, thus a drug-induced serum sickness reaction [22].

Cholesterol Embolism

Cholesterol embolism is a serious complication that may be seen in patients after invasive vascular procedures like coronary angiography, but is also described in patients who have been treated with thrombolytic agents like streptokinase and alteplase mainly for acute myocardial infarction [24–30]. Arterial circulation of different organs may be occluded by cholesterol crystals from an ulcerated atheromatous plaque as a result of lysis of the thrombus on the plaque caused by fibrinolytic therapy. Clinical cutaneous manifestations usually include livedo reticularis, cyanosis, purpura, ecchymoses, skin necrosis, ulcerations, or gangrene, mainly located at the toes or lower extremities, but may also involve the lower trunk, upper extremities, and hands [24–30].

Pruritus

Pruritus is a nonspecific cutaneous adverse reaction of drugs. It was reported in patients receiving thrombolytic therapy, mainly accompanying different types of drug eruptions [11, 16].

Other Reported Adverse Cutaneous Drug Reactions to Thrombolytic Agents

Maculopapular eruption has been reported in patients receiving anistreplase [31]. *Flushing* and *hyperhidrosis* were linked to some of the thrombolytic agents [2, 3].

References

1. Haire WD. Pharmacology of fibrinolysis. Chest. 1992;101:91S–7S.
2. Litt JZ. Drug eruption reference manual. 19th ed. Boca Raton: CRC Press (Taylor and Francis Group); 2013.
3. Frishman WH, Brosnan BD, Grossman M, Dasgupta D, Sun DK. Adverse dermatologic effects of cardiovascular drug therapy: part III. Cardiol Rev. 2002;10:337–48.
4. Smithson JE, Kennedy CT, Hughes S. A new skin lesion associated with intravenous streptokinase. BMJ. 1993;306:973.
5. Mirowska-Guzel D, Kobayashi A, Członkowska A. Widespread subcutaneous haematoma after thrombolytic therapy in stroke patients. Mild falls at stroke onset may be dangerous. Neurol Neurochir Pol. 2006;40:536–8.
6. Khanlou H, Malhotra G, Khanlou N, Eiger G, Frechie P. Massive subfascial hematoma after alteplase therapy for acute myocardial infarction. Am J Med Sci. 1999;317:53–4.
7. Cooper JP, Quarry DP, Beale DJ, Chappell AG. Life-threatening, localized angio-oedema associated with streptokinase. Postgrad Med J. 1994;70:592–3.
8. Cannas S, De Leo A, Marzari A. Anaphylactoid reaction during administration of tissue plasminogen activator (t-PA). G Ital Cardiol. 1997;27:278–80.
9. Massel D, Gill JB, Cairns JA. Anaphylactoid reaction during an infusion of recombinant tissue-type plasminogen activator for acute myocardial infarction. Can J Cardiol. 1991;7:298–302.
10. Vidovich RR, Heiselman DE, Hudock D. Treatment of urokinase-related anaphylactoid reaction with intravenous famotidine. Ann Pharmacother. 1992;26:782–3.
11. Pechlaner C, Knapp E, Wiedermann CJ. Hypersensitivity reactions associated with recombinant tissue-type plasminogen activator and urokinase. Blood Coagul Fibrinolysis. 2001;12:491–4.
12. Zarar A, Khan AA, Adil MM, Qureshi AI. Anaphylactic shock associated with intravenous thrombolytics. Am J Emerg Med. 2014;32:113.e3–5.
13. Ong AC, Handler CE, Walker JM. Hypersensitivity vasculitis complicating intravenous streptokinase therapy in acute myocardial infarction. Int J Cardiol. 1988;21:71–3.
14. Bucknall C, Darley C, Flax J, Vincent R, Chamberlain D. Vasculitis complicating treatment with intravenous anisoylated plasminogen streptokinase activator complex in acute myocardial infarction. Br Heart J. 1988;59:9–11.
15. Burrows N, Jones RR. Rash after treatment with anistreplase. Br Heart J. 1990;64:289–90.
16. Gupta S, Gupta S, Thomas M, Pandey P, Aggarwal M, Mahendra A, Jindal N. Streptokinase induced purpura-like lesions. Acta Med Indones. 2012;44:69–70.
17. Yerushalmi J, Zvulunov A, Halevy S. Serum sickness-like reactions. Cutis. 2002;69:395–7.
18. Al-Niaimi F. Drug eruptions in dermatology. Expert Rev Dermatol. 2011;6:273–86.
19. Schweitzer DH, van der Wall EE, Bosker HA, Scheffer E, Macfarlane JD. Serum-sickness-like illness as a complication after streptokinase therapy for acute myocardial infarction. Cardiology. 1991;78:68–71.
20. Creamer JD, McGrath JA, Webb-Peploe M, Smith NP. Serum sickness-like illness following streptokinase therapy. A case report. Clin Exp Dermatol. 1995;20:468–70.
21. Clesham GJ, Terry HJ, Jalihal S, Toghill PJ. Serum sickness and purpura following intravenous streptokinase. J R Soc Med. 1992;85:638–9.
22. Davies KA, Mathieson P, Winearls CG, Rees AJ, Walport MJ. Serum sickness and acute renal failure after streptokinase therapy for myocardial infarction. Clin Exp Immunol. 1990;80:83–8.
23. Patel A, Prussick R, Buchanan WW, Sauder DN. Serum sickness-like illness and leukocytoclastic vasculitis after intravenous streptokinase. J Am Acad Dermatol. 1991;24:652–3.
24. Schwartz MW, McDonald GB. Cholesterol embolization syndrome. Occurrence after intravenous streptokinase therapy for myocardial infarction. JAMA. 1987;258:1934–5.
25. Bucher A, Roald B. Cholesterol embolization after intravenous streptokinase therapy in acute myocardial infarction. Tidsskr Nor Laegeforen. 1993;113:1844–5.
26. Arora RR, Magun AM, Grossman M, Katz J. Cholesterol embolization syndrome after intravenous tissue plasminogen activator for acute myocardial infarction. Am Heart J. 1993;126:225–8.

27. Pettelot G, Bracco J, Barrillon D, Baudouy M, Morand P. Images in cardiovascular medicine. Cholesterol embolization: unrecognized complication of thrombolysis. Circulation. 1998;97:1522.
28. Bhardwaj M, Goldweit R, Erlebacher J, Kashani M, Levin D, Leber G. Tissue plasminogen activator and cholesterol crystal embolization. Ann Intern Med. 1989;111:687–8.
29. Wong FK, Chan SK, Ing TS, Li CS. Acute renal failure after streptokinase therapy in a patient with acute myocardial infarction. Am J Kidney Dis. 1995;26:508–10.
30. Queen M, Biem HJ, Moe GW, Sugar L. Development of cholesterol embolization syndrome after intravenous streptokinase for acute myocardial infarction. Am J Cardiol. 1990;65:1042–3.
31. Dykewicz MS, McMorrow NK, Davison R, Fintel DJ, Zull CC, Rutledge JL. Drug eruptions and isotypic antibody responses to streptokinase after infusions of anisoylated plasminogen-streptokinase complex (APSAC, anistreplase). J Allergy Clin Immunol. 1995;95:1020–8.

Chapter 14
Anticoagulants

Keywords Anticoagulants • Heparin • Low molecular weight heparin • Enoxaparin • Warfarin • Bleeding/purpura • Necrosis • Eczema • Angioedema/urticaria • Bullous hemorrhagic dermatosis • Vasculitis • Alopecia • Purple toe • Drug rash with eosinophilia and systemic symptoms

The adverse cutaneous reactions associated with injectable anticoagulants such as unfractionated (standard) heparin, low molecular weight heparins (LMWHs) (enoxaparin, nadroparin [fraxiparin], certoparin, ardeparin, dalteparin, tinzaparin, bemiparin), direct thrombin inhibitors (argatroban), hirudins (desirudin, lepirudin, bivalirudin), synthetic pentasaccharides (fondaparinux and idraparinux), heparinoids (danaparoid, pentosan polysulfate); and oral anticoagulants such as warfarin, acenocoumarol, fluindione, phenindione, direct thrombin inhibitor (dabigatran), and factor Xa inhibitors (rivaroxaban, apixaban, edoxaban) are reviewed in this section.

The adverse cutaneous drug reactions described below are meant to be sorted by starting from the well-known reactions of anticoagulants to the lesser known ones. The major ones are summarized in Table 14.1.

Bleeding/Purpura

As heparins predispose tendency to bleeding, ecchymoses or hematomas might occur during therapy [1]. In fact, this side effect would also be expected for other anticoagulants. Purpuric lesions might also occur due to heparin-induced thrombocytopenia that is classified into two types as type I and type II, the latter being an immunologic reaction as described below. Type I heparin-induced thrombocytopenia is stated to be more common, mild, and usually asymptomatic with early onset. The pathogenesis is suggested to be related with platelet proaggregating effect of heparin [2].

E. Özkaya, K.D. Yazganoğlu, *Adverse Cutaneous Drug Reactions to Cardiovascular Drugs*, DOI 10.1007/978-1-4471-6536-1_14

Table 14.1 Major adverse cutaneous drug reactions with anticoagulant drugs

Adverse cutaneous drug reaction	Main inducers
Bleeding/purpura	Class effect
Skin necrosis	Heparin, LMWHs, warfarin, acenocoumarol, fluindione
Eczematous eruption	Heparin, LMWHs, [a]danaparoid
Angioedema/urticaria	Heparin, LMWHs, lepirudin
Bullous eruption	
Bullous hemorrhagic dermatosis	LMWHs (enoxaparin, dalteparin, tinzaparin, and bemiparin), heparin calcium, idraparinux
Maculopapular eruption	Heparin, LMWHs, dabigatran
Vasculitis	LMWHs, warfarin, acenocoumarol
Alopecia	LMWHs, warfarin
Calcinosis cutis	Nadroparin calcium
Purple toe syndrome	Warfarin
DRESS	Phenindione, fluindione, acenocoumarol, enoxaparin, heparin
Acute generalized exanthematous pustulosis	Dalteparin, fluindione

LMWHs low molecular weight heparins, *DRESS* drug rash with eosinophilia and systemic symptoms
[a]Cross-reaction with heparin and low molecular weight heparins

Skin Necrosis

Skin necrosis associated with heparin, LMWHs, warfarin, acenocoumarol, and fluindione is a rare but serious adverse reaction [3–9]. Heparin- or LMWH-induced cutaneous necrosis usually develops after 2 days to 2 weeks of therapy. It commonly occurs at the injection site, although it can also develop at distant sites [3–5]. It generally starts as erythema and tenderness at the injection sites developing to erythematous, painful lesions and then to necrotic or ulcerated plaques, usually within 18–36 hours [3]. Histopathology shows occlusion of small dermal vessels along with epidermal necrosis [2–4]. The mechanisms underlying this disorder are not clarified. It was attributed to type II heparin-induced thrombocytopenia termed as "heparin-induced thrombocytopenia and thrombosis (HITT) syndrome" [4]. HITT syndrome is associated with the formation of platelet-activating antibodies induced by heparin. As a result of this immunologic response, the patient is at risk for thrombocytopenia (due to platelet consumption) and thrombotic complications such as deep vein thrombosis and pulmonary embolism [4]. Although there is an increased risk, these complications were stated to be uncommon in heparin-induced skin necrosis, and it is considered as a localized variant [4]. Immediate withdrawal of the anticoagulant therapy is required because of the risk of systemic thrombosis. The therapy was advised not to be changed to another heparin because of the possibility of cross-reactivity that can lead to sustained prothrombotic condition [2, 3]. Heparin-induced skin necrosis can also be associated with various other conditions such as protein S deficiency, antithrombin III deficiency, and antiphospholipid antibodies [2, 4].

Warfarin-induced skin necrosis is an uncommon adverse drug reaction clinically and histopathologically similar to heparin-induced skin necrosis [3]. It usually starts within 3–10 days of warfarin therapy [3]; however, earlier or later onset is also possible [6]. The predilection sites of skin necrosis are most commonly the areas of the body with high fat content such as the abdomen, thighs, and breasts [6]. This type of reaction due to warfarin is associated with underlying conditions like protein S, protein C, and antithrombin III deficiency [2, 3, 6]. Acenocoumarol was also reported to induce skin necrosis similar to warfarin. Interestingly, a biopsy taken within hours of the onset of necrosis showed leukocytoclastic vasculitis in a patient. The authors postulated that early lesion biopsies could reveal this result [7]. In patients with fluindione-induced skin necrosis, protein C deficiency was also present [8, 9].

Different from the classical, centrally located skin necrosis as described above, warfarin was also reported to be associated with gangrene of distal extremity or rarely digital necrosis of the toes and fingers, in the setting of hypercoagulability states like malignancy or heparin-induced thrombocytopenia [10, 11].

Eczematous Eruption

Delayed-type sensitization presenting as eczematous eruption to unfractionated heparin and LMWHs is a common problem. Pruritic eczematous plaques have been reported usually with heparin or LMWHs at the injection site [12–17]; rarely, generalized reactions may also occur [18, 19]. Obese individuals, women, and patients receiving long-term heparin therapy are at increased risk for developing this reaction [1, 16]. The reaction was reported to develop within 3–21 days after starting subcutaneous heparin therapy [13]. Previously sensitized individuals may experience early-onset reactions within 1 to several days [16]. In one patient, the reaction developed 11 days after stopping the therapy [14].

Epicutaneous (patch), intracutaneous (intradermal), or subcutaneous tests may be performed in these individuals both for diagnostic purpose and in order to determine a suitable alternative drug. However, patch tests have been reported to be rarely positive. Two cases with enoxaparin-induced eczematous drug eruption showed positive patch test reaction with the commercial product of enoxaparin [17]. One of them showed cross-reaction to the commercial product of nadroparin as well. The relatively low incidence of patch test positivity with LMWHs was attributed to the fact that low doses of LMWH may inhibit the elicitation of allergic contact dermatitis [15]. Subcutaneous provocation tests were reported to be more reliable for the diagnosis of delayed type hypersensitivity reaction against unfractionated heparin and LMWHs [13, 15, 20]. We have recently diagnosed a patient with enoxaparin-induced eczematous eruption partly showing a nummular pattern (Fig. 14.1) confirmed by subcutaneous provocation test. The patch test was negative. Flare-up of old lesions occurred during the provocation test and supported the clinical relevance (unpublished data).

Delayed-type cross-reactivity between unfractionated heparin and LMWHs as well as danaparoid is an important problem for patients who need thrombosis

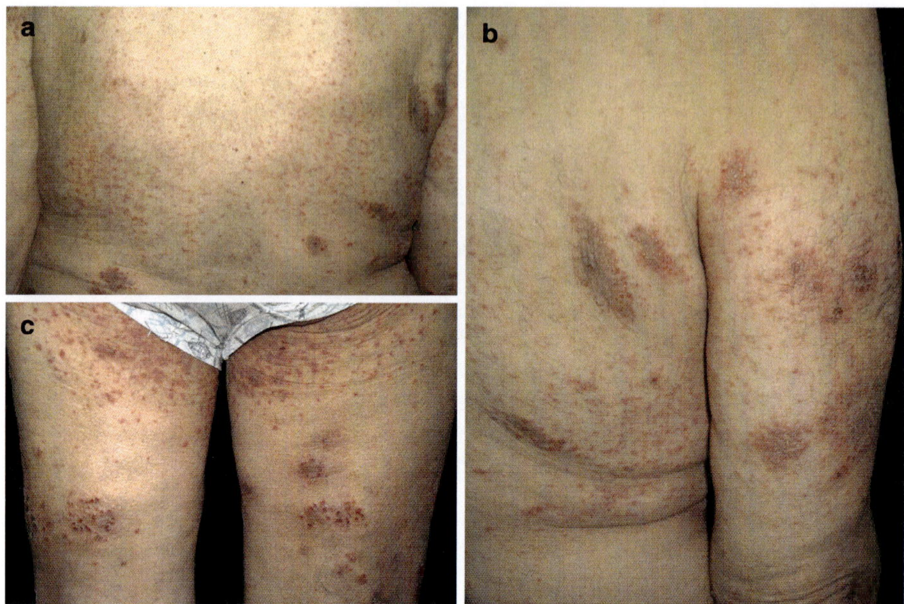

Fig. 14.1 Enoxaparin-induced eczematous eruption partly showing a nummular pattern involving the trunk (**a**, **b**), upper extremities (**b**), and the inguinal region and the lower extremities (**c**)

prophylaxis. Recombinant hirudins, such as desirudin, lepirudin, or fondaparinux, or in some cases subcutaneous pentosan polysulfate was recommended as alternatives in these patients [19–23]. Recombinant hirudins do not cross-react with low or high molecular weight heparins and heparinoids; however, hirudins themselves may also cause delayed-type sensitization [24, 25]. Moreover, intravenous lepirudin has the risk of eliciting anaphylactoid reactions as well [26, 27]. Fondaparinux was also shown to elicit eczematous reaction in a patient with dalteparin-induced exanthematous reaction [28]. Subcutaneous provocation tests were found to be most sensitive for excluding delayed-type cross-reactions and finding out a suitable alternative [19]. However, subcutaneous injection of pentosan polysulfate was reported to induce an erythematous reaction at the injection site in spite of negative subcutaneous test result in a patient [20]. On the other hand, intravenous administration of heparin and pentosan polysulfate was tolerated well without adverse effects in spite of positive patch test results to both drugs in a patient who was allergic to certoparin [12].

Angioedema/Urticaria

Immediate hypersensitivity reactions presenting as pruritus, urticaria, angioedema, or anaphylactoid reactions have been reported to occur with heparin, LMWHs, or lepirudin [16, 27, 29–31]. Fatal cases with lepirudin were also reported due to anaphylactoid reaction occurring concomitantly with acute cardiorespiratory arrest and acute myocardial infarction [27]. These cases were suggested to represent Kounis syndrome defined as concomitant occurrence of hypersensitivity reactions with acute coronary syndromes [26]. It was recommended to administer lepirudin therapy only then when the skills and equipment for the management of anaphylactic reaction are available. Urticarial eruptions can rarely occur with warfarin as well [2, 16].

In a patient with dalteparin-induced urticaria, cross-reactivity to other LMWHs (nadroparin, enoxaparin) and danaparoid was shown by skin prick or intradermal tests, while no sensitization to heparin, fondaparinux, and lepirudin was found [31]. The patient tolerated intravenous heparin and subcutaneous fondaparinux at full doses on rechallenge. The authors highlighted the role of skin tests in determining alternative anticoagulants in these patients and the importance of provocation tests [31].

Bullous Eruption

Bullous hemorrhagic dermatosis is a rare but well-described adverse cutaneous drug reaction of most LMWHs, such as enoxaparin being the most common inducer, but also dalteparin, tinzaparin, and bemiparin [32–37]. Heparin calcium [36] and idraparinux [38] were also reported to induce this reaction.

Bullous hemorrhagic dermatosis is described as the development of asymptomatic hemorrhagic intraepidermal bullae at skin areas that are distant from the injection sites. The bullae may be grouped in one region [34, 36, 37] or rarely distributed in a linear pattern [33]. Lesions may be covered with hemorrhagic crust [32, 33]. The bullous eruption was mostly reported to appear 2–21 days after starting therapy. However, it was described to occur in an average of 3 months in idraparinux-induced cases [38]. Histopathological examination of the lesions revealed no significant inflammatory infiltrate, capillary thrombosis, or vasculitis, but intraepidermal bullae containing red blood cells [32, 35–37]. The coagulation studies usually revealed normal results. Patients were occasionally using concomitant antiplatelet therapy that was considered to contribute to the hemorrhagic character of the lesions as well [34–36]. Resolution might occur after discontinuation of therapy [33, 37], but it was also reported to take place in several weeks despite continuing therapy [32, 34, 35].

Interestingly, instead of intraepidermal bullae, subepidermal bullae were reported in several patients [35, 39]. Two patients were reported to develop bullous eruption on an erythematous base from enoxaparin that was histopathologically consistent with subepidermal bullae with eosinophils suggesting bullous pemphigoid, whereas direct and indirect immunofluorescence examinations were negative [39].

Maculopapular Eruption

Erythema and local indurated plaques at the injection site and generalized maculopapular rash occurring in the same patient following subcutaneous or intravenous injections of either heparin or LMWH were reported in several cases [40, 41].

Dabigatran was also implicated as a probable cause of maculopapular eruption [42, 43]. The eruption started after 5 days of therapy with the drug and resolved 7 days after withdrawal in one patient. Intravenous heparin and warfarin were both used in this patient subsequently, without any further problems [42].

Vasculitis

Cutaneous vasculitis was reported to occur in association with LMWHs, warfarin, and acenocoumarol [44–48]. A case with delayed-type hypersensitivity to certoparin presenting with erythematous plaques on the injection site developed superficial leukocytoclastic vasculitis that was considered to be a local Arthus reaction at the injection site of subcutaneous provocation test with lepirudin starting 15 minutes after the application [12]. Another patient developed a localized leukocytoclastic vasculitis from nadroparin calcium as well, presenting as follicular purpura at the injection site that started a few hours after the injection [44].

Oral anticoagulants such as warfarin and acenocoumarol were reported to cause leukocytoclastic vasculitis with occasional renal involvement. The reaction was stated to occur within days to a month or even after years of therapy [46–48].

Alopecia

Nonscarring reversible alopecia, mainly telogen effluvium type, was reported with LMWHs (enoxaparin, dalteparin, tinzaparin) in several cases [49–51]. It was stated to develop usually within 3 weeks to 3 months of therapy and resolve in 2 weeks to 3 months after discontinuation of the drug [49, 51]. The reaction was attributed to the suspected LMWH because of the temporal relationship between the initiation of therapy and onset of the reaction and the fact that alopecia was reversible after discontinuation of the suspected anticoagulant [49]. Reexposure was very rarely experienced resulting in recurrence of alopecia [51]. Warfarin has also been reported to cause alopecia [52, 53].

Calcinosis Cutis

Calcinosis cutis has been reported to develop in several patients with acute or chronic renal failure after using subcutaneous injections of nadroparin calcium [54, 55]. The reaction developed at injection sites as asymptomatic or painful, erythematous to yellowish or whitish cutaneous and subcutaneous nodules. Central ulceration may be seen due to transepidermal elimination of calcified material clinically seen as a whitish or yellowish substance. The reaction was stated to develop usually within a few days (2–5 days) of therapy with nadroparin, but late occurrence after 40 days was also reported. The resolution of lesions may take quite a long time as reported between 5 and 18 weeks after discontinuation of the injections. Local trauma of injections was suggested to play a role in the development of the reaction that was considered to be caused by the calcium component of nadroparin preparation in the presence of elevated blood levels of calcium–phosphorus products due to renal failure [54, 55]. Calcifying panniculitis related with the use of nadroparin calcium was reported in a patient without an underlying renal disorder or elevated calcium–phosphate product but was associated with hyperparathyroidism due to osteomalacia [56].

Purple Toe Syndrome

Therapy with warfarin may cause purple toe syndrome which is described as the sudden onset of purple discoloration that is more prominent on the toes but may also involve the foot. It can be seen mostly bilaterally but also unilaterally [57–59]. It is a rare adverse cutaneous drug reaction. The lesions may be painful. It is stated to be more apparent when the legs are on a dependent position. Discontinuation of warfarin may lead to resolution of the lesions [57], but sometimes a mild discoloration may remain [58]. However, discoloration did not resolve in a patient who had accompanying antiphospholipid syndrome, and interestingly continuation of the drug did not cause any further problems [59]. The pathogenesis is considered to be related with cholesterol microemboli from an atheromatous plaque [58, 59].

Drug Rash with Eosinophilia and Systemic Symptoms

Acenocoumarol [60], fluindione [61, 62], enoxaparin [63], heparin [64], and phenindione [65–68] have been implicated as causative drugs in drug rash with eosinophilia and systemic symptoms (DRESS). In the acenocoumarol-induced case, a maculopapular eruption was observed on the trunk and limbs with accompanying blisters on distal parts of the legs [60]. Patch test with warfarin and dabigatran was performed in order to find an alternative oral anticoagulant and revealed negative results. The oral challenge test with both drugs was also negative, and dabigatran was used in further treatment of this patient without any problems [60]. DRESS presenting as erythroderma and maculopapular eruption was reported with the use of fluindione in two patients [61, 62]. The patient with maculopapular eruption showed positive patch test reaction to fluindione [62].

In phenindione-induced DRESS that might be fatal [68], there were various accompanying severe blood count anomalies like agranulocytosis, pancytopenia, and leukemoid reaction [65, 67, 68].

Acute Generalized Exanthematous Pustulosis

Acute generalized exanthematous pustulosis (AGEP) was reported to develop in a patient with the use of dalteparin [69]. The reaction started on the injection site as bullous eczematous lesions and progressed to generalized pustular eruption. Furthermore, subcutaneous provocation tests were performed with other LMWHs, danaparoid, pentosan polysulfate, and fondaparinux, revealing positive results with all of the tested drugs excluding pentosan polysulfate. Interestingly, a generalized pustular eruption has developed after 3 days following subcutaneous tests [69].

Two patients with fluindione-induced AGEP were reported [70, 71], one of them with a positive patch test reaction to fluindione [70].

Pruritus

Pruritus is a nonspecific cutaneous adverse reaction of drugs. It was reported in patients receiving anticoagulant therapy, mainly accompanying different types of drug eruptions [12, 16, 27, 29, 31, 63].

Other Reported Adverse Cutaneous Drug Reactions to Anticoagulants

Development of a delayed-type hypersensitivity reaction clinically occurring as erythema and induration on the injection site after extravasation of intravenous hirudin was reported in a patient [72]. It was compatible with a *granulomatous reaction* as the histopathology revealed an epithelioid granulomatous infiltrate. This reaction was closely related with extravasation of hirudin, as the patient continued to receive the intravenous treatment from another site without further reaction.

Fixed drug eruption has been reported to occur with heparin in two cases [73, 74].

Toxic epidermal necrolysis was reported to develop in a patient using iron protein succinylate and dabigatran, but the triggering drug was not defined [75].

A case of *Baboon syndrome* was reported with heparin [76].

Hyperpigmentation of the palm and fingertips was reported due to external contact from the broken phenindione tablets suggested to be possibly related with the skin's pH change and alkali neutralization after washing hands with a kind of soap [77].

References

1. Maldonado Cid P, de Alonso Celada RM, Noguera Morel L, Feito-Rodríguez M, Gómez-Fernández C, Herranz Pinto P. Cutaneous adverse events associated with heparin. Clin Exp Dermatol. 2012;37:707–11.

2. Frishman WH, Brosnan BD, Grossman M, Dasgupta D, Sun DK. Adverse dermatologic effects of cardiovascular drug therapy: part III. Cardiol Rev. 2002;10:337–48.
3. Patel GK, Knight AG. Generalised cutaneous necrosis: a complication of low-molecular-weight heparin. Int Wound J. 2005;2:267–70.
4. Toll A, Gallardo F, Abella ME, Fontcuberta J, Barranco C, Pujol RM. Low-molecular-weight heparin-induced skin necrosis: a potential association with pre-existent hypercoagulable states. Int J Dermatol. 2005;44:964–6.
5. Shelley WB, Sayen JJ. Heparin necrosis: an anticoagulant-induced cutaneous infarct. J Am Acad Dermatol. 1982;7:674–7.
6. Byrne JS, Abdul Razak AR, Patchett S, Murphy GM. Warfarin skin necrosis associated with protein S deficiency and a mutation in the methylenetetrahydrofolate reductase gene. Clin Exp Dermatol. 2004;29:35–6.
7. Valdivielso M, Longo I, Lecona M, Lázaro P. Cutaneous necrosis induced by acenocoumarol. J Eur Acad Dermatol Venereol. 2004;18:211–5.
8. Merklen-Djafri C, Mazurier I, Samama MM, Alhenc-Gelas M, Tortel MC, Cribier B, et al. Skin necrosis during long-term fluindione treatment revealing protein C deficiency. Ann Dermatol Venereol. 2012;139:199–203.
9. Beqqal K, Horellou MH, Philippe A, Alhene Gelas M, Flaujac C, Gorin I, et al. Skin necrosis due to fluindione treatment: a rare but serious complication. J Wound Care. 2014; 23(2 Suppl):S16–9.
10. Warkentin TE, Whitlock RP, Teoh KH. Warfarin-associated multiple digital necrosis complicating heparin-induced thrombocytopenia and Raynaud's phenomenon after aortic valve replacement for adenocarcinoma-associated thrombotic endocarditis. Am J Hematol. 2004;75:56–62.
11. Klein L, Galvez A, Klein O, Chediak J. Warfarin-induced limb gangrene in the setting of lung adenocarcinoma. Am J Hematol. 2004;76:176–9.
12. Jappe U, Reinhold D, Bonnekoh B. Arthus reaction to lepirudin, a new recombinant hirudin, and delayed-type hypersensitivity to several heparins and heparinoids, with tolerance to its intravenous administration. Contact Dermatitis. 2002;46:29–32.
13. Klein GF, Kofler H, Wolf H, Fritsch PO. Eczema-like, erythematous, infiltrated plaques: a common side effect of subcutaneous heparin therapy. J Am Acad Dermatol. 1989;21: 703–7.
14. Gupta S, Mishra P, Palaian S, Prabhu S, Bista D, Prabhu M. Probable cutaneous allergic response to subcutaneous heparin - a case report. Acta Dermatovenerol Alp Panonica Adriat. 2006;15:98–101.
15. Méndez J, Sanchís ME, de la Fuente R, Stolle R, Vega JM, Martínez C, et al. Delayed-type hypersensitivity to subcutaneous enoxaparin. Allergy. 1998;53:999–1003.
16. Bircher AJ, Harr T, Hohenstein L, Tsakiris DA. Hypersensitivity reactions to anticoagulant drugs: diagnosis and management options. Allergy. 2006;61:1432–40.
17. Enrique E, Alijotas J, Cistero A, san Miguel MM, Bartra J, Tresserra F. Patch-test positivity in cutaneous reactions to enoxaparin. Contact Dermatitis. 2000;42:43.
18. White JM, Munn SE, Seet JE, Adams N, Clement M. Eczema-like plaques secondary to enoxaparin. Contact Dermatitis. 2006;54:18–20.
19. Schiffner R, Glässl A, Landthaler M, Stolz W. Tolerance of desirudin in a patient with generalized eczema after intravenous challenge with heparin and a delayed-type skin reaction to high and low molecular weight heparins and heparinoids. Contact Dermatitis. 2000;42:49.
20. Koch P, Munssinger T, Rupp-John C, Uhl K. Delayed-type hypersensitivity skin reactions caused by subcutaneous unfractionated and low-molecular-weight heparins: tolerance of a new recombinant hirudin. J Am Acad Dermatol. 2000;42:612–9.
21. Grassegger A, Fritsch P, Reider N. Delayed-type hypersensitivity and cross-reactivity to heparins and danaparoid: a prospective study. Dermatol Surg. 2001;27:47–52.
22. Koch P. Delayed-type hypersensitivity skin reactions due to heparins and heparinoids. Tolerance of recombinant hirudins and of the new synthetic anticoagulant fondaparinux. Contact Dermatitis. 2004;49:276–80.

23. Jappe U, Juschka U, Kuner N, Hausen BM, Krohn K. Fondaparinux: a suitable alternative in cases of delayed-type allergy to heparins and semisynthetic heparinoids? A study of 7 cases. Contact Dermatitis. 2004;51:67–72.
24. Jappe U, Gollnick H. Allergy to heparin, heparinoids, and recombinant hirudin. Diagnostic and therapeutic alternatives. Hautarzt. 1999;50:406–11.
25. Zollner TM, Gall H, Völpel H, Kaufmann R. Type IV allergy to natural hirudin confirmed by in vitro stimulation with recombinant hirudin. Contact Dermatitis. 1996;35:59–60.
26. Koutsojannis CM, Kounis NG. Lepirudin anaphylaxis and Kounis syndrome. Circulation. 2004;109:315.
27. Greinacher A, Lubenow N, Eichler P. Anaphylactic and anaphylactoid reactions associated with lepirudin in patients with heparin-induced thrombocytopenia. Circulation. 2003;108: 2062–5.
28. Hohenstein E, Tsakiris D, Bircher AJ. Delayed-type hypersensitivity to the ultra-low-molecular-weight heparin fondaparinux. Contact Dermatitis. 2004;51:149–51.
29. Berkun Y, Haviv YS, Schwartz LB, Shalit M. Heparin-induced recurrent anaphylaxis. Clin Exp Allergy. 2004;34:1916–8.
30. Tejedor Alonso MA, Lopez Revuelta K, Garcia Bueno MJ, Casas Losada ML, Rosado Ingelmo A, Gruss Vergara E, et al. Thrombocytopenia and anaphylaxis secondary to heparin in a hemodialysis patient. Clin Nephrol. 2005;63:236–40.
31. Harr T, Scherer K, Tsakiris DA, Bircher AJ. Immediate type hypersensitivity to low molecular weight heparins and tolerance of unfractioned heparin and fondaparinux. Allergy. 2006;61:787–8.
32. Peña ZG, Suszko JW, Morrison LH. Hemorrhagic bullae in a 73-year-old man. Bullous hemorrhagic dermatosis related to enoxaparin use. JAMA Dermatol. 2013;149:871–2.
33. Dixit S, Fischer G, Lim A. Haemorrhagic purpura in an elderly man. BHD. Australas J Dermatol. 2013;54:228–9.
34. Villanueva CA, Nájera L, Espinosa P, Borbujo J. Bullous hemorrhagic dermatosis at distant sites: a report of 2 new cases due to enoxaparin injection and a review of the literature. Actas Dermosifiliogr. 2012;103:816–9.
35. Maldonado Cid P, de Moreno Alonso Celada R, Herranz Pinto P, Noguera Morel L, Feltes Ochoa R, Beato Merino MJ, et al. Bullous hemorrhagic dermatosis at sites distant from subcutaneous injections of heparin: a report of 5 cases. J Am Acad Dermatol. 2012;67:e220–2.
36. Perrinaud A, Jacobi D, Machet MC, Grodet C, Gruel Y, Machet L. Bullous hemorrhagic dermatosis occurring at sites distant from subcutaneous injections of heparin: three cases. J Am Acad Dermatol. 2006;54(2 Suppl):S5–7.
37. Beltraminelli H, Itin P, Cerroni L. Intraepidermal bullous haemorrhage during anticoagulation with low-molecular-weight heparin: two cases. Br J Dermatol. 2009;161:191–3.
38. Benatar J, Stewart RA. Cutaneous blood-filled vesicles on idraparinux. Lancet. 2008;372:1949.
39. Dyson SW, Lin C, Jaworsky C. Enoxaparin sodium-induced bullous pemphigoid-like eruption: a report of 2 cases. J Am Acad Dermatol. 2004;51:141–2.
40. Greiner D, Schofer H. Allergic drug exanthema to heparin. Cutaneous reactions to high molecular and fractionated heparin. Hautarzt. 1994;45:569–72.
41. Figarella I, Barbaud A, Lecompte T, De Maistre E, Reichert-Penetrat S, Schmutz JL. Cutaneous delayed hypersensitivity reactions to heparins and heparinoids. Ann Dermatol Venereol. 2001;128:25–30.
42. To K, Reynolds C, Spinler SA. Rash associated with dabigatran etexilate. Pharmacotherapy. 2013;33:e23–7.
43. Winkle RA, Mead RH, Engel G, Kong MH, Patrawala RA. The use of dabigatran immediately after atrial fibrillation ablation. J Cardiovasc Electrophysiol. 2012;23:264–8.
44. de Bats B, Rivard L, Bellemin B, Duflo F, Allaouchiche B, Chassard D. Leukocytoclastic vasculitis after injection of low-molecular-weight heparin (letter). Presse Med. 2000;29:1604.
45. Humeau-Commin A, Chatap G, Giraud K, Vincent JP. IgA vasculitis induced by low molecular weight heparin. Ann Dermatol Venereol. 2005;132:705–6.
46. Jiménez-Gonzalo FJ, Medina-Pérez M, Marín-Martín J. Acenocoumarol-induced leukocytoclastic vasculitis. Haematologica. 1999;84:462–3.

47. Aouam K, Gassab A, Khorchani H, Bel Hadj Ali H, Amri M, Boughattas NA, Zili JE. Acenocoumarol and vasculitis: a case report. Pharmacoepidemiol Drug Saf. 2007;16: 113–4.
48. Hsu CY, Chen WS, Sung SH. Warfarin-induced leukocytoclastic vasculitis: a case report and review of literature. Intern Med. 2012;51:601–6.
49. Wang YY, Po HL. Enoxaparin-induced alopecia in patients with cerebral venous thrombosis. J Clin Pharm Ther. 2006;31:513–7.
50. Sarris E, Tsele E, Bagiatoudi G, Salpigidis K, Stavrianaki D, Kaklamanis L, Siakotos M. Diffuse alopecia in a hemodialysis patient caused by a low-molecular-weight heparin, tinzaparin. Am J Kidney Dis. 2003;41:E15.
51. Apsner R, Horl WH, Sunder-Plassmann G. Dalteparin-induced alopecia in hemodialysis patients: reversal by regional citrate anticoagulation. Blood. 2001;97:2914–5.
52. Umlas J, Harken DE. Warfarin-induced alopecia. Cutis. 1988;42:63–4.
53. Nagao T, Ibayashi S, Fujii K, Sugimori H, Sadoshima S, Fujishima M. Treatment of warfarin-induced hair loss with ubidecarenone. Lancet. 1995;346:1104–5.
54. Eich D, Scharffetter-Kochanek K, Weihrauch J, Krieg T, Hunzelmann N. Calcinosis of the cutis and subcutis: an unusual nonimmunologic adverse reaction to subcutaneous injections of low-molecular-weight calcium-containing heparins. J Am Acad Dermatol. 2004;50: 210–4.
55. Boccara O, Prost-Squarcioni C, Battistella M, Brousse N, Rongioletti F, Fraitag S. Calcinosis cutis: a rare reaction to subcutaneous injections of calcium-containing heparin in patients with renal failure. Am J Dermatopathol. 2010;32:52–5.
56. Campanelli A, Kaya G, Masouyé I, Borradori L. Calcifying panniculitis following subcutaneous injections of nadroparin-calcium in a patient with osteomalacia. Br J Dermatol. 2005;153:657–60.
57. Al-Niaimi F, Clark C. A case of unilateral purple toes due to warfarin. Clin Exp Dermatol. 2009;34:527–8.
58. Dulíček P, Bártová J, Beránek M, Malý J, Pecka M. The purple toe syndrome in female with Factor V Leiden mutation successfully treated with enoxaparin. Clin Appl Thromb Hemost. 2013;19:100–2.
59. Talmadge DB, Spyropoulos AC. Purple toes syndrome associated with warfarin therapy in a patient with antiphospholipid syndrome. Pharmacotherapy. 2003;23:674–7.
60. Piñero-Saavedra M, Castaño MP, Camarero MO, Milla SL. DRESS syndrome induced by acenocoumarol with tolerance to warfarin and dabigatran: a case report. Blood Coagul Fibrinolysis. 2013;24:576–8.
61. Sparsa A, Bédane C, Benazahary H, De Vencay P, Gauthier ML, Le Brun V, et al. Drug hypersensitive syndrome caused by fluindione. Ann Dermatol Venereol. 2001;128:1014–8.
62. Frouin E, Roth B, Grange A, Grange F, Tortel MC, Guillaume JC. Hypersensitivity to fluindione (Previscan). Positive skin patch tests. Ann Dermatol Venereol. 2005;132:1000–2.
63. Ronceray S, Dinulescu M, Le Gall F, Polard E, Dupuy A, Adamski H. Enoxaparin-induced DRESS syndrome. Case Rep Dermatol. 2012;4:233–7.
64. Katoh S, Terashima S, Nakahara Y, Yamada H, Tatsukawa H, Ida K, Nakagawa M. Hypersensitivity to heparin; a case report. Nihon Jinzo Gakkai Shi. 1993;35:411–4.
65. Mohamed SD. Sensitivity reaction to phenindione with urticaria, hepatitis, and pancytopenia. Br Med J. 1965;2:1475–6.
66. Naisbitt DJ, Farrell J, Chamberlain PJ, Hopkins JE, Berry NG, Pirmohamed M, Park BK. Characterization of the T-cell response in a patient with phenindione hypersensitivity. J Pharmacol Exp Ther. 2005;313:1058–65.
67. Wright JS. Phenindione sensitivity with leukaemoid reaction and hepato-renal damage. Postgrad Med J. 1970;46:452–5.
68. Garnett ES, Pegrum GD, McDonald SJ. A fatal case of phenindione sensitivity. Br Med J. 1962;2:1032–3.
69. Komericki P, Grims R, Kränke B, Aberer W. Acute generalized exanthematous pustulosis from dalteparin. J Am Acad Dermatol. 2007;57:718–21.

70. Chtioui M, Cousin-Testard F, Zimmermann U, Amar A, Saiag P, Mahé E. Fluindione-induced acute generalised exanthematous pustulosis confirmed by patch testing. Ann Dermatol Venereol. 2008;135:295–8.
71. Thurot C, Reymond JL, Bourrain JL, Pinel N, Beani JC. Fluindione-induced acute exanthematous pustulosis with renal involvement. Ann Dermatol Venereol. 2003;130(12 Pt 1):1146–9.
72. Smith KJ, Rosario-Collazo J, Skelton H. Delayed cutaneous hypersensitivity reactions to hirudin. Arch Pathol Lab Med. 2001;125:1585–7.
73. Mohammed KN. Symmetric fixed eruption to heparin. Dermatology. 1995;190:91.
74. Shaheen S, Akhtar S. Fixed drug eruption due to heparin injection. JPMI. 2008;22:340–1.
75. Tsoumpris A, Tzimas T, Gkabrelas K, Akritidis N. Iron complex, dabigatran and toxic epidermal necrolysis syndrome: a case-report. J Clin Pharm Ther. 2013;38:177–8.
76. Pfeiff B, Pullmann H. Baboon-artiges Arzneiexanthem auf heparin. Dtsch Dermatologe. 1991;39:559–60.
77. Silverton NH. Skin pigmentation by phenindione. Br Med J. 1966;1:675.

Chapter 15
Other Cardiovascular Drugs

Keywords Digoxin • Pentoxifylline • Aminocaproic acid • Antianginal • Alpha-adrenergic receptor blockers • Prazosin • Lupus erythematosus • Adrenergic neuron blocker • Reserpine • Gangrene • Sympathomimetics • Injection site reaction

Other cardiovascular drugs not classified in the former sections include alpha-1 adrenergic receptor blockers, sympathomimetics, adrenergic neuron and ganglionic blockers, and drugs that are classified under the section of miscellaneous drugs, i.e., antiarrhythmic drugs like adenosine and digitalis glycosides, pentoxifylline, aminocaproic acid, protamine sulfate, and newer antianginal drugs such as ivabradine, ranolazine, and trimetazidine.

Alpha-Adrenergic Receptor Blockers

Alpha-1 adrenergic receptor blockers include doxazosin, prazosin, and terazosin. Phentolamine and phenoxybenzamine are combined alpha-1 and alpha-2 blockers.

Drug-Induced Lupus Erythematosus

Prazosin therapy was suggested to induce the formation of antinuclear antibody in some cases without the clinical presence of systemic lupus erythematosus [1]. However, some reports were not in favor of an increase in antinuclear antibody incidence with prazosin [2–4].

Erythroderma

Erythroderma has been observed in a patient after 3 days of terazosin therapy used for the treatment of benign prostatic hyperplasia, and it resolved with discontinuation of the drug and with systemic corticosteroid treatment within 2 weeks [5].

E. Özkaya, K.D. Yazganoğlu, *Adverse Cutaneous Drug Reactions to Cardiovascular Drugs*, DOI 10.1007/978-1-4471-6536-1_15

Oral Mucosal Reactions

In relation with their effect on salivary gland alpha-1 adrenoreceptors, these drugs are indicated to be responsible for the reduction of the production of saliva leading to xerostomia [6]. Xerostomia is stated to be an established class effect of alpha-1 adrenergic receptor blockers [6].

Pruritus

Pruritus is a nonspecific cutaneous adverse reaction of drugs. It is reported in patients receiving alpha-adrenergic receptor blockers mainly in the setting of different cutaneous eruptions [5, 7].

Other Reported Adverse Cutaneous Drug Reactions to Alpha-Adrenergic Receptor Blockers

Acute generalized exanthematous pustulosis with terazosin hydrochloride used for the treatment of benign prostatic hyperplasia [8], *lichenoid drug eruption* with terazosin used for the treatment of benign prostatic hyperplasia [7], *alopecia* or *hypertrichosis* in patients using doxazosin [9], and *angioedema/urticaria* from doxazosin [10, 11] were reported.

Other cutaneous side effects of alpha-adrenergic blockers include *diaphoresis* linked to doxazosin and terazosin, *edema/facial edema/peripheral edema* to doxazosin and terazosin, *flushing* to doxazosin [9, 11], phentolamine [11], and *purpura* and *xerosis* to doxazosin [11].

Sympathomimetics

Sympathomimetic (alpha-adrenergic) drugs include dopamine, dobutamine, midodrine, epinephrine, norepinephrine, isoproterenol, and phenylephrine.

The most common adverse cutaneous reactions to sympathomimetics occur as injection site reactions and peripheral gangrene. Cutaneous reactions to phenylephrine mostly include allergic contact dermatitis, usually presenting with blepharoconjunctivitis, due to its use as an eye drop [12].

Injection Site Reactions

Sympathomimetics, mainly dopamine, dobutamine, epinephrine, and norepinephrine were reported to cause injection site reactions such as erythema and pruritus with or without blisters, phlebitis, necrosis, and gangrene [13–16]. Injection site reactions mostly occur in association with intravenous administration of the drugs through a peripheral vein. Some may occur as a result of extravasation. Extravasation was reported to cause dermal necrosis around the injection sites at the elbow from dopamine [13], on the forearm from norepinephrine [14], and on the dorsum of the hands from dobutamine [13] and adrenaline [15].

In two patients, dobutamine caused erythema and pruritus around the injection site, phlebitis with or without bullae formation along the course of a vein, and peripheral eosinophilia [16]. The reaction was reported to recur with repeated injections. Skin tests (probably skin prick test) were performed with drug preparations, and revealed pruritic erythematous papules within 24–48 hours. The reaction was considered as a local hypersensitivity reaction probably from sulfites in the drug preparation [16].

Gangrene

Multiple extremity gangrenes including symmetrical peripheral gangrene have been described to occur after administration of dopamine, adrenaline, and noradrenaline [17–21]. Symmetrical peripheral gangrene is described as the gangrene of the hands and feet without large vessel obstruction or vasculitis. It is a serious side effect that can cause multiple-finger amputations and may be fatal. Peripheral gangrene is related with the vasoconstriction effects of the drugs that could be more intense in digital vascular beds leading to ischemia and progressively to gangrene. It is mainly associated with high doses of drugs but may also occur at low doses, especially in case of accompanying vascular disease or disseminated intravascular coagulation [17, 18, 21].

Other Reported Adverse Cutaneous Drug Reactions to Sympathomimetics

Fixed drug eruption from phenylephrine [22], *urticaria* and *anaphylaxis* with positive skin tests to multiple drugs including epinephrine and dopamine [23], *scalp pruritus* with the use midodrine [24] and dobutamine [25], and *piloerection* from midodrine [24] and dobutamine [26] have also been reported. Some sympathomimetics were linked to *flushing*, *hyperhidrosis*, and *xerostomia* [11]. Dobutamine was reported to cause a *rash* in a considerable number of patients in a study [27].

Adrenergic Neuron and Ganglionic Blockers

Adrenergic neuron and ganglionic blockers include reserpine, guanethidine, guanadrel, and mecamylamine.

The reported cutaneous adverse drug reactions are rare. Reserpine may cause *rash*, *flushing*, *peripheral edema*, *lupus erythematosus*, *pruritus*, and *xerostomia*

[28], whereas *alopecia*, *dermatitis*, *fixed drug eruption*, and *xerostomia* were reported due to guanethidine treatment [28, 29]. Mecamylamine was implicated to exacerbate *psoriasis* [28].

Miscellaneous

Adenosine and Digitalis Glycosides

Adenosine is a class IV antiarrhythmic drug. *Flushing* can be observed with adenosine, and is probably related to cutaneous vasodilatation induced by the drug. *Hyperhidrosis* may also occur with adenosine [30].

Generalized erythematous eruption has been observed during therapy with intravenous digoxin that resolved following withdrawal of the drug and additional systemic corticosteroid therapy, but the drug was readministered orally 48 hours following the first admission which led to the recurrence of the eruption within 72 hours [31]. The time between resolution of the reaction and readministration of the drug was rather short in this patient.

Psoriasiform eruption was reported to be caused by digoxin that was confirmed by a positive macrophage migratory inhibition factor test and recurrence of the reaction after drug readministration [32]. *Angioedema/urticaria, pruritus, gynecomastia, hyperhidrosis, vasculitis, maculopapular eruptions, bullous eruptions, alopecia*, and *shedding of fingernails and toenails* were stated to occur during therapy with digitalis glycosides [29, 30].

Thrombocytopenic purpura was reported to develop after 4 weeks of therapy with digitoxin [33]. The reaction resolved after the cessation of the drug, and substitution to digoxin was uneventful. However, readministration of digitoxin caused reappearance of the reaction [33].

Pentoxifylline

Pentoxifylline is a xanthine derivative. *Flushing* can be seen in patients receiving pentoxifylline [28]. Acute *urticaria* has been reported in a few patients using pentoxifylline [34, 35]. In one case, pentoxifylline was identified as the culprit agent by positive intradermal skin test and a positive oral rechallenge test [34]. In another case, prick test and intradermal test were negative with the drug, but oral rechallenge was positive, confirming that pentoxifylline was the causative factor [35].

A case of *acute generalized exanthematous pustulosis* was reported to develop 10 days after starting pentoxifylline treatment [36]. *Drug rash with eosinophilia and systemic symptoms* was reported in a patient following the use of pentoxifylline. This case was interesting as the patient had a history of intolerance to caffeine, another xanthine derivative, which was considered as a contraindication for pentoxifylline treatment [37].

Aminocaproic Acid

Epsilon-aminocaproic acid is an antifibrinolytic drug.

Maculopapular, generalized micropapular, purpuric maculopapular, and generalized erythematous eruptions with aminocaproic acid were observed [38–41]. Patch testing, performed in some of these cases, helped identify aminocaproic acid as the causative drug [38, 39].

Noninflammatory bullous eruptions limited to the legs following epsilon-aminocaproic acid infusion were observed in three patients [42]. Histopathological examination revealed subepidermal blister formation and fibrin thrombi in papillary dermal vessels, whereas direct immunofluorescence examination was nonspecific. The lesions were transient but one case required skin grafting. The authors suggested that the pathogenesis was related with cutaneous vascular thromboses caused by aminocaproic acid [42].

Contact dermatitis was reported with epsilon-aminocaproic acid-containing eye drops, confirmed by patch testing [43].

Epsilon-aminocaproic acid was considered as a possible inducer of an *anaphylactoid reaction* as well [44].

Protamine Sulfate

Anaphylactic/anaphylactoid reactions may occur with protamine sulfate, but the incidence was stated to be low (<1 %) [45]. Several factors including the use of neutral protamine Hagedorn (NPH) insulin, allergy to fish and to other medications, and prior exposure to protamine have been regarded as the risk factors for development of anaphylactic/anaphylactoid reactions to protamine [46, 47].

Newer Antianginal Drugs

Newer antianginal drugs include ivabradine, ranolazine, and trimetazidine [48]. In a study investigating the tolerability and clinical efficacy of ranolazine and ivabradine, ranolazine was found to have a better safety and tolerability profile than ivabradine [49]. Ivabradine was reported to be associated with hypersensitivity rash, probably compatible with a *maculopapular eruption*, with/without accompanying fever in occasional cases which was regarded as serum sickness-like reaction. The reaction occurred within 2–8 weeks of ivabradine therapy. However, it was stated that a causality establishment was needed to confirm this relationship [49]. We have recently seen a patient with maculopapular eruption probably induced by ivabradine (Fig. 15.1). The eruption started at the fourth week of therapy.

Ranolazine has been linked to *peripheral edema* and *xerostomia* [11].

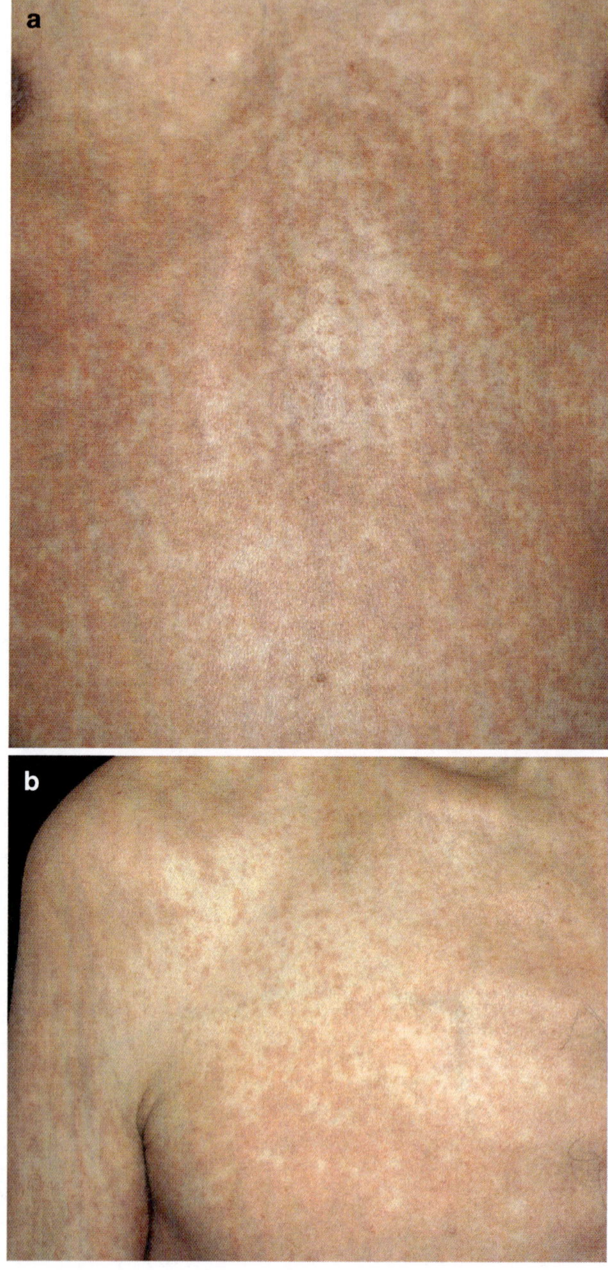

Fig. 15.1 Maculopapular eruption on the trunk (**a**, **b**) and upper extremity (**b**) that was developed on the fourth week of ivabradine therapy

References

1. Marshall AJ, McGraw ME, Barritt DW. Positive antinuclear factor tests with prazosin. Br Med J. 1979;1:165–6.
2. Wilson JD, Bullock JY, Booth RJ. Influence of prazosin on the development of antinuclear antibodies in hypertensive patients. Clin Pharmacol Ther. 1979;26:209–12.
3. Melkild A, Gaarder PI. Does prazosin induce formation of antinuclear factor? Br Med J. 1979;1:620–1.
4. Wilson JD, Booth RJ, Bullock JY. Antinuclear factor in patients on prazosin. Br Med J. 1979;1:553–4.
5. Hernandez-Cano N, Herranz P, Lazaro TE, Mayor M, Casado M. Severe cutaneous reaction due to terazosin. Lancet. 1998;352:202–3.
6. Torpet LA, Kragelund C, Reibel J, Nauntofte B. Oral adverse drug reactions to cardiovascular drugs. Crit Rev Oral Biol Med. 2004;15:28–46.
7. Koh MJ, Seah PP, Tay YK, Mancer K. Lichenoid drug eruption to terazosin. Br J Dermatol. 2008;158:426–7.
8. Speck LM, Wilkerson MG, Perri AJ, Kelly BC. Acute generalized exanthematous pustulosis caused by terazosin hydrochloride. J Drugs Dermatol. 2008;7:395–7.
9. The Treatment of Mild Hypertension Research Group. The treatment of mild hypertension study. A randomized, placebo-controlled trial of a nutritional-hygienic regimen along with various drug monotherapies. Arch Intern Med. 1991;151:1413–23.
10. Piller LB, Ford CE, Davis BR, Nwachuku C, Black HR, Oparil S, et al. Incidence and predictors of angioedema in elderly hypertensive patients at high risk for cardiovascular disease: a report from the Antihypertensive and Lipid-Lowering Treatment to Prevent Heart Attack Trial (ALLHAT). J Clin Hypertens (Greenwich). 2006;8:649–56; quiz 657–8.
11. Litt JZ. Drug eruption reference manual. 19th ed. Boca Raton: CRC Press (Taylor and Francis Group); 2013.
12. Raison-Peyron N, Du Thanh A, Demoly P, Guillot B. Long-lasting allergic contact blepharoconjunctivitis to phenylephrine eyedrops. Allergy. 2009;64:657–8.
13. Bhosale GP, Shah VR. Extravasation injury due to dopamine infusion leading to dermal necrosis and gangrene. J Anaesthesiol Clin Pharmacol. 2012;28:534–5.
14. Kim SM, Aikat S, Bailey A. Well recognised but still overlooked: norepinephrine extravasation. BMJ Case Rep. 2012. doi:10.1136/bcr-2012-006836.
15. van der Rijt R, Martin-Smith JD, Clover AJ. Reversal of hand peripheral ischaemia due to extravasation of adrenaline during cardiopulmonary resuscitation. J Plast Reconstr Aesthet Surg. 2013;66:e260–3.
16. Wu CC, Chen WJ, Cheng JJ, Hsieh YY, Lien WP. Local dermal hypersensitivity from dobutamine hydrochloride (Dobutrex solution) injection. Chest. 1991;99:1547–8.
17. Tsai Pai MA, Chien SW, Kuo YC, Wu TK, Chen CH, Lim PS. Symmetrical peripheral gangrene after using high-dose inotropes. Acta Nephrologica. 2013;27:48–51.
18. Colak T, Erdogan O, Yerebakan O, Arici C, Gurkan A. Symmetrical peripheral gangrene and dopamine. Ulus Travma Acil Cerrahi Derg. 2003;9:222–4.
19. Hayes MA, Yau EH, Hinds CJ, Watson JD. Symmetrical peripheral gangrene: association with noradrenaline administration. Intensive Care Med. 1992;18:433–6.
20. Joynt G, Doedens L, Lipman J, Bothma P. High-dose adrenaline with low systemic vascular resistance and symmetrical peripheral gangrene. S Afr J Surg. 1996;34:99–101.
21. Winkler MJ, Trunkey DD. Dopamine gangrene. Association with disseminated intravascular coagulation. Am J Surg. 1981;142:588–91.

22. López Abad R, Iriarte Sotés P, Castro Murga M, Gracia Bara MT, Sesma Sánchez P. Fixed drug eruption induced by phenylephrine: a case of polysensitivity. J Investig Allergol Clin Immunol. 2009;19:322–3.
23. Tsuchimoto T, Miyazaki H, Suzuki E, Maekawa N. Case report: severe anaphylactic shock followed by positive skin-prick-test to multiple vasoconstrictors. Masui. 2010;59: 788–91.
24. Parsaik AK, Singh B, Altayar O, Mascarenhas SS, Singh SK, Erwin PJ, Murad MH. Midodrine for orthostatic hypotension: a systematic review and meta-analysis of clinical trials. J Gen Intern Med. 2013;28:1496–503.
25. McCauley CS, Blumenthal MS. Dobutamine and pruritus of the scalp. Ann Intern Med. 1986;105:966.
26. Ross M. Dopamine-induced localized cutaneous vasoconstriction and piloerection. Arch Dermatol. 1991;127:586–7.
27. Baumgart D, Buck T, Leischik R, Oelert H, Farahati J, Reiners C, Erbel R. Enoximon-echocardiography. A new diagnostic approach for the detection of viable myocardium comparison to dobutamin-echocardiography. Herz. 1994;19:227–34.
28. Frishman WH, Brosnan BD, Grossman M, Dasgupta D, Sun DK. Adverse dermatologic effects of cardiovascular drug therapy: part III. Cardiol Rev. 2002;10:337–48.
29. Almeyda J, Levantine A. Cutaneous reactions to cardiovascular drugs. Br J Dermatol. 1973;88:313–9.
30. Frishman WH, Brosnan BD, Grossman M, Dasgupta D, Sun DK. Adverse dermatologic effects of cardiovascular drug therapy: part II. Cardiol Rev. 2002;10:285–300.
31. Martin SJ, Shah D. Cutaneous hypersensitivity reaction to digoxin. JAMA. 1994;271: 1905.
32. David M, Livni E, Stern E, Feuerman EJ, Grinblatt J. Psoriasiform eruption induced by digoxin: confirmed by re-exposure. J Am Acad Dermatol. 1981;5:702–3.
33. Berger H. Thrombopenic purpura following use of digitoxin. J Am Med Assoc. 1952;148:282–3.
34. Gonzalez-Mahave I, Del Pozo MD, Blasco A, Lobera T, Venturini M. Urticaria due to pentoxyfylline. Allergy. 2005;60:705.
35. Seoane-Lestón FJ, Añibarro-Bausela MB, Mugíca-García MV, Aguilar-Martínez A. Urticaria caused by pentoxifylline. J Investig Allergol Clin Immunol. 2009;19:74–5.
36. Patrizi A, Tabanelli M, Antonucci A, Neri I. Acute generalized exanthematous pustulosis induced by pentoxifylline. Int J Dermatol. 2007;46:1310–2.
37. Saunderson RB, Garsia R, Headley AP, McCaughan GW, O'Toole S, Strasser SI. Pentoxifylline-induced drug rash with eosinophilia and systemic symptoms (DRESS) in a patient with caffeine intolerance. J Dermatol Case Rep. 2013;7:77–81.
38. Gonzalez Gutierrez ML, Esteban Lopez MI, Ruiz Ruiz MD. Positivity of patch tests in cutaneous reaction to aminocaproic acid: two case reports. Allergy. 1995;50: 745–6.
39. Villarreal O. Systemic dermatitis with eosinophilia due to epsilon-aminocaproic acid. Contact Dermatitis. 1999;40:114.
40. Cunha D, Carvalho R, Santos R, Cardoso J. Systemic allergic dermatitis to epsilon-aminocaproic acid. Contact Dermatitis. 2009;61:303–4.
41. Chakrabarti A, Collett KA. Purpuric rash due to epsilon-aminocaproic acid. Br Med J. 1980;281:197–8.
42. Brooke CP, Spiers EM, Omura EF. Noninflammatory bullae associated with epsilon-aminocaproic acid infusion. J Am Acad Dermatol. 1992;27:880–2.
43. Miyamoto H, Okajima M. Allergic contact dermatitis from epsilon-aminocaproic acid. Contact Dermatitis. 2000;42:50.
44. Yien HW, Hseu SS, Chan KH, Lee TY. Suspected anaphylactoid shock to aminocaproic acid (plaslloid) during operation. Zhonghua Yi Xue Za Zhi (Taipei). 1992;50:415–9.

45. Nybo M, Madsen JS. Serious anaphylactic reactions due to protamine sulfate: a systematic literature review. Basic Clin Pharmacol Toxicol. 2008;103:192–6.
46. Ford SA, Kam PC, Baldo BA, Fisher MM. Anaphylactic or anaphylactoid reactions in patients undergoing cardiac surgery. J Cardiothorac Vasc Anesth. 2001;15:684–8.
47. Roelofse JA, van der Bijl P. An anaphylactic reaction to protamine sulfate. Anesth Prog. 1991;38:99–100.
48. Jones DA, Timmis A, Wragg A. Novel drugs for treating angina. BMJ. 2013;347:f4726.
49. Chaturvedi A, Singh Y, Chaturvedi H, Thawani V, Singla S, Parihar D. Comparison of the efficacy and tolerability of ivabradine and ranolazine in patients of chronic stable angina pectoris. J Pharmacol Pharmacother. 2013;4:33–8.

Part III
Patch Testing in Drug Eruptions

Chapter 16
Patch Testing in Drug Eruptions

Keywords Drug eruption • Patch test • Photopatch test • Cardiovascular drugs • Commercial drug • Patch testing in loco • Serial dilution • Tape stripping • Prick/scratch/intradermal tests with late readings • Clinical relevance

Patch testing is a method carried out by dermatologists to evaluate type IV hypersensitivity reactions. It is the gold standard in the diagnosis of allergic contact dermatitis. Based on the recent knowledge on the involvement of different subtypes of type IV hypersensitivity reactions in the immunopathogenesis of drug eruptions (Table 1.1), patch testing is also of particular value in determining the responsible drug in certain drug eruptions such as eczematous eruption, maculopapular/morbilliform eruption, fixed drug eruption (FDE), photoallergic drug eruption, drug-induced Baboon syndrome (BS)/symmetrical drug-related intertriginous and flexural exanthema (SDRIFE), and acute generalized exanthematous pustulosis (AGEP) as a first-step diagnostic method [1–4]. It is also helpful in identifying the possible cross-reactive drugs and safe alternatives. Photopatch testing should be performed if there is suspicion of photoallergic drug eruptions.

It is generally not recommended to perform patch testing in case of a clinical suspicion of type I hypersensitivity reactions. However, open patch testing or classical patch testing with early readings at 20 minutes may also be useful for the investigation of immediate-type hypersensitivity reactions.

Classical (Occlusive) Patch Testing

Optimum Time for Patch Testing in Drug Eruptions

According to the guidelines of the European Society of Contact Dermatitis, drug patch testing is recommended to be performed 6 weeks to 6 months after complete healing of the lesions and at least 1 month following the cessation of therapy with systemic corticosteroids [4]. Patch testing should be avoided in the presence of active lesions and conditions that would suppress the patch test reaction, e.g., use of corticosteroids, immunosuppressives, immunomodulators, and exposure to UV radiation.

E. Özkaya, K.D. Yazganoğlu, *Adverse Cutaneous Drug Reactions to Cardiovascular Drugs*, DOI 10.1007/978-1-4471-6536-1_16

In spite of the published guidelines for drug patch testing, there is still a need for establishing an optimum method of patch testing with systemic drugs along with the appropriate test vehicles and test concentrations.

Test Vehicles

Concerning that the epidermal penetration of the drugs would be variable according to their lipophilic or hydrophilic character, it would be best to choose at least two different vehicles such as petrolatum and aqua (Fig. 16.1). This would help reduce the number of false-negative reactions. Epidermal penetration of lipophilic drugs is better. For hydrophilic drugs and for drugs with a molecular weight >500 Da, the "tape stripping" method is recommended to reduce the stratum corneum layer and to increase the penetration [3, 5].

In order to avoid false-negative patch test results, it was recommended to use petrolatum as vehicle for beta-lactam antibiotics, carbamazepine, celecoxib, and other nonsteroidal antiinflammatory drugs (NSAIDs); water for acyclovir; ethanol for corticosteroids; and dimethyl sulphoxide (DMSO) for co-trimoxazole [6–8].

Vehicles should also be tested as negative controls.

Test Concentrations

As for contact allergens, there is a need for determining the optimum test concentrations of drugs that would not cause an irritant patch test reaction. Testing with serial dilutions of the suspected drugs is always superior to testing with a single test concentration. This would help differentiate positive patch test reactions from irritant reactions, thus reducing the need for control groups. The onset of erythema confined to the test area of the highest serial dilution is consistent with an irritant patch test reaction. Increasing degree of patch test reactions in test areas with increasingly higher serial dilutions, however, would speak for a positive reaction (Figs. 16.1b and 16.2). Moreover, serial dilutions might also help identify the threshold concentration of allergens for eliciting an allergic reaction.

Serial dilutions are usually started from 1 % of the drug or if necessary, from lower concentrations such as 0.1 or 0.01 %. It might be recommended to test at least with a twofold or, preferably, with a threefold serial dilution.

Test Allergens

Only a limited number of systemic drugs including antibiotics, e.g., amoxicillin and ampicillin; NSAIDs, e.g., diclofenac, piroxicam, and ketoprofen; antiepileptics such as carbamazepine; antihistamines (hydroxyzine); antivirals (acyclovir); antihypertensives such as diltiazem and captopril; and the diuretic hydrochlorothiazide are available as patch test allergens [9]. Carbamazepine, diclofenac, ketoprofen, piroxicam, and hydroxyzine are available at 1 %, captopril at 5 %, and the remaining at 10 % concentrations in petrolatum.

Most of the systemic drugs have to be prepared freshly and applied within 24 hours. It is recommended to test with the commercial product as well as with its active and inactive ingredients. Cross-reactive allergens may also be tested; however, cross-sensitivities in patch tests may sometimes lack clinical relevance.

The commercialized form of the drug is recommended to be tested in a serial dilution up to 30 %, usually starting from 1 %, preferably both in petrolatum and in aqua [4], for example, in concentrations of 1 %, 5 %, 10 %, 30 %. On the other hand, it is advisable to test the active and inactive ingredients in a serial dilution up to 10 %, again both in petrolatum and in aqua [4].

In severe drug eruptions and when testing with certain drugs such as acyclovir, carbamazepine, and pseudoephedrine, it is advised to start with lower concentrations such as 0.1 %, in order to avoid strong positive patch test reactions as well as

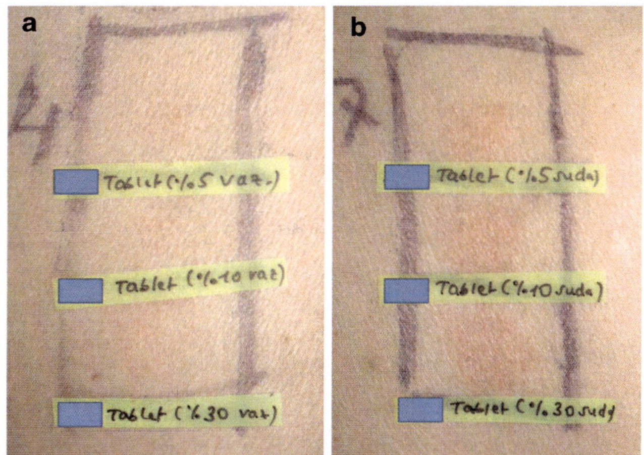

Fig. 16.1 (**a**). Negative patch test reactions with a serial dilution of a drug in petrolatum. (**b**). Positive patch test reactions with a serial dilution of the same drug in aqua (*suda*)

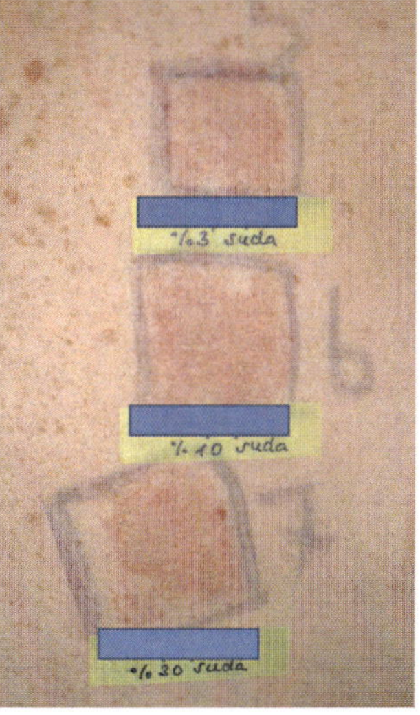

Fig. 16.2 Positive patch test reactions with a serial dilution of the suspected drug in aqua (*suda*)

relapses of the drug eruption [4]. If necessary, test concentrations might then eventually be increased up to 10 %. The appropriate patch test concentrations for carbamazepine, ampicillin, and amoxicillin were defined as 1 or 5 % [10]. In fixed drug eruption, there is usually a need for higher test concentrations [8].

Commercial drug preparations include many inactive ingredients including emulgators, preservatives, dyes, and others. Most of them are available as standardized patch test allergens. Sometimes, there is a need for asking the manufacturer to provide them. Although rare, positive patch test reactions have been reported with inactive drug ingredients such as benzyl alcohol, chlorocresol, and parabens [11]. Positive patch test reactions with the commercialized forms of the drugs might be mistakenly attributed to the active ingredients if the inactive ingredients are not tested.

Preparation of Systemic Drugs for Patch Testing

Tablets, capsules, or liquid drugs may be easily prepared for patch testing. A pH measurement is required for liquid drugs.

The outer dye layer of a tablet, if there is any, should be rinsed off in water. After that, the tablet is allowed to dry and, then, crushed into powder in a mortar. It may then easily be mixed with appropriate amounts of petrolatum or water to obtain a specific test concentration (Figs. 16.3, 16.4, 16.5, and 16.6). The dye can also be tested separately.

The powder ingredient of capsules may also be prepared for patch testing by mixing it with appropriate amounts of petrolatum or water to obtain a specific test concentration (Figs. 16.7, 16.8, 16.9, and 16.10). The outer shell of the capsules can be wetted and tested separately.

Drug preparations in petrolatum are directly applied to the patch test chambers, whereas those in aqua should be dropped to the filter paper in the test chamber.

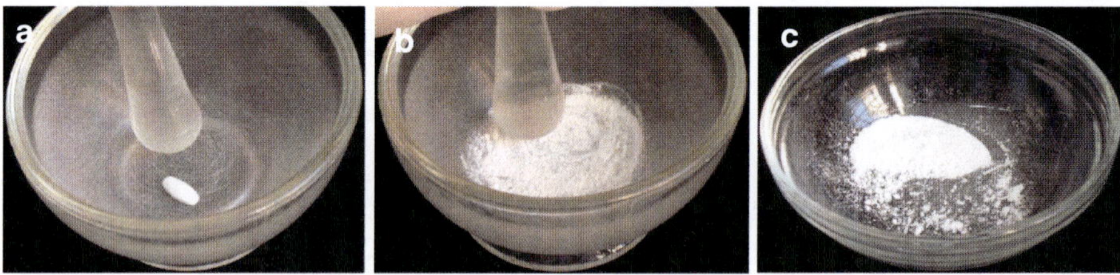

Fig. 16.3 Preparation of a tablet for patch testing using petrolatum as vehicle: after removal of the outer dye layer of the tablet, it is crushed into powder in a mortar (**a**–**c**)

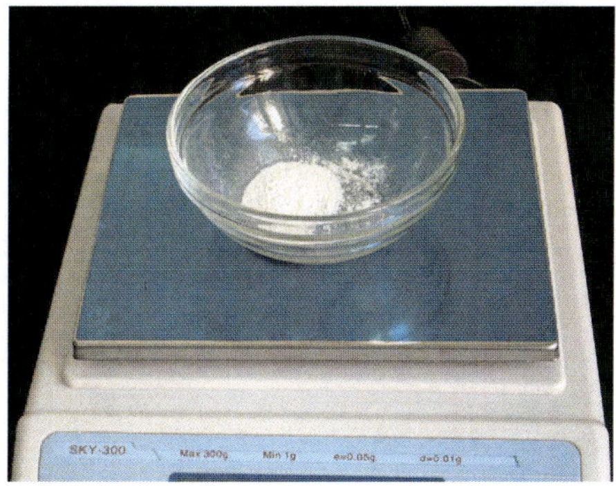

Fig. 16.4 The powder is weighed out using a digital scale

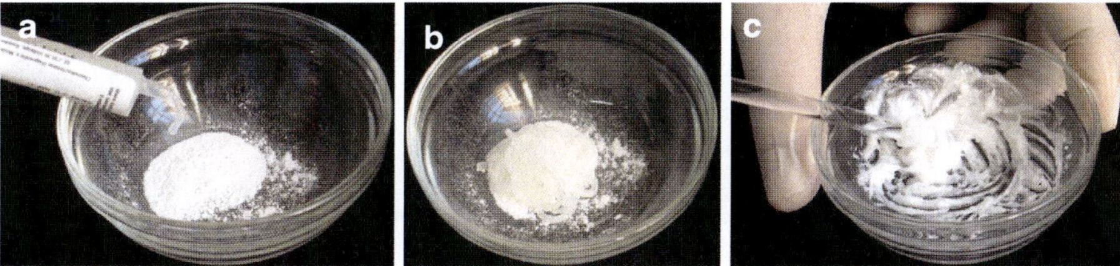

Fig. 16.5 It is then mixed with appropriate amounts of petrolatum to obtain a specific test concentration (**a**–**c**)

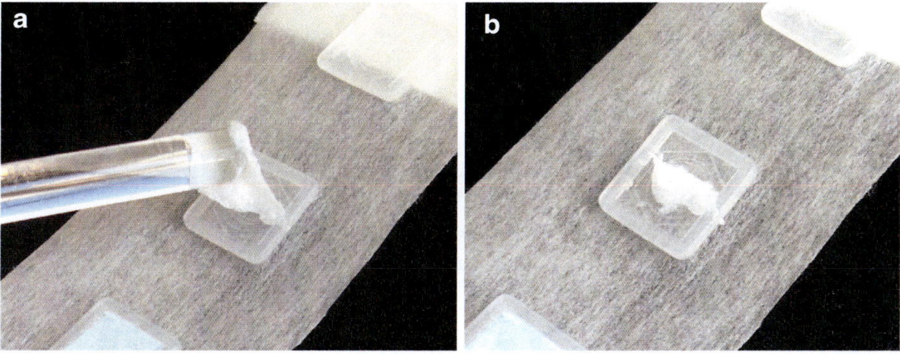

Fig. 16.6 Patch test chamber is filled with appropriate amount of the homogeneous mixture of drug and petrolatum (**a**, **b**)

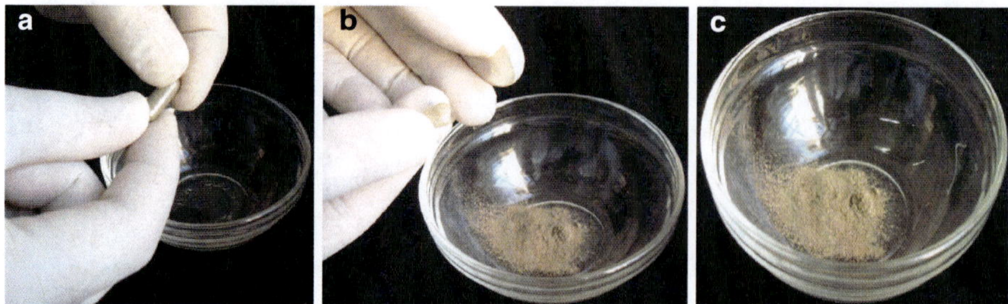

Fig. 16.7 Preparation of a capsule for patch testing using petrolatum as vehicle: the powder ingredient of the capsule is emptied (**a**–**c**)

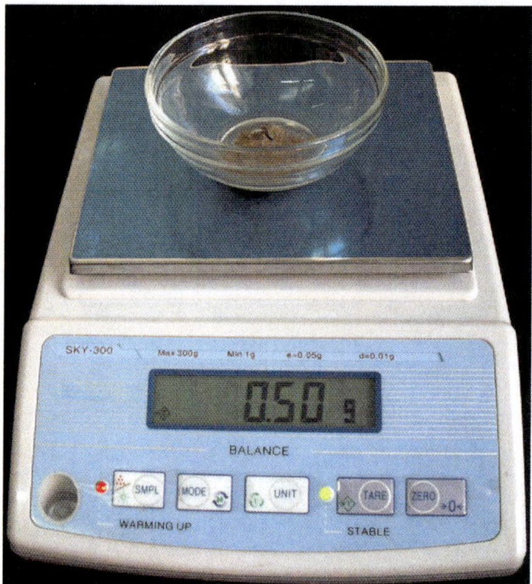

Fig. 16.8 The powder is weighed out using a digital scale

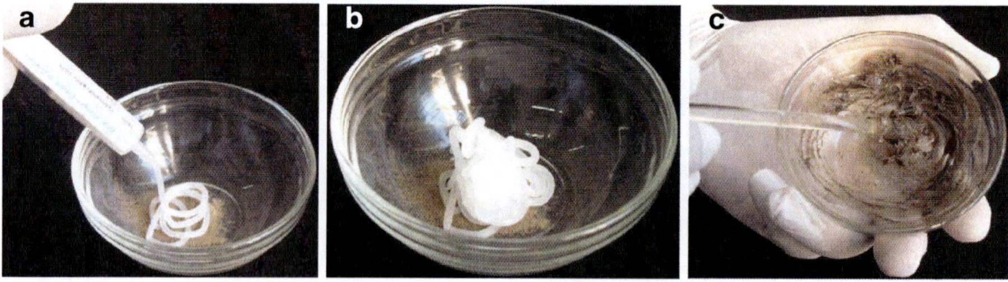

Fig. 16.9 It is then mixed with appropriate amounts of petrolatum to obtain a specific test concentration (**a**–**c**)

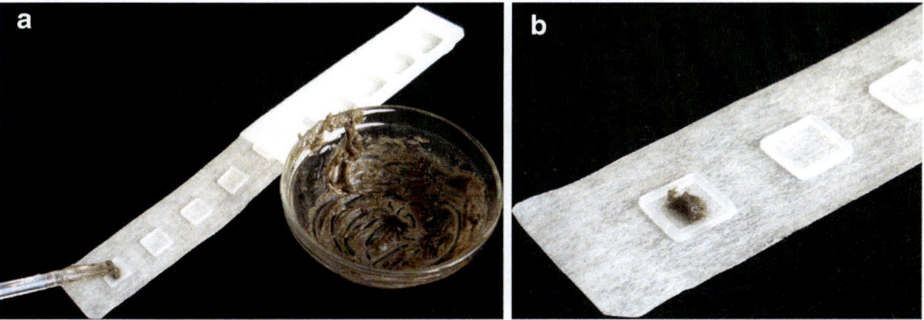

Fig. 16.10 Patch test chamber is filled with appropriate amount of the homogeneous mixture of drug and petrolatum (**a**, **b**)

Test Area

Patch test allergens are applied to the unlesional upper back and the outer surface of the upper arms according to the methods used in allergic contact dermatitis. In drug eruptions, it was also suggested to test on the most affected site of the initial eruption [1, 4]. In fixed drug eruption and in some drug-related BS/SDRIFE, patch test will only be positive if it is applied to previously involved skin (patch testing *in loco*) [8, 12–15]. The test area should be free of lesion and excessive hair, and it should be clean and dry.

Test Method

Patch test is a practical tool with negligible side effects. Informed consent of patients is necessary. Drug patch testing is not standardized and is performed according to the methods used in patch testing for the investigation of allergic contact dermatitis. Therefore, it requires further validation [16].

When testing systemic drugs, it is recommended to perform open tests first, preferably on the volar forearm skin, in order to exclude the immediate type of reactions such as immunologic or non-immunologic contact urticaria with the suspected drugs like beta-lactam antibiotics, neomycin, bacitracin, diclofenac, and gentamicin [6]. If the open test is negative after 20–60 minutes, it might be continued with occlusive patch testing.

Occlusive patch testing is performed using specific patch test strips with patch test chambers (Fig. 16.11). After the chambers are filled with the suspected allergens (Fig. 16.12), the test strips are applied to the test area, i.e., the back skin or the outer parts of the upper arms for 48 hours (Figs. 16.13 and 16.14). Test strips are usually covered with a second, hypoallergenic plaster (Figs. 16.13 and 16.14). Patients should avoid removing, rubbing, or wetting them as well as showers, exercise, and sunbathing.

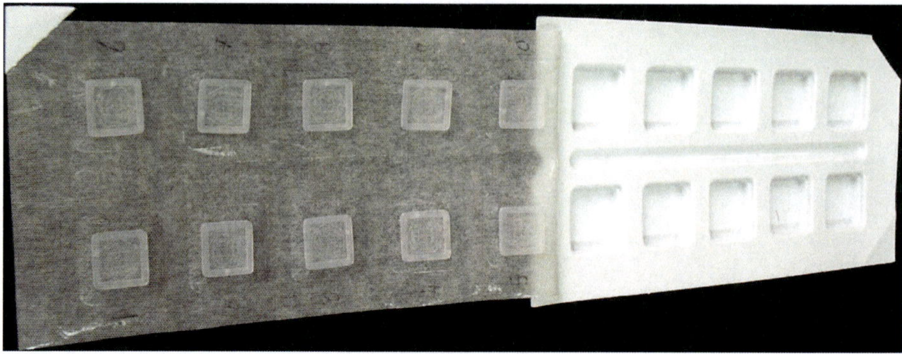

Fig. 16.11 Occlusive patch testing is performed using specific patch test strips with patch test chambers

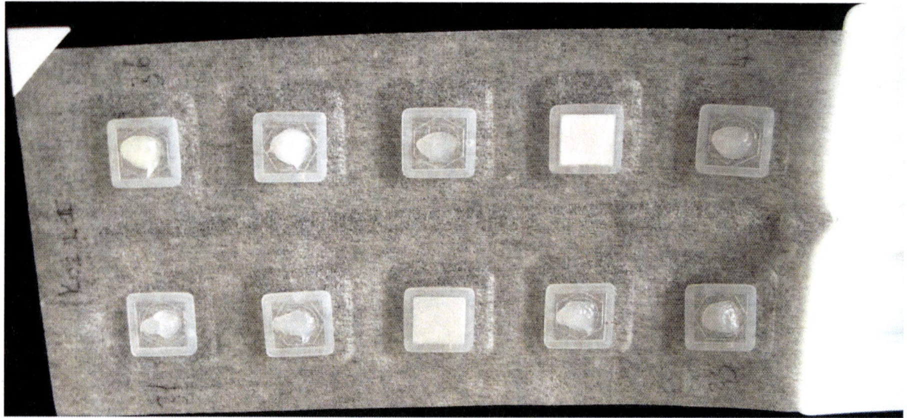

Fig. 16.12 Patch test chambers are filled with the suspected allergens

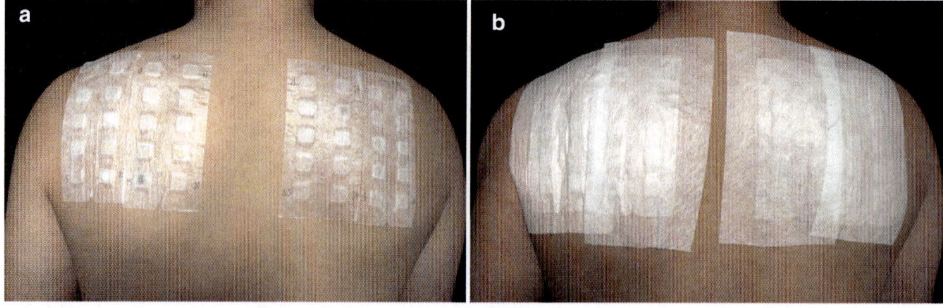

Fig. 16.13 The back skin is the major patch test area. Test strips are applied to the unlesional upper back (**a**) and then covered with a second, hypoallergenic plaster (**b**)

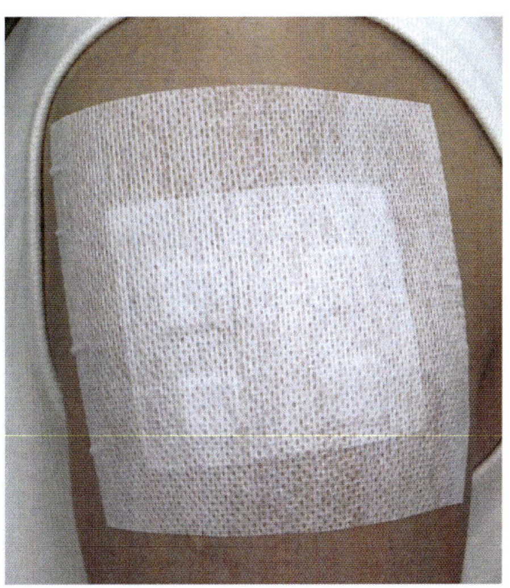

Fig. 16.14 Patch test strips can also be applied to the outer parts of the upper arms

As an alternative to the classical occlusive patch testing for 48 hours, a thin layer of the test preparation may be applied to the test area every 12 hours up to four times [17]. Repeated open tests are preferred for the investigation of the causative drug in FDE and when DMSO is used as test vehicle as DMSO might cause irritancy in occlusive testing [17].

Evaluation of the Results of Patch Test Reactions

Occlusive patch testing with drugs should be first evaluated after 20 minutes with regard to immediate-type hypersensitivity reactions, especially when testing with drugs such as beta-lactam antibiotics, aminoglycosides, and diclofenac. If there is no reaction after 20 minutes, test strips may remain on the test area for 48 hours.

Test strips are removed after 48 hours and marked clearly. An immediate reflex erythema might occur; therefore, it is recommended to wait at least for 30 minutes before the first reading. Test areas are evaluated at 2, 3, 4, and 7 days with regard to delayed-type hypersensitivity reactions.

Results of patch testing should be reported according to the International Contact Dermatitis Research Group criteria [18]. Positive reactions are eczematous in nature. Reactions of + to +++ are regarded as positive. Erythema and infiltration with/without papules are considered as + reaction (Fig. 16.15), whereas erythema, infiltration, and multiple vesicles speak for a ++ reaction (Fig. 16.16). A +++ reaction is defined as erythema, infiltration, coalescing vesicles, and occasional formation of bullae (Fig. 16.17). Erythema in the test area without infiltration is a doubtful reaction. Irritant patch test reactions, e.g., erythema with sharp margins, soap effect, and pustules, should be differentiated from true-positive reactions.

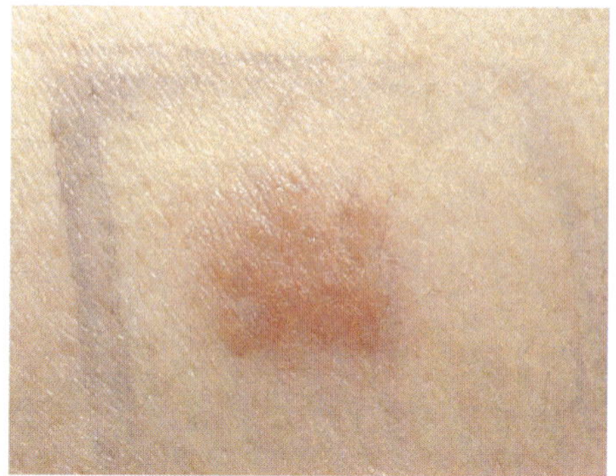

Fig. 16.15 A + patch test reaction showing erythema, infiltration, and sparse papules

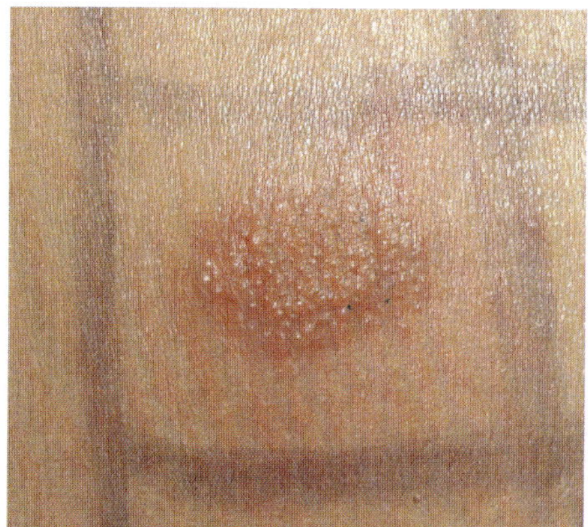

Fig. 16.16 A ++ patch test reaction showing erythema, infiltration, and multiple vesicles

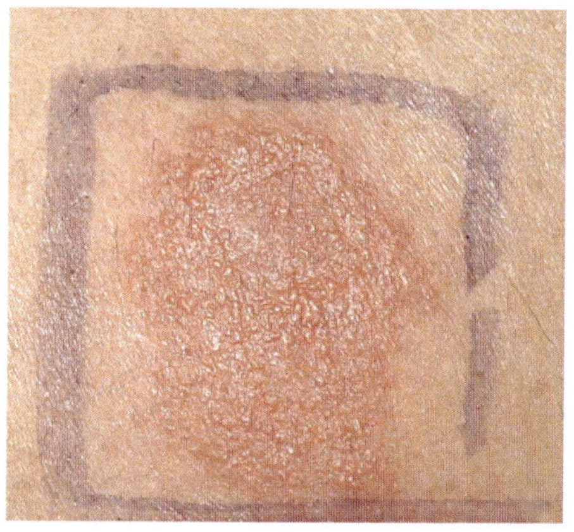

Fig. 16.17 A +++ patch test reaction showing erythema, infiltration, and coalescing vesicles

Positive patch test reactions in drug eruptions are usually eczematous, regardless of the clinical morphology of the eruption that might be variable showing macules, papules, vesicules, or pustules. In FDE, however, the patch test reaction is rarely eczematous. The appearance of erythema with or without induration in the patch test area, i.e., in an old FDE site, starting within 24 hours and lasting at least 6 hours, is defined as a positive test reaction, in the presence of a negative test reaction in the uninvolved skin [19].

Positive Patch Test Reactions to Multiple Drugs

Positive patch test reactions to multiple drugs might result from cross-reaction against chemically related drugs or from multiple drug allergy (polysensitivity) against chemically unrelated drugs [20, 21].

Cross-sensitivities may occur among aromatic anticonvulsants such as carbamazepine and phenytoin, among beta-lactam antibotics, between acyclovir, valacyclovir, and famciclovir, among corticosteroids, and among oxicams. Cross-reaction between sulfonamide antibiotics and sulfonamide nonantibiotics is controversial, as only a minority of sulfonamide nonantibiotics have the arylamine group (para-amino group) that is suggested to be responsible for cross-reactions [22, 23].

In a recent study, multiple delayed drug sensitizations were found in 12 % of patients with positive results in drug patch testing [24]. Patch tests were positive mainly in maculopapular-type multiple drug allergy but also in drug rash with eosinophilia and systemic symptoms (DRESS) and toxic epidermal necrolysis (TEN) according to previous reports [24, 25].

Site-specific polysensitivity to multiple drugs has been reported in FDE [26, 27].

Interpretation of the Patch Test Results

The clinical relevance of positive patch test reactions should be established as some of the reactions might be of past relevance or not related to the present dermatitis [4]. It is also necessary to compare all positive test results with those obtained in negative controls [4].

False-Positive Patch Test Reactions

The main reason for false-positive patch test reactions in drug patch testing is irritant reactions due to inappropriate patch test concentration or vehicle, a low or high pH of the test preparation, the presence of sodium lauryl sulfate in the commercialized form of some drugs such as spironolactone [28], the irritant nature of the drug itself, or an angry back reaction against marginal irritant allergens. An angry back reaction is suspected if more than five chemically unrelated patch test allergens became "false positive." Testing with the wrong drug, or a cross-reactive drug, and sensitivity to inactive ingredients of the drug preparations, such as propylene glycol or parabens [28], are other reasons for false-positive reactions.

Some systemic drugs with positive patch test reaction may be well tolerated due to the so called "oral tolerance" [4, 28, 29]. This occurs mainly if the sensitization is against the inactive ingredients of the drug.

If there is suspect of false-positive test reactions, it may be recommended to test with serial dilutions of the drug preparations or testing in control groups.

False-Negative Patch Test Reactions

On the other hand, negative patch test reactions do not necessarily imply the absence of a sensitization as patch testing with drugs is still not standardized, and false-negative results may occur due to various factors, e.g., the insufficient bioavailability of the test material; testing with the inappropriate test concentration or vehicle; testing when the skin immunity was impaired, e.g., by corticosteroids or UV exposure; testing with the wrong drug; testing with the right drug but when a drug metabolite or photometabolite was the allergen and not the drug itself; and testing only with the commercialized form of the drug [30]. Compound allergy, where patch test is negative with the individual constituents of a drug and only positive with the end product, is another reason for false-negative patch test results [31]. Connubial allergy to a drug used by the partner of the patient should also be borne in mind [32].

Drug patch testing might be negative if there is a pseudoallergic reaction where the immune mechanisms do not play a role and if there was a transient drug intolerance as in the presence of a coexisting viral infection [4].

In drug-induced BS, it is recommended to perform prick/intradermal tests with delayed readings when the patch test results are negative. Positive results might be achieved exclusively with delayed readings of prick/intradermal tests in some cases.

If necessary, photopatch test or patch test with "tape stripping" should also be applied. Finally, systemic provocation tests may be performed if skin tests are negative with the suspected drug.

Complications of Drug Patch Testing

The main complications of drug patch testing include immediate-type reactions such as contact urticaria on the test area or, in rare instances, a more generalized reaction leading to anaphylaxis, reactivation of the old lesions, and an active sensitization.

Contact urticaria may be seen with beta-lactams, aminoglycosides, and diclofenac, whereas penicillins, bacitracin, and neomycin may cause anaphylaxis. Patients should therefore be observed for at least 30 minutes following the patch test application [33].

Flare-up reactions in the old lesions have been reported with drugs, e.g., pseudoephedrine [34].

Patch testing with penicillins or other drugs may rarely cause an active sensitization with the tested drug [35].

Factors Influencing the Success of Patch Testing in Drug Eruptions

Positive patch test reactions have been reported in up to 50 % of patients tested with drugs. The specificity and the negative predictive value of drug patch testing have not yet been established [1].

There are various factors that would influence the success of drug patch testing such as the drug that was tested, the type of the eruption, the test concentration and the vehicle, and even the test area [4, 36]. In a recent study, positive patch test findings depended mainly on the causative drug rather than the clinical features of the drug eruption [16].

A high percent of positive results have been reported with beta-lactam antibiotics such as amoxicillin, antiepileptics such as carbamazepine, contrast media, co-trimoxazole, corticosteroids, and pseudoephedrine on patch testing [1, 3, 16, 37]. The molecular weight and solubility of drugs are important factors influencing the skin penetration and thus the success of drug patch testing. For example, patch testing has been shown not to be useful with allopurinol and its active metabolite oxypurinol due to their poor penetration into the skin [38].

Drug patch testing was most successful in eczematous drug eruption, maculopapular/morbilliform eruption, drug-induced BS/SDRIFE, FDE, AGEP, and DRESS [3, 8, 16, 37, 39, 40].

In eczematous drug eruption, positive patch test reactions are mainly reported with beta-lactams, pseudoephedrine, and carbamazepine [20, 37, 41–43].

In maculopapular/morbilliform drug eruption, positive patch test reactions are mainly reported with amoxicillin and other beta-lactam antibiotics [44–47], whereas beta-lactam antibiotics, contrast media, and pseudoephedrine were frequently positive in drug-induced BS/SDRIFE [12, 14, 34, 48–51].

In a Turkish series of patients with FDE, the success of drug patch testing in previous FDE sites was 93 % with co-trimoxazole and 60 % with NSAIDs. As a test vehicle, DMSO was superior to petrolatum [17, 52].

In pustular drug eruptions/AGEP, patch testing was mainly positive with beta-lactam antibiotics and pseudoephedrine [39, 53–56]. Terbinafine, a common cause of AGEP, has been rarely found positive in patch testing [57]. Positive patch test reactions in AGEP have an eczematous pattern both clinically and histopathologically [58].

In a multicenter study, patch testing was positive in 64 % of patients with DRESS [40]. Carbamazepine and proton pump inhibitors were among the main inducers. Recent reports supported the usefulness of patch testing in the diagnosis of carbamazepine- and phenytoin-induced DRESS [38, 59, 60]. However, patch testing was not found to be beneficial in allopurinol-induced DRESS due to its poor penetration into the skin [38].

Positive patch test reactions with carbamazepine have also been reported in erythema multiforme (EM)-like drug eruption [61, 62] and in drug-induced erythroderma [62], all showing an eczematous morphology.

Patch testing is not recommended in severe conditions like Stevens Johnson syndrome (SJS) and TEN. However, there are studies investigating the usefulness of patch testing in these conditions. A previous study stated that patch testing had a weak sensitivity for SJS and TEN [53]. On the other hand, a recent study suggested that patch testing might be safe and useful in carbamazepine-induced severe drug eruptions [63].

Patch Testing in Control Group

In case of positive patch test reactions with drugs, testing in an appropriate control group of 15–20 individuals is necessary to differentiate irritant reactions from positive reactions. An individual might be regarded as a negative control for a specific drug, if he or she was patch tested with this drug previously and showed negative reactions [4].

Testing with serial dilutions of drugs reduces the need for control groups.

Photopatch Test

Photopatch test is most useful in the investigation of photoallergic contact dermatitis. It may also be performed if there is suspicion of photoallergic drug eruption. However, its effectiveness in drug-induced photosensitivity is not yet validated.

Test allergens are applied in double sets, with only one being irradiated with UV light after 24–48 hours. Steps of photopatch testing are shown in Figs. 16.18, 16.19, 16.20, 16.21, and 16.22. Test areas are usually irradiated with 5–10 J/cm^2 UVA according to skin type and for some drugs like hydrochlorothiazide (Fig. 16.23), sulfonamides, and diphenhydramine also with 10 mJ/cm^2 UVB [64, 65]. Low doses are usually recommended to avoid phototoxic reactions. A 50 % of UVA minimal erythema dose or 50–75 % of UVB minimal erythema dose would also be appropriate. The minimal erythema dose is the lowest dose of radiation required to produce uniform erythema on the irradiated skin site [66].

Results of photopatch testing is evaluated according to the International Contact Dermatitis Research Group criteria as described for patch test reactions [18] at 2, 3, 4, and 7 days following UV irradiation. A photoallergy is diagnosed if there is a positive reaction to an allergen only in the irradiated test area and not in the control area. Immediate erythema on photopatch test areas (Fig. 16.23b), seen within 20 minutes following irradiation, is usually an irritant reaction that would fade away during its course.

Photopatch test was successful especially in eczematous- or lichenoid-type photoallergic drug eruptions [67–69]. Positive results have been reported mainly with piroxicam, carbamazepine, isoniazid, triflusal, and hydrochlorothiazide [67–69].

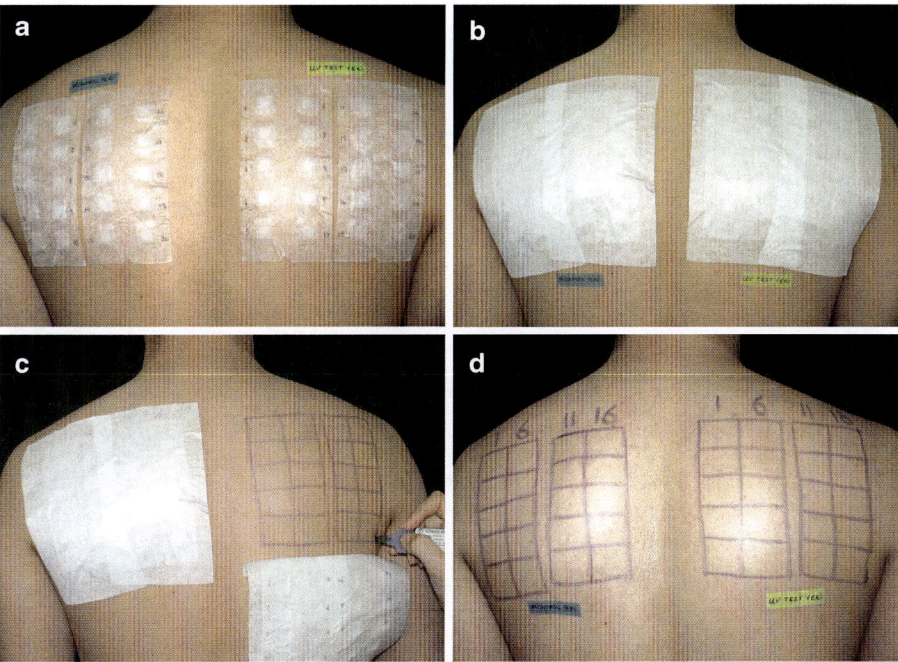

Fig. 16.18 Photopatch test allergens are applied in double sets to the back skin, one set as control area and the other one as test area to be irradiated with UV (**a**). Test strips are covered with a second, hypoallergenic plaster and allowed to remain there for 24–48 hours (**b**). Test strips are removed after 24–48 hours, and test areas are marked clearly (**c**–**d**)

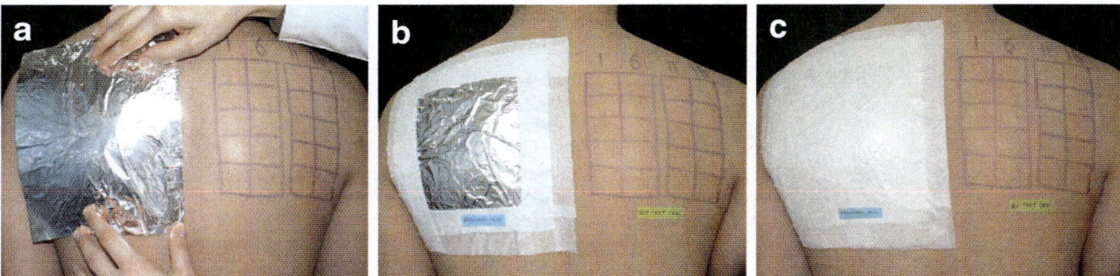

Fig. 16.19 The control area is covered with an opaque material (**a**–**c**) prior to UV irradiation of the test area

Photopatch test might be negative, if the photoallergen is a drug metabolite and not the drug itself, which would require to rechallenge the patient with the suspected drug first and to irradiate a small test area after then. Systemic phototest, on the other side, might be performed if there is suspect of drug-induced phototoxicity [70]. A positive phototest, showing a decrease in the minimal dose of the UVA and UVB radiation required to induce an erythema in a patient while taking the suspected drug, would suggest a drug-induced phototoxic reaction.

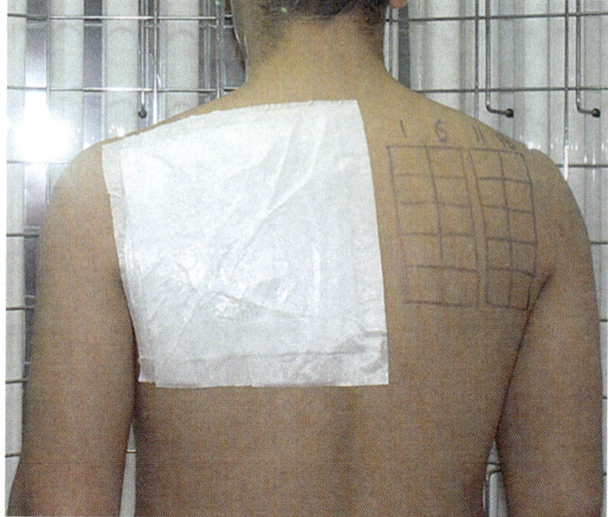

Fig. 16.20 The test area is irradiated with UV (usually UVA, 5–10 J/cm² according to skin type) using an appropriate UV light source. For some drugs like hydrochlorothiazide, it is recommended to irradiate another set of test allergens with 10 mJ/cm² UVB as well

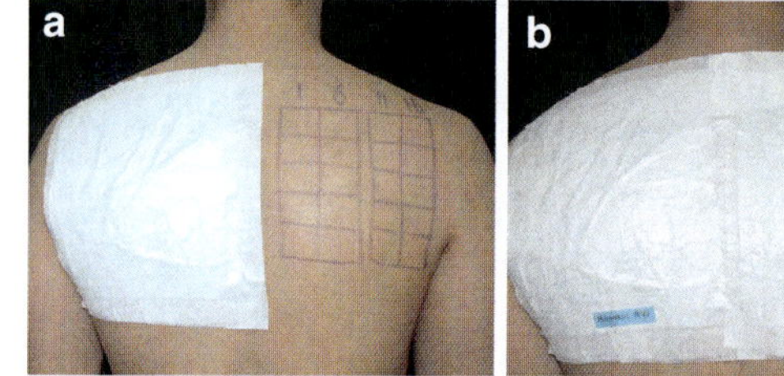

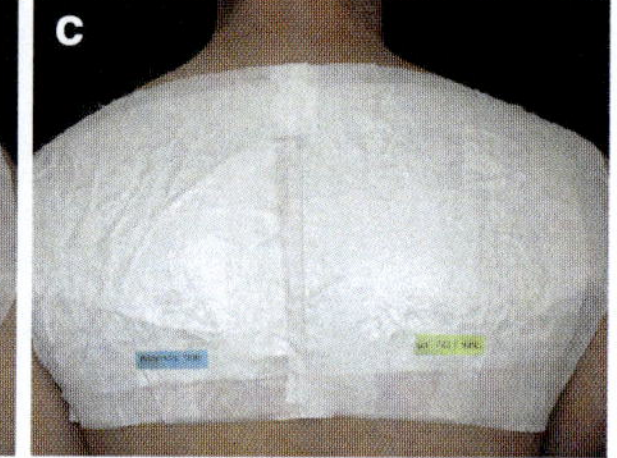

Fig. 16.21 Test areas are evaluated 20 minutes following UV irradiation with regard to immediate-type hypersensitivity reactions or irritant reactions (**a**). After that, the irradiated test area is covered with an opaque material as well and remained so for 48 hours (**b**, **c**)

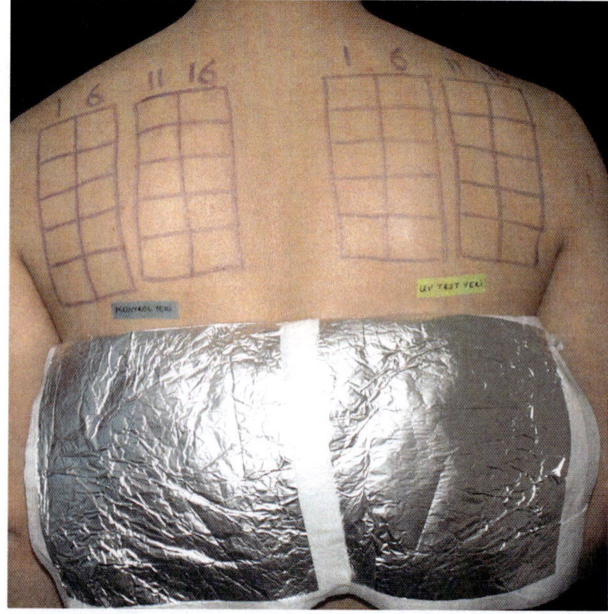

Fig. 16.22 Forty-eight hours following irradiation, plasters and opaque material are removed both from the test area and the control area. After the first reading at 48 hours, test and control areas are further evaluated at 3, 4, and 7 days with regard to delayed-type hypersensitivity reactions

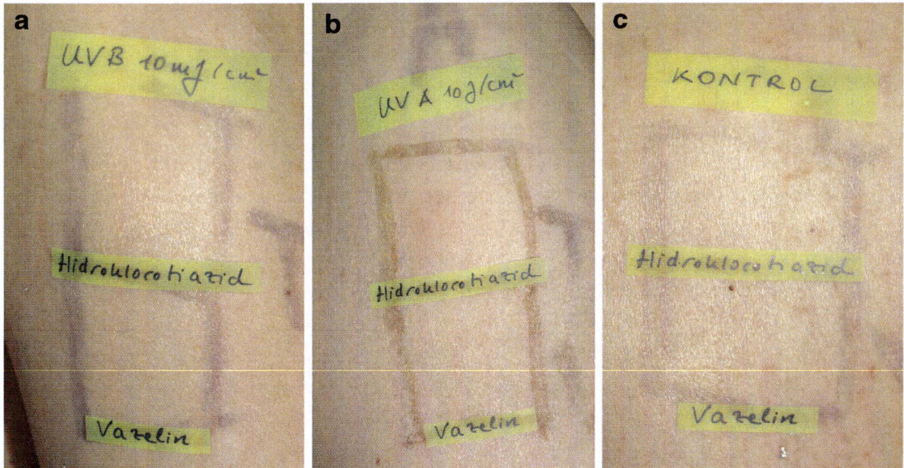

Fig. 16.23 If there is suspect of photoallergic drug eruption from hydrochlorothiazide, it is usually recommended to irradiate another set of drug preparation with UVB (**a**), in addition to UVA (**b**). Test vehicle such as petrolatum (*Vazelin*) is tested as negative control as well. The control site remains unirradiated (**c**). Note the immediate erythema on the photopatch test area (**b**) that developed within 20 minutes following irradiation with UVA, which is usually an irritant reaction that would fade away during its course

Alternative Tests with Systemic Drugs

Classical occlusive patch testing may be inadequate for high molecular weight haptens with a poor epidermal penetration. Therefore, late readings of prick/scratch/intradermal tests up to 1 week or scratch-patch (scratch-chamber) test are recommended for identifying the culprit drug in these cases [2, 4, 20]. Indeed, the success of delayed readings of intradermal tests or scratch-patch tests was high with high molecular weight heparins [4, 71].

Similarly, photoscratch test may be performed to enhance the epidermal penetration of drugs, if there is suspicion of false-negative photopatch test reaction due to poor penetration of the tested drug. However, there is high risk for false-positive irritant reactions with photoscratch tests, and it was shown that they do not change the sensitivity of phototesting [72].

In case of a negative patch test reaction to a suspected drug, systemic provocation, e.g., oral challenge, might be performed in order to confirm the relationship between the drug and the eruption, if there is no risk of triggering a severe drug eruption.

Examples of Patch/Photopatch Testing with Cardiovascular Drugs and Possible Cross-Reactions

Our knowledge on patch/photopatch testing with cardiovascular drugs is mainly based on case reports and occasionally case series in the literature. Positive patch test results were mainly achieved with diltiazem, heparinoids, and captopril [4, 36, 73–76], the latter also known to induce irritant patch test reactions [28]. Irritant patch test reactions have also been reported with spironolactone, probably due to sodium lauryl sulfate in the drug preparation [28].

Patch testing was mainly performed with the commercialized form of the drugs in previous reports. Serial dilutions of the same drug were tested in occasional cases. Control groups were usually tested to exclude irritant test reactions. Patch test results were frequently confirmed by oral provocation tests.

Patch/Photopatch Testing with Angiotensin-Converting Enzyme Inhibitors

Among angiotensin-converting enzyme inhibitors (ACEIs), captopril is the most frequently reported drug with positive patch test results. In a study investigating the usefulness of skin tests to prove drug hypersensitivity, patch testing revealed positive reactions to captopril in 4 of the 11 tested patients and to quinapril in 1 of 3 tested patients [73].

The captopril-associated drug eruption was usually maculopapular or eczematous [73, 77–79], but positive patch test reactions have also been reported in DRESS [77, 80] or even in cutaneous eruption histopathologically consistent with lymphocytic vasculitis [81].

It was recommended to perform patch testing with captopril at concentrations between 1 and 10 % in petrolatum [82]. The commercially available patch test preparation of captopril contains 5 % of the drug in petrolatum [9].

Photoallergic drug eruption has also been reported with ACEIs, the reported cases showing positive photopatch test findings with captopril 1 % in petrolatum [83], ramipril [84], or quinapril [85].

Interestingly, patch testing in cases of captopril-induced maculopapular or eczematous eruptions revealed positive reactions to captopril, but negative to several other ACEIs such as enalapril, lisinopril, fosinopril, ramipril, quinapril, and benazepril [77–79]. Lack of cross-reactivity with other ACEIs was also confirmed with negative oral challenge tests in some cases. Captopril is the only ACEI drug with a sulfhydryl group, which was regarded to be responsible for selective captopril hypersensitivity and the lack of cross-reactions with other ACEIs [74, 82, 86].

Patch/Photopatch Testing with Angiotensin II Receptor Blockers

Patch testing with angiotensin II receptor blockers has been rarely reported in the literature. In one case with irbesartan + hydrochlorothiazide-induced lichenoid eruption, patch testing with irbesartan and hydrochlorothiazide as single substances revealed negative results, but it was positive for the combination drug suggesting that the reaction was a "compound allergy" [87].

Patch/Photopatch Testing with Alpha-2 Adrenergic Receptor Agonists

Positive photopatch testing was reported with methyldopa in a patient with drug-induced photosensitivity [88].

Patch/Photopatch Testing with Class I Antiarrhythmic Drugs

Among class I antiarrhythmic drugs, quinidine is well known to induce photoallergic drug eruption, occasionally confirmed by positive photopatch test findings [89, 90]. The action spectrum was found to be in the UVA range.

In a study investigating the usefulness of skin tests to prove drug hypersensitivity, patch testing revealed positive reactions to quinidine in 1 of the 3 tested patients [73].

Mexiletine, another class I antiarrhythmic drug, has been frequently reported to show positive patch test finding, especially in cases with drug hypersensitivity syndrome/DRESS [91–94] and in one case with AGEP [95]. Serial dilutions with the commercial form of mexiletine revealed positive patch test reactions at concentrations of 5 %, 10 %, and 20 % in petrolatum [93], and with mexiletine hydrochloride at concentrations of 10 and 20 % in petrolatum in previous reports [95].

Patch/Photopatch Testing with Beta-Blockers

Allergic contact dermatitis from beta-blockers in eye drops [96] or in patients working in pharmaceutical industry [97] is a well-known phenomenon, mainly confirmed by patch testing.

However, there are only a few reports on patch testing with beta-blockers in drug eruptions. In a study investigating the usefulness of skin tests to prove drug hypersensitivity, no positive reactions were seen with beta-blockers [73]. Beta-blocker-induced FDE is very rarely reported in the literature. Propranolol was the culprit drug in one patient [98], bisoprolol in another one [99], and atenolol in two patients [100, 101]. In one of the cases, atenolol was confirmed to be the causative drug by patch testing in the previously affected skin site at a concentration of 10 % in petrolatum [101].

Photosensitivity was reported with tilisolol in a patient and confirmed by positive rechallenge and photopatch testing [102].

Patch/Photopatch Testing with Class III Antiarrhythmics

Amiodarone is one of the best known drugs for its photosensitizing property. However, a literature review gave no results for positive photopatch test results with amiodarone. Both UVA and UVB irradiation play a role in amiodarone-induced photosensitivity [103, 104].

Patch/Photopatch Testing with Calcium Channel Blockers

Diltiazem is most frequently reported to elicit positive patch test reactions, followed by nifedipine and verapamil, all belonging to three different subgroups of calcium channel blockers (CCBs), namely, benzothiazepines, dihydropyridines, and phenylalkylamines, respectively. The type of the drug eruption was usually maculopapular in the reported cases [73, 105]. Patch testing was found useful for identifying the culprit drug in diltiazem-induced AGEP as well [53, 58, 106–111] and also in diltiazem-induced erythroderma in occasional cases [112]. Lymphocyte activation/proliferation tests, performed in some cases, correlated well with positive patch test results to diltiazem in diltiazem-induced maculopapular eruption [105] or AGEP [58].

CCBs were usually patch tested with commercialized forms of the drugs at 30 % and/or with the pure drug at 10 % in petrolatum and water [105].

Cross-reactivity among CCBs has not yet been established clearly. While reactions suggesting cross-sensitivity between different subgroups of CCBs can be observed, it may not always be seen among the same subgroup. For example, patch testing with diltiazem was positive in three patients with erythroderma. One patient showed an additional patch test positivity to nifedipine, and another one to verapamil, suggesting a cross-reactivity between different subgroups of CCBs [112]. On the other hand, another patient with nimodipine-induced maculopapular eruption progressing to generalized eczema reacted positively to nimodipine in patch testing, but test results were negative for amlodipine and nifedipine [113]. It was suggested that the structural differences in lateral chains of amlodipine and nifedipine, two further drugs belonging to dihydropyridine subgroup, might be responsible for the lack of cross-reaction with nimodipine [113].

Although photosensitivity reactions have been described with nifedipine and diltiazem, no reports on positive photopatch test results with these drugs could be found in the literature. One study showed positive UVA photopatch and photoscratch test results with nicardipine [72].

Patch/Photopatch Testing with Diuretics

Among diuretic drugs, thiazides are well known to induce photosensitivity. Photopatch testing might be useful for identifying the culprit drug [68, 84]. As both the UVA and UVB wavebands were found to be responsible for thiazide-induced photosensitivity [114], it was recommended to perform both UVA and UVB photopatch testing with thiazides [65]. Positive photopatch test with UVA was reported with a combination drug of hydrochlorothiazide and losartan, tested with 30 % of the drug in petrolatum, suggesting a photoallergic drug eruption from hydrochlorothiazide as losartan has only rarely been reported to induce photosensitivity [115].

In a patient with photosensitivity from a combination drug of triamterene and xipamide, photopatch test was negative, but systemic photochallenge test with the drug was found to be positive, suggesting a photoallergic drug eruption [116]. The patient reacted with chlortalidone as well, suggesting that xipamide was the inducer drug as xipamide and chlortalidone have a structural similarity [116, 117].

Photopatch test was also reported to be positive with triamterene, a potassium-sparing diuretic, in a single patient [118]. One study showed positive UVA and UVB photopatch and photoscratch test results with spironolactone [72].

In a study investigating the usefulness of skin tests to prove drug hypersensitivity, patch testing revealed positive reactions to hydrochlorothiazide + amiloride in 1 of 2 tested patients [73]. No positive reactions were seen with other diuretics. Patch testing was found to be more useful, when the patient had a maculopapular drug eruption [73]. Positive patch test results have also been reported with a combination drug containing hydrochlorothiazide and irbesartan [87], and with spironolactone [119] in lichenoid drug eruptions. As patch testing was not positive to single substances in the former case, a compound allergy was suggested. One patient with lichenoid eruption probably induced by hydrochlorothiazide was administered furosemide that caused reappearance of the lesions which resolved upon discontinuation of furosemide, suggesting cross-sensitivity between the two drugs [120]. Positive patch test reaction to spironolactone was also reported in a patient with maculopapular eruption, confirmed by positive oral rechallenge [121]. However, patch test reactions to spironolactone should be evaluated carefully as irritant patch test reactions may occur, probably due to sodium lauryl sulfate in the drug preparation [28].

Patch testing or, if negative, delayed reading of prick/intradermal testing with acetazolamide, another sulfonamide diuretic, was reported to be positive in all of the nine tested patients with maculopapular eruption or AGEP [122]. Patch testing was performed with 30 % of the commercial acetazolamide in petrolatum.

Cross-reactivity between sulfonamide antibiotics and sulfonamide diuretics is controversial. It is generally not expected, because sulfonamide diuretics contain a sulfonamide moiety but not an arylamine group [123], which is thought to be responsible for the common delayed-type hypersensitivity reactions and the possible cross-reactions of sulfonamide antibiotics [124]. Indeed, in a study investigating 28 patients with FDE caused by sulfonamide antibiotics, no cross-reactivity was found between sulfonamide antibiotics and other sulfonamide derivatives including sulfonamide diuretics, confirmed by oral challenge testing [125].

On the other hand, a cross-reaction between sulfonamide antibiotics and other sulfonamides lacking an arylamine group would be theoretically possible, presuming that other yet undefined functional groups might also play a role in sulfonamide hypersensitivity [126]. Indeed, in a patient with FDE due to indapamide, a nontiazidic sulfonamide diuretic, cross-reaction with sulfonamide antibiotics, i.e., sulfamethoxazole and sulfadiazine, was reported and confirmed by positive controlled oral challenge [127].

Moreover, there might also be a theoretical risk for patients who are sensitized with p-phenylenediamine, a contact allergen containing an arylamine group, to develop a drug eruption with sulfonamides including thiazide diuretics, due to possible formation of some unknown intermediate substances during their metabolic process, as was reported before [128].

Patch/Photopatch Testing with Vasodilatory Drugs

In a patient with bosentan-induced maculopapular eruption, patch test and delayed reading of intradermal skin test with bosentan were negative, but lymphocyte transformation test was positive [129]. Moreover, rechallenge with bosentan caused DRESS [129].

Another patient with bosentan-induced DRESS had a history of previous allergy to co-trimoxazole and several other drugs, and the authors suspected that the sulfonamide moiety of bosentan could have a contributing effect on the cutaneous reaction [130].

Patch/Photopatch Testing with Lipid-Lowering Drugs

Among statins, pravastatin was reported to show a positive patch test reaction in a patient with nummular eczematous drug eruption [131]. Occupational airborne contact dermatitis was reported with simvastatin in patients working in pharmaceutical companies and was proven by patch testing [97, 132, 133].

Photosensitivity reactions have been rarely reported with statins. Simvastatin was the cause in one patient, confirmed by positive photopatch testing and rechallenge with phototesting [134].

Regarding fibrates, eczematous or lichenoid photosensitivity reactions were reported mainly with fenofibrate [72, 135–138]. Fenofibrate was confirmed to be the culprit drug by systemic photochallenge or photopatch testing either with UVA or UVB radiation or both [135–138] and also by photoscratch testing [72]. It was suggested that the test concentration should be higher than 1–5 % in order to avoid false-negative reactions [135]. On the other hand, systemic photochallenge was regarded as a more appropriate test to determine the fenofibrate-induced photosensitivity [136, 139]. In case of negative photopatch test results, it might be suggested that the drug metabolite could have caused the reaction [72, 136].

Cross-photosensitization might occur between fenofibrate and other benzophenone-containing drugs [137]. There is a well-known association between photocontact sensitivity to ketoprofen, which is also a benzophenone-containing drug, and systemic photosensitivity to fenofibrate, confirmed by positive photopatch testing [140].

Patch/Photopatch Testing with Anticoagulants

Eczematous eruption may develop with anticoagulants, usually starting from the injection sites. However, positive patch test reactions have rarely been reported with unfractionated heparin or low molecular weight heparins (LMWHs) such as enoxaparin [141, 142]. Patch tests after tape stripping have been tried for better antigen penetration when testing with heparin [143]. Intradermal testing was also found to be useful to confirm heparin as the causative agent [141]. Subcutaneous provocation tests were reported to be more reliable than other tests for the diagnosis of delayed-type hypersensitivity to LMWHs [144]. The relatively low incidence of patch test positivity with LMWHs was attributed to the fact that low doses of LMWH may inhibit the elicitation of allergic contact dermatitis [144].

Delayed-type cross-reactivity between unfractionated heparin and LMWHs as well as heparinoids such as danaparoid is an important problem for patients who need thrombosis prophylaxis [145]. In a study investigating cross-reactivity between bemiparin and several other LMWHs by means of subcutaneous testing, bemiparin had the highest cross-reactivity with enoxaparin [146]. One patient with a positive patch test reaction to the commercial product of enoxaparin showed cross-reaction to the commercial product of nadroparin as well [142]. Fondaparinux, a synthetic pentasaccharide, or recombinant hirudins were suggested as alternatives, but unfortunately, both of these agents may cause type IV hypersensitivity reactions themselves [147, 148]. Fondaparinux was also shown to elicit eczematous reaction in a patient with dalteparin-induced exanthematous reaction [148].

Previous reports suggested that lepirudin might be a good alternative in patients with delayed-type hypersensitivity to heparins and heparinoids [145, 149].

On the other hand, intravenous administration might be safe in patients with hypersensitivity reactions to subcutaneously injected heparin [149]. Intravenous administration of heparin and pentosan polysulfate was tolerated well in spite of positive patch test results to both drugs in a patient allergic to certoparin [150].

Positive patch test reactions were also reported with fluindione in a patient with DRESS presenting as maculopapular eruption [151], and another one with AGEP [152].

Patch/Photopatch Testing with Sympathomimetic Drugs

Allergic reaction to systemically administered sympathomimetic drugs is rare. Lesional patch test was positive with phenylephrine (1 % in aqua) in a patient with FDE [153]. It was stated that inappropriate test concentration and vehicle might lead to false-negative patch test results with sympathomimetics.

Cross-reactivity between phenylephrine and other sympathomimetic drugs belonging to the phenylamine family is controversial. In a study investigating cross-reactivity among sympathomimetics by means of patch testing, nearly all of the tested patients showed cross-reactions to at least one other sympathomimetic drug except epinephrine [154].

Patch/Photopatch Testing with Platelet Inhibitors

Among platelet inhibitors, delayed-type hypersensitivities are mainly reported with clopidogrel presenting as exanthematous (maculopapular) eruption. Patch testing showed cross-reactivity between clopidogrel, ticlopidine, and prasugrel in some of these patients [155].

Lesional patch test revealed positive results with ticlopidine at 1 and 5 % in petrolatum in a patient with FDE and was confirmed by oral challenge as well [156].

Positive patch test reaction helped to determine ticlopidine as the causative agent in a patient with AGEP [157].

Patch testing with the combination drug of dipyridamole and acetylsalicylic acid, at a concentration of 30 % in petrolatum, was positive in a patient with generalized eczematous drug eruption. Testing in unexposed controls was negative. Oral rechallenge with acetylsalicylic acid was negative, suggesting dipyridamole as the culprit agent [158].

Aspirin was confirmed to be the culprit drug in a patient with DRESS by means of patch testing and lymphocyte stimulation test [159]. Patch test was positive with aspirin at concentrations of 10 and 20 % in petrolatum.

Patch/Photopatch Testing with Other Cardiovascular Drugs

Contact dermatitis from epsilon-aminocaproic acid, mainly due to eye drops containing it, is a well-known phenomenon and is usually confirmed by patch testing [160, 161].

On the other hand, drug eruptions from systemic use of aminocaproic acid as antifibrinolytic drug are rare. Aminocaproic acid was confirmed as the culprit drug in a patient with DRESS [162], and in two patients with maculopapular eruption by means of patch testing [161].

References

1. Barbaud A. Drug patch testing in systemic cutaneous drug allergy. Toxicology. 2005;209: 209–16.
2. Hug K, Yawalkar N, Helbling A, Pichler WJ. Scratch-patch and patch testing in drug allergy-an assessment of specificity. J Investig Allergol Clin Immunol. 2003;13:12–9.
3. Friedmann PS. Patch testing in drug allergy. Curr Opin Allergy Clin Immunol. 2010;10:291–6. doi:10.1097/ACI.0b013e32833aa54d.
4. Barbaud A, Gonçalo M, Bruynzeel D, Bircher A. European society of contact dermatitis. Guidelines for performing skin tests with drugs in the investigation of cutaneous adverse drug reactions. Contact Dermatitis. 2001;45:321–8.
5. Dickel H, Goulioumis A, Gambichler T, Fluhr JW, Kamphowe J, Altmeyer P, et al. Standardized tape stripping: a practical and reproducible protocol to uniformly reduce the stratum corneum. Skin Pharmacol Physiol. 2010;23:259–65. doi:10.1159/000314700.
6. Mahajan VK, Handa S. Patch testing in cutaneous adverse drug reactions: methodology, interpretation, and clinical relevance. Indian J Dermatol Venereol Leprol. 2013;79:836–41. doi:10.4103/0378-6323.120751.
7. Isaksson M, Bruze M. Contact allergen of the year: corticosteroids. Dermatitis. 2005;16:3–5.
8. Özkaya E. Fixed drug eruption: state of the art. J Dtsch Dermatol Ges. 2008;6:181–8.
9. Chemotechnique Diagnostics. Patch test products 2013. http://www.chemotechnique.se/Catalogue.htm. Brial katalog. Accessed 26 Apr 2014.
10. Gonçalo M, Fernandes B, Oliveira HS, Figueiredo A. Epicutaneous patch testing in drug eruptions. Contact Dermatitis. 2000;42(Suppl 2):22.
11. Cham PMH, Warshaw EM. Patch testing for evaluating drug reactions due to systemic antibiotics. Dermatitis. 2007;18:63–77.
12. Häusermann P, Harr T, Bircher AJ. Baboon syndrome resulting from systemic drugs: is there strife between SDRIFE and allergic contact dermatitis syndrome? Contact Dermatitis. 2004;51:297–310.
13. Barbaud A, Tréchot P, Granel F, Lonchamp P, Faure G, Schmutz JL, et al. A baboon syndrome induced by intravenous human immunoglobulins: report of a case and immunological analysis. Dermatology. 1999;199:258–60.
14. Sánchez-Morillas L, Reaño Martos M, Rodríguez Mosquera M, Iglesias Cadarso A, Pérez Pimiento A, Domínguez Lázaro AR. Baboon syndrome due to pseudoephedrine. Contact Dermatitis. 2003;48:234.
15. Schultz ES, Diepgen TL. Clinical characteristics and the causes of the baboon syndrome. Dermatosen. 1996;44:266–9.
16. Ohtoshi S, Kitami Y, Sueki H, Nakada T. Utility of patch testing for patients with drug eruption. Clin Exp Dermatol. 2014;39:279–83. doi:10.1111/ced.12239.
17. Ozkaya E. Topical provocation in fixed drug eruption due to metamizol and naproxen. Clin Exp Dermatol. 2004;29:419–22.
18. Wilkinson DS, Fregert S, Magnusson B, Bandmann HJ, Calnan CD, Cronin E, et al. Terminology of contact dermatitis. Acta Derm Venereol. 1970;50:287–92.
19. Alanko K, Stubb S, Reitamo S. Topical provocation of fixed drug eruption. Br J Dermatol. 1987;116:561–7.
20. Özkaya E, Yazganoglu KD. Sequential development of eczematous type multiple drug allergy to unrelated drugs. J Am Acad Dermatol. 2011;65:e26–9.
21. Özkaya E. Eczematous-type multiple drug allergy from isoniazid and ethambutol with positive patch test results. Cutis. 2013;92:121–4.

22. Lee AG, Anderson R, Kardon RH, Wall M. Presumed "sulfa allergy" in patients with intracranial hypertension treated with acetazolamide or furosemide: cross-reactivity, myth or reality? Am J Ophthalmol. 2004;138:114–8.
23. Wulf NR, Matuszewski KA. Sulfonamide cross-reactivity: is there evidence to support broad cross-allergenicity? Am J Health Syst Pharm. 2013;70:1483–94. doi:10.2146/ajhp120291.
24. Liippo J, Pummi K, Hohenthal U, Lammintausta K. Patch testing and sensitization to multiple drugs. Contact Dermatitis. 2013;69:296–302. doi:10.1111/cod.12076.
25. Gex-Collet C, Helbling A, Pichler WJ. Multiple drug hypersensitivity–proof of multiple drug hypersensitivity by patch and lymphocyte transformation tests. J Investig Allergol Clin Immunol. 2005;15:293–6.
26. Ozkaya E. Independent lesions of fixed drug eruption due to cotrimoxazole and tenoxicam in the same patient: A rare case of polysensitivity. J Am Acad Dermatol. 2004;51(2Suppl):S102–4.
27. Özkaya E. Polysensitivity in fixed drug eruption due to a novel drug combination: independent lesions due to piroxicam and cotrimoxazole. Eur J Dermatol. 2006;16:591–2.
28. Barbaud A, Trechot P, Reichert-Penetrat S, Commun N, Schmutz JL. Relevance of skin tests with drugs in investigating cutaneous adverse drug reactions. Contact Dermatitis. 2001;45:265–8.
29. Barbaud A, Béné MC, Faure G, Schmutz JL. Skin tests in the study of drug eruptions with suspected immuno-allergic mechanism. Bull Acad Natl Med. 2000;184:775–91.
30. Özkaya E. Current understanding of Baboon Syndrome. Expert Rev Dermatol. 2009;4:163–75.
31. Kellett JK, King CM, Beck MH. Compound allergy to medicaments. Contact Dermatitis. 1986;14:45–8.
32. Zawar V, Kirloskar M, Chuh A. Fixed drug eruption – a sexually inducible reaction? Int J STD AIDS. 2004;15:560–3.
33. Gonçalo M, Bruynzeel DP. Patch testing in adverse drug reactions. In: Johansen JD, Frosch PJ, Lepoittevin J-P, editors. Contact dermatitis. 5th ed. Berlin: Springer; 2011. p. 475–91.
34. Sánchez TS, Sánchez-Pérez J, Aragüés M, García-Díaz A. Flare-up reaction of pseudoephedrine baboon syndrome after positive patch test. Contact Dermatitis. 2000;42:312–3.
35. van Ketel WG. Patch testing in penicillin allergy. Contact Dermatitis. 1975;1:253–4.
36. Sasseville D. The role of skin testing in drug eruptions. http://www.dermatologyrounds.ca/crus/dermaeng_050602.pdf. Accessed 26 Apr 2014.
37. Barbaud A. Drug skin tests and systemic drug reactions: an update. Expert Rev Dermatol. 2007;2:481–95.
38. Santiago F, Gonçalo M, Vieira R, Coelho S, Figueiredo A. Epicutaneous patch testing in drug hypersensitivity syndrome (DRESS). Contact Dermatitis. 2010;62:47–53. doi:10.1111/j.1600-0536.2009.01659.x.
39. Mayo-Pampín E, Flórez A, Feal C, Conde A, Abalde MT, De la Torre C, et al. Acute generalized exanthematous pustulosis due to pseudoephedrine with positive patch test. Acta Derm Venereol. 2006;86:542–3.
40. Barbaud A, Collet E, Milpied B, Assier H, Staumont D, Avenel-Audran M, et al. A multicentre study to determine the value and safety of drug patch tests for the three main classes of severe cutaneous adverse drug reactions. Br J Dermatol. 2013;168:555–62. doi:10.1111/bjd.12125.
41. Moreno-Escobosa MC, de las Heras M, Figueredo E, Umpiérrez A, Bombin C, Cuesta J. Generalized dermatitis due to pseudoephedrine. Allergy. 2002;57:753.
42. Terui T, Tagami H. Eczematous drug eruption from carbamazepine: coexistence of contact and photocontact sensitivity. Contact Dermatitis. 1989;20:260–4.
43. Özkaya E, Güngör H. Carbamazepine induced eczematous eruption clinically resembling atopic dermatitis. J Eur Acad Dermatol Venereol. 1999;12:182–3.
44. Yawalkar N, Hari Y, Frutig K, Egli F, Wendland T, Braathen LR, et al. T cells isolated from positive epicutaneous test reactions to amoxicillin and ceftriaxone are drug specific and cytotoxic. J Invest Dermatol. 2000;115:647–52.
45. Bruynzeel DP, Van Ketel WG. Skin tests in the diagnosis of maculopapular drug eruptions. Semin Dermatol. 1987;6:119–24.

46. Barbaud AM, Béné MC, Schmutz JL, Ehlinger A, Weber M, Faure GC. Role of delayed cellular hypersensitivity and adhesion molecules in maculopapular rashes induced by amoxicillin. Arch Dermatol. 1997;133:481–6.
47. Padial A, Antunez C, Blanca-Lopez N, Fernandez TD, Cornejo-Garcia JA, Mayorga C, et al. Non-immediate reactions to betalactams: diagnostic value of skin testing and drug provocation test. Clin Exp Allergy. 2008;38:822–8. doi:10.1111/j.1365-2222.2008.02961.x.
48. Duve S, Worret W, Hofmann H. The baboon syndrome: a manifestation of haematogenous contact-type dermatitis. Acta Derm Venereol. 1994;74:480–1.
49. Wakelin SH, Sidhu S, Orton DI, Chia Y, Shaw S. Amoxycillin-induced flexural exanthem. Clin Exp Dermatol. 1999;24:71–3.
50. Köhler LD, Schönlein K, Kautzky F, Vogt HJ. Diagnosis at first glance: the baboon syndrome. Int J Dermatol. 1996;35:502–3.
51. Arnold AW, Häusermann P, Bach S, Bircher AJ. Recurrent flexural exanthema (SDRIFE or baboon syndrome) after administration of two different iodinated radio contrast media. Dermatology. 2007;214:89–93.
52. Ozkaya E, Bayazit H, Ozarmagan G. Topical provocation in 27 cases of cotrimoxazole-induced fixed drug eruption. Contact Dermatitis. 1999;41:185–9.
53. Wolkenstein P, Chosidow O, Fléchet ML, Robbiola O, Paul M, Dumé L, et al. Patch testing in severe cutaneous adverse drug reactions, including Stevens-Johnson syndrome and toxic epidermal necrolysis. Contact Dermatitis. 1996;35:234–6.
54. Harries MJ, McIntyre SJ, Kingston TP. Co-amoxiclav-induced acute generalized exanthematous pustulosis confirmed by patch testing. Contact Dermatitis. 2006;55:372.
55. Padial MA, Alvarez-Ferreira J, Tapia B, et al. Acute generalized exanthematous pustulosis associated with pseudoephedrine. Br J Dermatol. 2004;150:139–42.
56. Assier-Bonnet H, Viguier M, Dubertret L, Revuz J, Roujeau JC. Severe adverse drug reactions due to pseudoephedrine from over-the-counter medications. Contact Dermatitis. 2002;47:165–82.
57. Kempinaire A, De Raeve L, Merckx M, De Coninck A, Bauwens M, Roseeuw D. Terbinafine-induced acute generalized exanthematous pustulosis confirmed by a positive patch-test result. J Am Acad Dermatol. 1997;37:653–5.
58. Girardi M, Duncan KO, Tigelaar RE, Imaeda S, Watsky KL, McNiff JM. Cross-comparison of patch test and lymphocyte proliferation responses in patients with a history of acute generalized exanthematous pustulosis. Am J Dermatopathol. 2005;27:343–6.
59. Elzagallaai AA, Knowles SR, Rieder MJ, Bend JR, Shear NH, Koren G. Patch testing for the diagnosis of anticonvulsant hypersensitivity syndrome: a systematic review. Drug Saf. 2009;32:391–408.
60. Chauhan A, Anand S, Thomas S, Subramanya HC, Pradhan G. Carbamazepine induced DRESS syndrome. J Assoc Physicians India. 2010;58:634–6.
61. Liao HT, Hung KL, Wang CF, Chen WC. Patch testing in the detection of cutaneous reactions caused by carbamazepine. Zhonghua Min Guo Xiao Er Ke Yi Xue Hui Za Zhi. 1997;38:365–9.
62. Alanko K. Patch testing in cutaneous reactions caused by carbamazepine. Contact Dermatitis. 1993;29:254–7.
63. Lin YT, Chang YC, Hui RC, Yang CH, Ho HC, Hung SI, Chung WH. A patch testing and cross-sensitivity study of carbamazepine-induced severe cutaneous adverse drug reactions. J Eur Acad Dermatol Venereol. 2013;27:356–64. doi:10.1111/j.1468-3083.2011.04418.x.
64. Emmett EA. Drug photoallergy. Int J Dermatol. 1978;17:370–9.
65. Schwarze HP, Albes B, Marguery MC, Loche F, Bazex J. Evaluation of drug-induced photosensitivity by UVB photopatch testing. Contact Dermatitis. 1998;39:200.
66. Drucker AM, Rosen CF. Drug-induced photosensitivity: culprit drugs, management and prevention. Drug Saf. 2011;34:821–37. doi:10.2165/11592780-000000000-00000.
67. Lee AY, Joo HJ, Chey WY, Kim YG. Photopatch testing in seven cases of photosensitive drug eruptions. Ann Pharmacother. 2001;35:1584–7.

68. White IR. Photopatch test in a hydrochlorothiazide drug eruption. Contact Dermatitis. 1983;9:237.
69. Lee AY, Jung SY. Two patients with isoniazid-induced photosensitive lichenoid eruptions confirmed by photopatch test. Photodermatol Photoimmunol Photomed. 1998;14:77–8.
70. Marguery MC, Chouini-Lalanne N, Drugeon C, Gadroy A, Bayle P, Journe F, et al. UV-B phototoxic effects induced by atorvastatin. Arch Dermatol. 2006;142:1082–4.
71. Nino M, Patruno C, Zagaria O, Balato N. Allergic contact dermatitis from heparin-containing gel: use of scratch patch test for diagnosis. Dermatitis. 2009;20:171–2.
72. Conilleau V, Dompmartin A, Michel M, Verneuil L, Leroy D. Photoscratch testing in systemic drug-induced photosensitivity. Photodermatol Photoimmunol Photomed. 2000;16:62–6.
73. Lammintausta K, Kortekangas-Savolainen O. The usefulness of skin tests to prove drug hypersensitivity. Br J Dermatol. 2005;152:968–74.
74. Gaig P, San Miguel-Moncin MM, Bartra J, Bonet A, García-Ortega P. Usefulness of patch tests for diagnosing selective allergy to captopril. J Investig Allergol Clin Immunol. 2001;11:204–6.
75. Watanabe K, Nishimura K, Shiode M, Sekiya M, Ikeda S, Inoue Y, et al. Captopril, an angiotensin-converting enzyme inhibitor, induced pulmonary infiltration with eosinophilia. Intern Med. 1996;35:142–5.
76. Knowles S, Gupta AK, Shear NH. The spectrum of cutaneous reactions associated with diltiazem: three cases and a review of the literature. J Am Acad Dermatol. 1998;38:201–6.
77. Cnudde F, Leynadier F, Dry J. Cutaneous reaction to captopril: value of patch tests. Contact Dermatitis. 1990;23:375–6.
78. Pfützner W, Rueff F, Przybilla B. Systemic contact dermatitis due to captopril without cross-sensitivity to fosinopril, quinapril and benazepril. Acta Derm Venereol. 2004;84:91–2.
79. Martinez JC, Fuentes MJ, Armentia A, Vega JM, Fernandez A. Dermatitis to captopril. Allergol Immunopathol (Madr). 2001;29:279–80.
80. Chaabane A, Fadhl NB, Chadly Z, Fredj NB, Boughattas NA, Aouam K. Captopril-induced DRESS: first reported case confirmed by patch test. Dermatitis. 2013;24:255–7.
81. Smit AJ, Van der Laan S, De Monchy J, Kallenberg CG, Donker AJ. Cutaneous reactions to captopril. Predictive value of skin tests. Clin Allergy. 1984;14:413–9.
82. Balieva F, Steinkjer B. Contact dermatitis to captopril. Contact Dermatitis. 2009;61:177–8.
83. Pérez-Ferriols A, Martínez-Menchón T, Fortea JM. Follicular mucinosis secondary to captopril-induced photoallergy. Actas Dermosifiliogr. 2005;96:167–70.
84. Wagner SN, Welke F, Goos M. Occupational UVA-induced allergic photodermatitis in a welder due to hydrochlorothiazide and ramipril. Contact Dermatitis. 2000;43:245–6.
85. Rodríguez Granados MT, Abalde T, García Doval I, De la Torre C. Systemic photosensitivity to quinapril. J Eur Acad Dermatol Venereol. 2004;18:389–90.
86. Lluch-Bernal M, Novalbos A, Umpierrez A, Figueredo E, Bombin C, Sastre J. Cutaneous reaction to captopril with positive patch test and lack of cross-sensitivity to enalapril and benazepril. Contact Dermatitis. 1998;39:316–7.
87. Pfab F, Athanasiadis GI, Kollmar A, Ring J, Ollert M. Lichenoid drug eruption due to an antihypertonic drug containing irbesartan and hydrochlorothiazide. Allergy. 2006;61:786–7.
88. Vaillant L, Le Marchand D, Grognard C, Hocine R, Lorette G. Photosensitivity to methyldopa. Arch Dermatol. 1988;124:326–7.
89. Lang Jr PG. Quinidine-induced photodermatitis confirmed by photopatch testing. J Am Acad Dermatol. 1983;9:124–8.
90. Schürer NY, Lehmann P, Plewig G. Quinidine-induced photoallergy. A clinical and experimental study. Hautarzt. 1991;42:158–61.
91. Higa K, Hirata K, Dan K. Mexiletine-induced severe skin eruption, fever, eosinophilia, atypical lymphocytosis, and liver dysfunction. Pain. 1997;73:97–9.
92. Yagami A, Yoshikawa T, Asano Y, Koie S, Shiohara T, Matsunaga K. Drug-induced hypersensitivity syndrome due to mexiletine hydrochloride associated with reactivation of human herpesvirus 7. Dermatology. 2006;213:341–4.

93. Lee SP, Kim SH, Kim TH, Sohn JW, Shin DH, Park SS, et al. A case of mexiletine-induced hypersensitivity syndrome presenting as eosinophilic pneumonia. J Korean Med Sci. 2010;25:148–51.
94. Morito H, Ogawa K, Kobayashi N, Fukumoto T, Asada H. Drug-induced hypersensitivity syndrome followed by persistent arthritis. J Dermatol. 2012;39:178–9. doi:10.1111/j.1346-8138.2011.01236.x.
95. Sasaki K, Yamamoto T, Kishi M, Yokozeki H, Nishioka K. Acute exanthematous pustular drug eruption induced by mexiletine. Eur J Dermatol. 2001;11:469–71.
96. Jappe U, Uter W, Menezes de Pádua CA, Herbst RA, Schnuch A. Allergic contact dermatitis due to beta-blockers in eye drops: a retrospective analysis of multicentre surveillance data 1993–2004. Acta Derm Venereol. 2006;86:509–14.
97. Neumark M, Moshe S, Ingber A, Slodownik D. Occupational airborne contact dermatitis to simvastatin, carvedilol, and zolpidem. Contact Dermatitis. 2009;61:51–2. doi:10.1111/j.1600-0536.2009.01555.x.
98. Zaccaria E, Gualco F, Drago F, Rebora A. Fixed drug eruption due to propranolol. Acta Derm Venereol. 2006;86:371.
99. Giner Esparza MA, Miedes Pitarch E, Miquel Miquel FJ, Palop Larrea V. Fixed drug eruption and bisoprolol. Aten Primaria. 2009;41:351.
100. Palungwachira P, Palungwachira P. Fixed drug eruption due to atenolol: a case report. J Med Assoc Thai. 1999;82:1158–61.
101. Belhadjali H, Trimech O, Youssef M, Elhani I, Zili J. Fixed drug eruption induced by atenolol. Clin Cosmet Investig Dermatol. 2009;1:37–9.
102. Miyauchi H, Horiki S, Horio T. Clinical and experimental photosensitivity reaction to tilisolol hydrochloride. Photodermatol Photoimmunol Photomed. 1994;10:255–8.
103. Zachary CB, Slater DN, Holt DW, Storey GC, MacDonald DM. The pathogenesis of amiodarone-induced pigmentation and photosensitivity. Br J Dermatol. 1984;110: 451–6.
104. Ferguson J, Addo HA, Jones S, Johnson BE, Frain-Bell W. A study of cutaneous photosensitivity induced by amiodarone. Br J Dermatol. 1985;113:537–49.
105. Cholez C, Trechot P, Schmutz JL, Faure G, Bene MC, Barbaud A. Maculopapular rash induced by diltiazem: allergological investigations in four patients and cross reactions between calcium channel blockers. Allergy. 2003;58:1207–9.
106. Wakelin SH, James MP. Diltiazem-induced acute generalised exanthematous pustulosis. Clin Exp Dermatol. 1995;20:341–4.
107. Vicente-Calleja JM, Aguirre A, Landa N, Crespo V, Gonzalez-Perez R, Diaz-Perez JL. Acute generalized exanthematous pustulosis due to diltiazem: confirmation by patch testing. Br J Dermatol. 1997;137:837–9.
108. Jan V, Machet L, Gironet N, Martin L, Machet MC, Lorette G, et al. Acute generalized exanthematous pustulosis induced by diltiazem: value of patch testing. Dermatology. 1998;197:274–5.
109. Gesierich A, Rose C, Brocker EB, Trautmann A, Leverkus M. Acute generalised exanthematous pustulosis with subepidermal blisters of the distal extremities induced by diltiazem. Dermatology. 2006;213:48–9.
110. Gensch K, Hodzic-Avdagic N, Megahed M, Ruzicka T, Kuhn A. Acute generalized exanthematous pustulosis with confirmed type IV allergy. Report of 3 cases. Hautarzt. 2007;58(250–2):254–5.
111. Serrão V, Caldas Lopes L, Campos Lopes JM, Lobo L, Ferreira A. Acute generalized exanthematous pustulosis associated with diltiazem. Acta Med Port. 2008;21:99–102.
112. Gonzalo Garijo MA, Perez Calderon R, de Argila Fernandez-Duran D, Rangel Mayoral JF. Cutaneous reactions due to diltiazem and cross reactivity with other calcium channel blockers. Allergol Immunopathol (Madr). 2005;33:238–40.
113. Nucera E, Schavino D, Roncallo C, de Pasquale T, Buonomo A, Pollastrini E, et al. Delayed-type allergy to oral nimodipine. Contact Dermatitis. 2002;47:246–7.
114. Addo HA, Ferguson J, Frain-Bell W. Thiazide-induced photosensitivity: a study of 33 subjects. Br J Dermatol. 1987;116:749–60.

115. Masuoka E, Bito T, Shimizu H, Nishigori C. Dysfunction of melanocytes in photoleukomelanoderma following photosensitivity caused by hydrochlorothiazide. Photodermatol Photoimmunol Photomed. 2011;27:328–30.
116. Lehmann P, Hölzle E, Plewig G. Photoallergy to Neotri and cross reaction to tenoretic–detection by systemic photoprovocation. Hautarzt. 1988;39:38–41.
117. Prichard BN, Brogden RN. Xipamide. A review of its pharmacodynamic and pharmacokinetic properties and therapeutic efficacy. Drugs. 1985;30:313–32.
118. Fernández de Corres L, Bernaola G, Fernández E, Leanizbarrutia I, Muñoz D. Photodermatitis from triamterene. Contact Dermatitis. 1987;17:114–5.
119. Schon MP, Tebbe B, Trautmann C, Orfanos CE. Lichenoid drug eruption induced by spironolactone. Acta Derm Venereol. 1994;74:476.
120. Aouam K, Ali HB, Youssef M, Chaabane A, Hamdi MH, Boughattas NA, et al. Lichenoid eruption associated with hydrochlorothiazide and possible cross reactivity to furosemide. Therapie. 2009;64:344–7.
121. Alonso JC, Ortega FJ, Gonzalo MJ, Palla PS. Cutaneous reaction to oral spironolactone with positive patch test. Contact Dermatitis. 2002;47:178–9.
122. Jachiet M, Bellon N, Assier H, Amsler E, Gaouar H, Pecquet C, et al. Cutaneous adverse drug reaction to oral acetazolamide and skin tests. Dermatology. 2013;226:347–52. doi:10.1159/000350939.
123. Garg A, Smith W. Sulfur allergies can be misleading. J Pharm Pract Res. 2013;43:332.
124. Lee AG, Johnson KK, Green DL, Rife JP, Limon L. Sulfonamide cross-reactivity: fact or fiction? Ann Pharmacother. 2005;39:290–301.
125. Tornero P, De Barrio M, Baeza ML, Herrero T. Cross-reactivity among p-amino group compounds in sulfonamide fixed drug eruption: diagnostic value of patch testing. Contact Dermatitis. 2004;51:57–62.
126. Brackett CC, Singh H, Block JH. Likelihood and mechanisms of cross-allergenicity between sulfonamide antibiotics and other drugs containing a sulfonamide functional group. Pharmacotherapy. 2004;24:856–70.
127. De Barrio M, Tornero P, Zubeldia JM, Sierra Z, Matheu V, Herrero T. Fixed drug eruption induced by indapamide. Cross-reactivity with sulfonamides. J Investig Allergol Clin Immunol. 1998;8:253–5.
128. Jacob SE, Zapolanski T, Chayavichitsilp P. Sensitivity to para-phenylenediamine and intolerance to hydrochlorothiazide. Dermatitis. 2008;19:E44–5.
129. Romano A, Giovannetti A, Caruso C, Rosato E, Pierdominici M, Salsano F. Delayed hypersensitivity to bosentan. Allergy. 2009;64:499–501. doi:10.1111/j.1398-9995.2008.01927.x.
130. Allanore Y, Moachon L, Maury E, Isvy A, Kahan A. Bosentan-induced drug reaction with eosinophilia and systemic symptoms (DRESS) syndrome. J Rheumatol. 2010;37:1077–8. doi:10.3899/jrheum.091266.
131. de Boer EM, Bruynzeel DP. Allergy to pravastatin. Contact Dermatitis. 1994;30:238.
132. Peramiquel L, Serra E, Dalmau J, Vila AT, Mascaró JM, Alomar A. Occupational contact dermatitis from simvastatin. Contact Dermatitis. 2005;52:286–7.
133. Field S, Bourke B, Hazelwood E, Bourke JF. Simvastatin - occupational contact dermatitis. Contact Dermatitis. 2007;57:282–3.
134. Granados MT, de la Torre C, Cruces MJ, Piñeiro G. Chronic actinic dermatitis due to simvastatin. Contact Dermatitis. 1998;38:294–5.
135. Machet L, Vaillant L, Jan V, Lorette G. Fenofibrate-induced photosensitivity: value of photopatch testing. J Am Acad Dermatol. 1997;37:808–9.
136. Leenutaphong V, Manuskiatti W. Fenofibrate-induced photosensitivity. J Am Acad Dermatol. 1996;35:775–7.
137. Hong JB, Wang SH, Chu CY. Fenofibrate-induced photosensitivity-a case report and literature review. Dermatol Sin. 2009;27:37–43.
138. Gardeazabal J, Gonzalez M, Izu R, Gil N, Aguirre A, Diaz-Perez JL. Phenofibrate-induced lichenoid photodermatitis. Photodermatol Photoimmunol Photomed. 1993;9:156–8.

139. Leenutaphong V. Reply: Fenofibrate-induced photosensitivity: value of photopatch testing. J Am Acad Dermatol. 1997;37:809.
140. Serrano G, Fortea JM, Latasa JM, Millan F, Janes C, Bosca F, et al. Photosensitivity induced by fibric acid derivatives and its relation to photocontact dermatitis to ketoprofen. J Am Acad Dermatol. 1992;27(2 Pt 1):204–8.
141. Carrozza P, Gabutti L, Gilliet F, Marone C. Heparin-induced systemic inflammatory response syndrome with progressive skin necrosis in haemodialysis. Nephrol Dial Transplant. 1997;2:2424–7.
142. Enrique E, Alijotas J, Cistero A, san Miguel MM, Bartra J, Tresserra F. Patch-test positivity in cutaneous reactions to enoxaparin. Contact Dermatitis. 2000;42:43.
143. Oldhoff JM, Bihari IC, Knol EF, Bruijnzeel-Koomen CA, de Bruin-Weller MS. Atopy patch test in patients with atopic eczema/dermatitis syndrome: comparison of petrolatum and aqueous solution as a vehicle. Allergy. 2004;59:451–6.
144. Méndez J, Sanchís ME, de la Fuente R, Stolle R, Vega JM, Martínez C, et al. Delayed-type hypersensitivity to subcutaneous enoxaparin. Allergy. 1998;53:999–1003.
145. Koch P, Münssinger T, Rupp-John C, Uhl K. Delayed-type hypersensitivity skin reactions caused by subcutaneous unfractionated and low-molecular-weight heparins: tolerance of a new recombinant hirudin. J Am Acad Dermatol. 2000;42:612–9.
146. Grims RH, Weger W, Reiter H, Arbab E, Kränke B, Aberer W. Delayed-type hypersensitivity to low molecular weight heparins and heparinoids: cross-reactivity does not depend on molecular weight. Br J Dermatol. 2007;157:514–7.
147. Zollner TM, Gall H, Volpel H, Kaufmann R. Type IV allergy to natural hirudin confirmed by in vitro stimulation with recombinant hirudin. Contact Dermatitis. 1996;35:59–60.
148. Hohenstein E, Tsakiris D, Bircher AJ. Delayed-type hypersensitivity to the ultra-low-molecular-weight heparin fondaparinux. Contact Dermatitis. 2004;51:149–51.
149. Trautmann A, Seitz CS. Heparin allergy: delayed-type non-IgE-mediated allergic hypersensitivity to subcutaneous heparin injection. Immunol Allergy Clin North Am. 2009;29:469–80.
150. Jappe U, Reinhold D, Bonnekoh B. Arthus reaction to lepirudin, a new recombinant hirudin, and delayed-type hypersensitivity to several heparins and heparinoids, with tolerance to its intravenous administration. Contact Dermatitis. 2002;46:29–32.
151. Frouin E, Roth B, Grange A, Grange F, Tortel MC, Guillaume JC. Hypersensitivity to fluindione (Previscan). Positive skin patch tests. Ann Dermatol Venereol. 2005;132(12 Pt 1):1000–2.
152. Chtioui M, Cousin-Testard F, Zimmermann U, Amar A, Saiag P, Mahé E. Fluindione-induced acute generalised exanthematous pustulosis confirmed by patch testing. Ann Dermatol Venereol. 2008;135:295–8.
153. López Abad R, Iriarte Sotés P, Castro Murga M, Gracia Bara MT, Sesma Sánchez P. Fixed drug eruption induced by phenylephrine: a case of polysensitivity. J Investig Allergol Clin Immunol. 2009;19:322–3.
154. Barranco R, Rodríguez A, de Barrio M, Trujillo MJ, de Frutos C, Matheu V, et al. Sympathomimetic drug allergy: cross-reactivity study by patch test. Am J Clin Dermatol. 2004;5:351–5.
155. Cheema AN, Mohammad A, Hong T, Jakubovic HR, Parmar GS, Sharieff W, et al. Characterization of clopidogrel hypersensitivity reactions and management with oral steroids without clopidogrel discontinuation. J Am Coll Cardiol. 2011;58:1445–54.
156. Garcia CM, Carmena R, Garcia R, Berges P, Camacho E, Cotter MP, et al. Fixed drug eruption from ticlopidine, with positive lesional patch test. Contact Dermatitis. 2001;44:40–1.
157. Cannavo SP, Borgia F, Guarneri F, Vaccaro M. Acute generalized exanthematous pustulosis following use of ticlopidine. Br J Dermatol. 2000;142:577–8.
158. Salava A, Alanko K, Hyry H. Dipyridamole-induced eczematous drug eruption with positive patch test reaction. Contact Dermatitis. 2012;67:103–4. doi:10.1111/j.1600-0536.2012.02066.x.

159. Kawakami T, Fujita A, Takeuchi S, Muto S, Soma Y. Drug-induced hypersensitivity syndrome: drug reaction with eosinophilia and systemic symptoms (DRESS) syndrome induced by aspirin treatment of Kawasaki disease. J Am Acad Dermatol. 2009;60:146–9. doi:10.1016/j.jaad.2008.07.044.
160. Miyamoto H, Okajima M. Allergic contact dermatitis from epsilon-aminocaproic acid. Contact Dermatitis. 2000;42:50.
161. González Gutiérrez ML, Esteban López MI, Ruíz Ruíz MD. Positivity of patch tests in cutaneous reaction to aminocaproic acid: 2 case reports. Allergy. 1995;50:745–6.
162. Villarreal O. Systemic dermatitis with eosinophilia due to epsilon-aminocaproic acid. Contact Dermatitis. 1999;40:114.

Index

E. Özkaya, K.D. Yazganoğlu, *Adverse Cutaneous Drug Reactions to Cardiovascular Drugs*, DOI 10.1007/978-1-4471-6536-1

Q

R

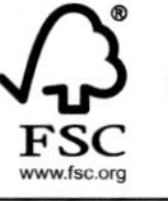

MIX
Papier aus verantwortungsvollen Quellen
Paper from responsible sources
FSC® C105338

Printed by Books on Demand, Germany